Generalization Strategies in the Treatment of Communication Disorders

Generalization Strategies in the Treatment of Communication Disorders

Leija V. McReynolds, Ph.D.

Professor
Hearing and Speech Department
University of Kansas Medical Center
Kansas City, Kansas

Joseph E. Spradlin, Ph.D.

Senior Scientist
Bureau of Child Research
University of Kansas
Lawrence, Kansas

1989
B.C. Decker Inc • Toronto • Philadelphia

Publisher

B.C. Decker Inc
3228 South Service Road
Burlington, Ontario L7N 3H8

B.C. Decker Inc
320 Walnut Street
Suite 400
Philadelphia, Pennsylvania 19106

Sales and Distribution

United States and Possessions
The C.V. Mosby Company
11830 Westline Industrial Drive
Saint Louis, Missouri 63146

Canada
The C.V. Mosby Company, Ltd.
5240 Finch Avenue East, Unit No. 1
Scarborough, Ontario M1S 5P2

United Kingdom, Europe and the Middle East
Blackwell Scientific Publications, Ltd.
Osney Mead, Oxford OX2 OEL, England

Australia and New Zealand
Harcourt Brace Jovanovich Group (Australia) Pty Limited
30–52 Smidmore Street
Marrickville, N.S.W. 2204
Australia

Japan
Igaku-Shoin Ltd.
Tokyo International P.O. Box 5063
1–28–36 Hongo, Bunkyo-ku, Tokyo 113, Japan

Asia
Info-Med Ltd.
802–3 Ruttonjee House
11 Duddell Street
Central Hong Kong

South Africa
Libriger Book Distributors
Warehouse Number 8
"Die Ou Looiery"
Tannery Road
Hamilton, Bloemfontein 9300

South America
Inter-Book Marketing Services
Rua das Palmeriras, 32
Apto. 701
222–70 Rio de Janeiro
RJ, Brazil

NOTICE

The authors and publisher have made every effort to ensure that the patient care recommended herein, including choice of drugs and drug dosages, is in accord with the accepted standards and practice at the time of publication. However, since research and regulation constantly change clinical standards, the reader is urged to check the product information sheet included in the package of each drug, which includes recommended doses, warnings, and contraindications. This is particularly important with new or infrequently used drugs.

Generalization Strategies in the Treatment of Communication Disorders ISBN 1–55664–069–2

Library of Congress catalog card number: 88–71396

10 9 8 7 6 5 4 3 2 1

CONTRIBUTORS

PHIL J. CONNELL, Ph.D.

Associate Professor, Department of Communication Sciences and Disorders, Northwestern University, Evanston, Illinois

Facilitating Generalization Through Induction Teaching

MARY ELBERT, Ph.D.

Professor, Department of Speech and Hearing Sciences, Indiana University, Bloomington, Indiana

Generalization in the Treatment of Phonological Disorders

JANIS COSTELLO INGHAM, Ph.D.

Professor, Department of Speech and Hearing Sciences, University of California, Santa Barbara, California

Generalization in the Treatment of Stuttering

KEVIN P. KEARNS, Ph.D.

Adjunct Assistant Professor of Neurology and Psychiatry and Behavioral Sciences, University of Health Sciences/Chicago Medical School; Chief, Audiology and Speech Pathology, Veterans Administration Medical Center, North Chicago, Illinois

Methodologies for Studying Generalization

LYNN KERN KOEGEL, M.A., CCC–SP

Associate Specialist, Facial Process Research Institute and Clinical Supervisor, Autism Research Center, University of California, Santa Barbara, California

Generalization in the Treatment of Autism

ROBERT L. KOEGEL, Ph.D.

Professor, Department of Speech and Hearing Sciences and Director, Autism Research Center, University of California, Santa Barbara, California

Generalization in the Treatment of Autism

LEIJA V. McREYNOLDS, Ph.D.

Professor, Hearing and Speech Department, University of Kansas Medical Center, Kansas City, Kansas

Generalization Issues in the Treatment of Communication Disorders

ROBERT E. O'NEILL, Ph.D.

Research Associate, Specialized Training Program, University of Oregon, Eugene, Oregon

Generalization in the Treatment of Autism

JOSEPH E. SPRADLIN, Ph.D.

Professor, Human Development and Family Life and Senior Scientist, Bureau of Child Research, University of Kansas, Lawrence; Director, University Affiliated Facility and Parsons Research Center, Parsons, Kansas

Model of Generalization

CYNTHIA K. THOMPSON, Ph.D.

Associate Professor, Department of Speech, University of Florida, Gainesville, Florida

Generalization in the Treatment of Aphasia

PREFACE

The goal of speech-language remediation is to teach clients communication skills that will be useful for the clients as they go about their daily activities. This goal has been a major problem for speech-language clinicians. The clinician typically teaches a set of speech or language skills within the confines of a clinic. Often, clients fail to exhibit those skills in nonclinic settings. In summary, clients do not commonly generalize skills taught in the clinic to their natural environments. The chapters of this book address this fundamental clinical problem of generalization as it relates to teaching speech and language to people exhibiting communication disorders. Although the content is directed to speech-language pathologists in particular, it also has relevance to teachers, special educators, students, and researchers interested in generalization.

As readers progress through the book they will become aware that the term generalization is used in two distinct ways; as a desired treatment outcome and as a behavioral process. Discussions of both of these content areas are important. Discussions of how to obtain generalization of taught skills to the person's daily activities are important because that is the goal of treatment. Discussions of generalization as a behavioral process are important because, if the principles drawn from the rather extensive literature on generalization as a process are considered, they may lead to procedures that will aid in the goal of getting taught communication skills used in the natural environment. For the teacher and clinician, such considerations are critical to selecting valid procedures for implementation.

The majority of the chapters in the book address generalization in terms of specific communication disorders, i.e., a chapter about generalization in treatment of articulation and phonological disorders, others about treatment of child language disorders, stuttering, aphasia, and autism. Each of these chapters presents conceptual issues related to generalization as a process. Critical research is presented and evaluated. Finally, each chapter includes a set of practical suggestions concerning how to achieve the use of taught communication skills in clients' daily lives.

Preceding the specific disorders chapters are two introductory chapters. In Chapter 1, the issues involved in defining and obtaining generalization in the treatment of communication disorders are presented. Practical suggestions for ways to study and to measure generalization during intervention are found in Chapter 2.

There are numerous areas of agreement across the authors of all chapters. First, there is agreement that the appropriate goal for treatment is demonstration of the taught communication skill in the clients' daily activities. Second, all of the writers believe that important speech and language skills can be taught. Third, all of the authors agree that some sort of inductive training procedure is effective for promoting generalization into new situations. This induction is brought about by a training procedure similar to Stokes and Baer's (1977) Train Multiple Exemplars procedure. This is not to suggest that there is total conceptual agreement across the various authors or that one needs to read only the chapter relating to a particular communication disorder to obtain all of the useful information relevant to that disorder.

There are major issues that separate the authors of the various chapters. For some of the authors, generalization of speech and language skills to natural settings is a matter of teaching the skill across a number of representative contexts in the hope that the skill would then come under the control of the appropriate environmental stimuli. For others, the issue is teaching a rule or the discovery of a rule that is internalized. When this occurs it is assumed that the speaker can apply the rule when appropriate. For these authors, generalization is a function of internal stimuli controlling generalization. Readers will be attracted to the various conceptualizations according to their own theoretical view.

This book is unique in several ways. First, it is devoted entirely to the topic of generalization in the treatment of communication disorders. Second, the book supplies information on methods used to study and measure generalization throughout treatment. Third, the book is unique in that it is an attempt to bring together in a systematic, organized manner the variables identified in the study of generalization in the various specific disorders. The organization results in a preliminary model of generalization that contains principles that can be used in developing and implementing treatment programs across all communication disorders as well as other problem behaviors.

It is hoped that the information in this book has practical value for clinicians and teachers for developing treatments or educational programs for specific problems in clinics and schools. Although each chapter is directed to discussion of a specific communication problem, it is suggested that readers do not restrict their reading to specific chapters devoted to a particular communication disorder that may be of special interest to them. Procedures and variables that have been identified as useful for one problem often have application to others as well. That is, some variables that may be relevant to several disorders may only have been explored in the treatment of one and so be described in only the chapter devoted to that specific disorder. That does not necessarily mean, however, that the variable can only be applied to that particular treatment for that particular problem. It is likely to have greater generality, or at least the possibility for greater generality. Thus, clinicians and teachers are encouraged to read all of the chapters. Undoubtedly, there is overlap, but there are also specific topics that are discussed in only one or two chapters.

It is hoped that the information in this book will result in an increased interest and research in generalization. Ideally, clinicians and teachers give consideration to generalization in the planning stages of developing treatments. The earlier that generalization is considered, the sooner and more extensive the generalization obtained when training starts. As for research, an entire chapter is devoted to descriptions of generalization issues and suggestions for methods that can be used to examine them. In addition, each specific chapter includes descriptions of the procedures used to study generalization in treatment of a specific disorder. All of this information from both sources can be used by students, clinicians, academicians, and researchers to design a variety of methods and measures for obtaining data on generalization throughout a treatment program and across any situation and context. The more data on generalization we obtain, the more we know about how behaviors develop and the more we can do to improve our treatments.

Leija V. McReynolds, Ph.D.
Joseph E. Spradlin, Ph.D.

CONTENTS

Chapter One

GENERALIZATION ISSUES IN THE TREATMENT OF COMMUNICATION DISORDERS

LEIJA V. McREYNOLDS, Ph.D.

A question of prime importance in the treatment of communication disorders is whether generalization of the treated behavior will occur. Although the question is at least as important as questions concerning whether the behavior will be acquired with the treatment administered, it has received less attention in research and in the communication disorders literature.

The lack of attention may be attributed, at least partly, to two beliefs or attitudes on the part of speech-language pathologists. The first is that if a behavior is trained adequately in the clinic, it will automatically generalize to situations in which no training is provided. The second attitude reflects a lack of knowledge concerning how best to obtain generalization and what variables clinicians can manipulate to ensure that generalization will be attained. Clinicians do not plan for generalization because they do not know how to accomplish it. These two factors result in treatment programs that emphasize how to plan for acquisition of a behavior, but not how to achieve generalization of the behavior.

The emphasis on variables and procedures that can facilitate acquisition of appropriate behaviors has resulted in the development of some successful treatments for communication disorders. At the same time, the success in teaching acquisition has revealed the weaknesses in most of the treatments in obtaining generalization of the newly acquired behavior. The client performs well in training, is dismissed, and the newly acquired behavior is not produced outside the clinic. In other words, contrary to expectations, acquisition does not ensure generalization, and this lack of generalization is of serious concern to researchers and clinicians.

The problems in obtaining generalization in treatment have led to a shift in attention by some investigators from research in acquisition to research in generalization and the variables that influence it. More studies are now directed to trying to understand what generalization is all about, and to identifying variables and procedures that appear to influence generalization, hopefully in a facilitative manner.

Although many questions remain to be explored and the data are incomplete, the information base is growing. The chapters in this book were written to present the information available on generalization in the treatment of various communication disorders, and to bring as much order as possible to the information gathered. The goal is to organize the information so that a model of generalization, and principles of generalization, can emerge if they are present.

The chapter sequence is as follows. This first chapter presents an introduction to the topic of generalization and identifies some of the relevant issues needing to be addressed. The second chapter, by Kevin Kearns, discusses methods for studying and for measuring generalization. It also provides information on some of the approaches to understanding generalization and obtaining it in treatment. The third chapter, by Mary Elbert, contains information on some of the variables that promise to be important to generalization in phonological disorders. The chapter on articulation is followed by a chapter on child language in relation to generalization, by Phil Connell. The fifth chapter, by Janis Costello Ingham, reviews factors that influence or are related to generalization in stuttering; and Cynthia Thompson, in chapter six, covers the research in generalization in treatment of aphasia. The current status of generalization in the treatment of autism is covered in chapter seven by Robert Koegel, Lynn Koegel, and Rob O'Neill. And finally, in chapter eight, Joseph Spradlin brings together the information from the preceding chapters in an attempt to determine if a model of generalization in treatment or principles for facilitating generalization have emerged. He looks for order and lawfulness in the variables discussed in treating communication disorders in the hope that some important factors can be discovered and be taken into consideration when planning treatment for any communication disorder.

The rest of this first chapter is devoted to the following topics: how generalization is viewed from theoretical and atheoretical approaches to treatment, and philosophical and practical issues that need to be attended to by researchers and clinicians. The discussion here is somewhat brief, because the authors of the subsequent chapters address the issues in greater detail.

GENERALIZATION DEFINED

The topic of this book is generalization. More specifically, it is about generalization during and after intervention in the treatment of a variety of communication disorders. Generalization is defined in various ways by individuals who come from different views of learning and intervention strategies.

Strictly speaking, generalization can be defined procedurally (Blough, 1966). In experimental research, the procedure is to reinforce responses in the presence of a specific stimulus until responding has stabilized. Then stimuli similar and dissimilar in a particular dimension to the training stimulus are presented in the presence of extinction, to determine which stimuli will function to evoke the trained response. The result is a generalization gradient in which responses decrease in frequency as the test stimulus moves farther away from the training stimulus in the targeted parameter. When the test stimulus is very dissimilar to the training stimulus, responding stops altogether; it is extinguished. In the laboratory experiment the stimulus can be defined physically, and the parameters composing the stimuli are identified (e.g., the training stimulus is a 1,000 Hz tone presented at 50 dB and the first test tone is an 1,100 Hz tone at 50 dB).

Definitions are not as easy when the stimuli and responses consist of communication behavior in the natural environment. The stimuli that evoke a response are complex and sometimes subtle, so they are not readily identified or defined. Consequently, the procedural and laboratory definition of generalization probably does not capture the human behavioral event accurately. Because of this, the definition of generalization has been modified in intervention and is tested in complex and not always clearly specified contexts. Thus, we find definitions such as, "Generalization is defined as the accurate production and use of trained target sounds in other untrained contexts or environments" (Elbert and Gierut, 1986, p. 121) and "... the generic term 'generalization' has come to be used most commonly to describe the extension of some learning to new instances" (Hughes, 1985, p. 2). Hegde (1985) suggests that "generalization has a stimulus dimension and a response dimension. It is the basis upon which some new learning is demonstrated without additional conditioning" (p. 177). One of the most comprehensive definitions in behavioral terms has been offered by Stokes and Baer (1977): ..."the occurrence of relevant behavior under different, nontraining conditions (i.e., across subjects, settings, people, behaviors, and/or time) without the scheduling of the same events in those conditions as had been scheduled in the training conditions" (p. 350). They offer qualifications to the definition by proposing that generalization occurs "...when no extratraining manipulations are needed... or, when some extratraining manipulations are necessary, but their cost or extent is clearly less than that of the direct intervention" (p. 350). Several authors have taken issue with the qualification, suggesting either that if manipulations are required, the behavior observed cannot be described as generalization (Hegde, 1985) or that generalization needs more than one definition (Hughes, 1985).

Different versions of the above definitions can be found, but essentially, the term *generalization* is used here simply to describe the occurrence of a specific behavior or related behaviors in contexts in which that behavior has never been trained. The term is a description of what is observed; it is not an explanation of it. Definitions are included in the individual chapters in the book as they address the different communication disorders. Therefore, no in-depth discussion of definitions is offered in this introduction.

It should be noted that some other terms are used to describe what is defined as generalization in this discussion. They include *transfer, carry-over, induction, rules, concept formation*, and *spread of effect*. Although the terms have specific meaning for some individuals in the context of their theoretical formulation, others use them interchangeably. Those who accept all the terms interchangeably suggest that all of the terms present a similar concept, that what is occurring in training can be observed in nontraining conditions as well when an individual is treated for a communication disorder. As more cognitive approaches are introduced into views concerning the nature of disorders, they affect our conceptualizations of intervention. Thus, for those who believe in innate structures and rules, the term generalization has less meaning (Johnston, 1983); in fact, it has no meaning. The premise is that once the client has induced a rule in the clinic situation, the rule is applied in all situations, and generalization is not necessarily an issue. In fact, the term is not used. However, it should be noted that generalization and rule acquisition are tested in the same way. That is, procedures are designed to determine if a particular behavior acquired in training will be produced in untrained situations and in the natural environment.

BASES FOR TREATMENT PLANS

Two issues in planning intervention in the hope that it facilitates generalization are often discussed. One issue has more to do with language-impaired and phonologically disordered children; the second issue applies to both children and adults and to various communication disorders. The first issue is concerned with whether target behaviors for treatment should be selected on the basis of normal developmental information obtained from normative studies (Guess, Sailor, and Baer, 1978; Hegde, 1985). Usually the question is raised in regard to acquisition. The issue raised is whether a developmental sequence should be followed in selecting targets in treatment. However, equally relevant in using developmental sequences may be questions concerning characteristics of the generalization behavior observed in intervention and characteristics in normal acquisition. Do the same variables influence generalization in normal acquisition and in intervention? Are the patterns during normal language acquisition similar to, or different from, the patterns observed in intervention as children begin to generalize the behaviors learned in training?

The second issue also has to do with criteria used to select behaviors to be trained in the clinic and the context in which the behavior is to be trained if generalization is to be facilitated. Should functional behaviors or responses be selected and trained, and should they be trained in a natural environment; or, should targets be selected from other sources and be taught in structured clinical environments?

In the first discussion a comparison between normal acquisition patterns and the generalization patterns exhibited by children in intervention is addressed. The purpose is to explore similarities and dissimilarities to determine whether normal acquisition patterns have any implications for the generalization patterns to be expected in treatment of communication disorders (Ferguson, 1978; Ferguson and Farwell, 1975; Ferguson and Macken, 1983; Vihman and Associates, 1985).

Normal Development As a Standard

For children with language and phonological disorders, target behaviors for treatment have traditionally been selected on the basis of normative developmental data from descriptive studies (Templin, 1957; Leonard, 1982). Since this is the case, one way to examine the selection is to compare the behaviors of normal children with those of impaired children when new forms are first acquired and begin to be produced in new contexts in the normal environment and in intervention.

The behaviors that are compared may be considered to be evidence for generalization, although in normal acquisition the evidence may be difficult to identify. In normal acquisition a child may produce the /k/ correctly for the first time in a word such as "candy." Subsequently, he may be observed to produce it correctly for the first time in the word "kitty." That production may or may not be generalization depending on the events surrounding the /k/ production in "kitty."

On the other hand, the evidence for generalization may be more obvious in intervention. During treatment a phonologically disordered child may be taught to produce /k/ correctly for the first time in a word such as "cat." Subsequently, during a probe for generalization, he may produce the /k/ correctly in the word "car" where it had previously been produced incorrectly. Because the events surrounding that production are known and no consequent events are administered for the correct production, the response is probably correctly labeled generalization. Despite these differences, it may be worthwhile to examine the behaviors in the two populations to determine if they are similar or different. It is particularly intriguing because in general there are considerable differences in the two learning environments for the two populations of children.

In the natural environment during normal acquisition, a specific construction or form is not targeted for teaching. The child appears to be learning a variety of structures simultaneously. In some ways the learning environment appears to offer haphazard opportunities for acquisition. For example, perhaps the first time a child produces /k/ correctly is when he requests "candy." That correct production may be punished when the mother responds to the request with a "no." At another time, the request might be reinforced because the mother gives candy to the child.

In both situations reinforcement may be occurring, but possibly it is stronger in one than in the other. If the request is denied, the response is punished because it is denied, but it is reinforced because the mother understood the request. When candy is offered, the response is reinforced because the request was understood and also because the request was fulfilled. Thus, the consequences of speaking may be quite complex.

Sometimes overt models are offered to the child to imitate with, "say candy," but that is not a consistent procedure in normal acquisition. In fact, it is most customary only in very early stages of language acquisition, when newly produced words are first recognized, and is not always pursued later by the adults in the child's environment. Moreover, the various individuals in the child's surroundings might react quite differently to his productions of "candy." In addition, in between productions of "candy" many other responses occur and are acted upon in the environment. Thus, the word "candy" might be produced only intermittently. Without doubt the environment in which normal language is learned varies considerably from day to day and from item to item. Yet, in this kind of an unstructured milieu the normal child learns to produce /k/ in one or two words and later produces it in all appropriate words.

Contrast this environment with the environment in which a phonologically impaired child usually learns to produce /k/. Prior to training, the impaired child, like the normal child, has either substituted another sound for /k/ or has omitted it in words. When training is initiated, the child is placed in a restricted environment in a therapy room with a table and chairs. The clinician faces the child across the table and usually presents the /k/ alone or in a simple context, asking the child to imitate it. Treatment progresses in carefully structured steps from simple to complex linguistic contexts in which /k/ is the only constant element in each stimulus–response trial. The child's responses are followed frequently by verbal praise and some concrete token when they are correct, and with other consequent events if incorrect. In a ½ hour of training the child may have produced /k/ as many as 100 times with careful monitoring and feedback from the clinician, and with minimal distraction from the task.

The differences between the two learning environments could result in very different patterns of behavior when new forms are acquired and generalized. Yet, there appear to be more similarities than there are differences. One similarity often noted is that both normal and impaired children tend to "overgeneralize" a form they have learned (Ferguson and Macken, 1983). In language the most obvious example is extension of the regular past tense to irregular verbs. For example, after a child learns the past tense for "mend" (mended) he might produce it in such words as "bend" in which it would be inappropriate. Such overgeneralization has been observed in language-impaired children when they are tested in articulation for generalization to appropriate and inappropriate contexts (McLean, 1970).

Another pattern that has been observed in the behaviors of both groups of children is the nonlinear nature of acquisition and generalization. The pattern shows stops and starts, progressions and regressions, asymptotes and spurts, as well as unexpected gaps. Generalization in normal acquisition is never precipitous; one day a behavior is absent, and the next day it is produced consistently and appropriately in all obligatory contexts. In the same way, generalization is piecemeal, not precipitous, in intervention. It cannot be expected to be different in the two contexts. For example, during normal acquisition a child may produce the form correctly in a specific context on a specific day but produce it incorrectly in the same context the next day. Sometimes the newly acquired correct form is replaced by the old incorrect form, even though the new form has been produced a number of times. New forms are not acquired gradually in a linear fashion, but rather, the child may use the new form in many new contexts on one occasion and then not produce it in any new contexts for a period of time. In other cases the child may produce a new form in an unexpectedly complex context without ever having produced it in contexts that were less complex.

It is the same in language-impaired children (Coggins and Olswang, 1987) and phonologically impaired children (McReynolds, 1987) undergoing treatment. When generalization is tested, the new form may be produced in an erratic manner from one test to another. Children may produce the new form correctly on only one item for several probes and then suddenly produce twice as many correctly. Sometimes, when generalization is tested in what appears to be increasingly complex linguistic contexts and the experimenter expects a gradient of generalization, the gradient does not show up because the child responds correctly in unexpected ways. The general pattern of acquisition in normal development resembles that of generalization in language intervention. Eventually, for both groups of children, all the appropriate forms are produced in appropriate contexts, but the path to that goal is not smooth or linear for either group.

Apparently the unstructured nature of the natural environment is insufficient for some children to acquire language. They require a structured environment directed to teaching the forms missing from their repertoires. Thus, the initial teaching environments for the two populations need to be different. However, when the acquired forms are extended to new contexts or related structures, the patterns for extension are similar. It is possible, then, that clinicians can shift from a highly structured environment to an environment more similar to the normal environment without sacrificing generalization. In fact, such a shift might facilitate generalization.

A puzzling similarity between normal development and generalization in intervention is the variability observed across individual children. Variability has also been documented within children and that variability was discussed in the previous paragraphs. Equally puzzling, however has been the differences observed across children. In normal acquisition the differences are attributed to differences in the strategies children use to acquire language. For example, some children imitate often during acquisition, whereas other children seldom imitate. Some children verbalize a great deal, producing many errors in the process, whereas other children are rather quiet and seldom practice orally. When they finally produce a structure, they may produce it correctly the first time. Some children need to learn a structure in only a few exemplars before they extend it to new contexts; others appear to require many exemplars before a structure is stabilized and used appropriately in new contexts. In normal acquisition then, children exhibit a variety of learning patterns. In general, the differences are attributed to characteristics within the children themselves, not to the environment in which language is learned (Ferguson and Farwell, 1975; Vihman et al, 1985). When similar discrepancies are observed in remediation, they are occasionally attributed to different learning histories among children. An equally likely possibility is that they may simply represent accidental differences in momentary probabilities of stimulus control, because intervention environments contain many stimuli, any one of which may control responding at different times for brief periods. (See Spradlin's discussion of this factor in this volume.) The research indicates that in normal acquisition, part of the variability observed within and across children may be due to a shift from the stimuli controlling the response, a shift in children's attention. On one occasion the child might attend to the frication at the end of the word "fish," so that the final consonant is produced, but on the next occasion the frication in /f/ assumes control of the response so that the child produces the /f/, but not the /sh/. The specific stimulus controlling children's responses from day to day is not identical either within or across children; consequently, variability is observed. In the same way, control of responses in the clinic may shift from one occasion to another so that response variability occurs, and the controlling stimuli differ across children. Because the control may be accidental and fleeting, it is difficult to identify which stimulus of the many that are present is operating on any one occasion. For example, different clinicians may offer varying degrees of stimulus control.

Generalization in intervention that resembles the variability in normal acquisition has been observed across children (McReynolds, 1981). Some children begin to generalize after a structure is learned in only a few exemplars in training, whereas others do not begin to generalize until many exemplars are learned. When generalization is tested in a variety of items, some children produce the trained structure in many of the items; others produce it in only a few items. Often these differences across children are obtained even when they have all reached identical training criterion. That is, the trained structure has the same status in the repertoires of the children when they are tested, in that they have learned the structure to the same degree and are producing it at the same criterion level in the training contexts.

However, the generalization patterns reflect considerable discrepancies across children. The amount of training, as in trials to criterion before generalization begins, also varies considerably across children. Some children reach criterion and begin to generalize in a minimum number of trials, whereas other children require the maximum number offered before generalization occurs.

Explanations for the differences across children are difficult to find. Primarily, as in normal acquisition, it is recognized that children learn differently and generalize differently, but what accounts for the differences is not clear. Explanations have been sought in variables present in the environment, the contexts in which structures are learned, the procedures used to teach the structures, and the contexts in which generalization is tested. All of these variables contribute a partial explanation, but much still remains a mystery. Although no firm explanations have been forthcoming, the research looks promising.

Because the variability is still an enigma, two approaches to contending with the puzzle have been offered. In one approach the source of the variability is sought within the child. In normal acquisition the source has been suspected to be internal to the child, as mentioned earlier, and this source has been suggested as a way of explaining disordered children's generalization patterns (Elbert, Dinnsen, and Weismer, 1984). In this approach, it is suggested that a conventional assessment examines a child's surface performance only. In such evaluations the children appear to be similar in regard to the errors and inadequacies discovered in the evaluation. Only a more in-depth analysis of the children's repertoires reveals the differences among them, particularly in regard to what they know about the language of their community, that is, their level of competence. These differences in levels of knowledge may account for some of the differences in generalization patterns. For example, children who show a high level of knowledge may show a different pattern of generalization from children with little knowledge. Thus, generalization patterns may reflect what children know about their language before intervention. If so, it behooves the clinician to learn as much as possible about the child's characteristics, the content of his language repertoire, and the status of the specific behaviors to be trained, before developing remediation plans. Again, this approach may help to describe some of the differences found across children, but it still does not explain why the differences occurred in the first place. That is, it does not explain why some children come to treatment with more knowledge of their language than others.

The other approach is to accept the differences without attempting to explain or account for them (Baer, 1981; Costello, 1983). Instead, training is conducted with an eye to generalization from the very beginning of treatment. In this approach, as many of the variables as possible that have been identified or suggested as facilitating generalization are incorporated into the treatment in the planning stages. (These variables are discussed in several of the remaining chapters.) The intent is to use the facilitating variables from the beginning and throughout treatment to increase the probability that generalization will occur for all the children treated (Hughes, 1985). Thus, often the stimuli from the natural environment that are thought to be relevant to generalization are introduced into treatment gradually, as soon as the clinician thinks it feasible. Or, in a gradual manner the client is introduced into the environment outside the clinic.

Regardless of which approach is adopted, generalization within and across children continues to evidence considerable individual variability. That variability is not accounted for by in-depth analysis of children's knowledge or by introducing variables that facilitate generalization early in treatment. Generalization may be facilitated by both, but it is not complete for any child, and children demonstrate variability when tested. Thus, variability within and across children remains an issue in attempting to understand and to predict generalization in intervention.

Theoretical Constructs

Perhaps the second most frequent rationale for selecting targets for training comes from the theoretical framework within which the clinician functions in planning treatment (Johnston, 1983; McReynolds, 1987). However, theories probably dictate interpretations of what the behaviors trained signify, more than the selection of behaviors to be trained. That is, the same behaviors may be selected for training by clinicians who adhere to a behavioral approach as by clinicians who adhere to a cognitive theory or a structural linguistic theory. The behaviors may be the same, but what they represent is open to various interpretations that depend on the theory in which each clinician believes. By the same token, generalization of similar behaviors is tested in similar ways, but what the test results represent is interpreted differently by clinicians who hold different views. For example, if generative theory forms the basis for data interpretation, correct responses on untrained items signify to the clinician that the child is applying a rule that was learned in treatment. If a behavioral framework is the basis for a clinician's interpretation of data, correct responses on untrained items demonstrate stimulus–response generalization or formation of response classes.

Not only do rationales vary, but the targets for treatment also vary as a function of theory. Nevertheless, the actual behaviors taught in intervention may not vary much across theories. For example, in phonology, the target might be establishment of a perceptual-motor skill, learning a distinctive feature contrast, acquiring a phonological rule, eliminating a phonological process, or producing a sound that developmentally should already be in the client's repertoire. However, for all of these theoretical targets, the behavior most likely to be trained is correct articulation of a target sound, and the target sound may be the same sound. This is not to say that the targets could not be different as a function of the theory used to select target sounds, but they often are not. Similarly, theories may dictate the kind of generalization test that is constructed, particularly if a theory has been tested to the extent that it can be used to predict generalization. Not many theories have been evaluated for their usefulness for predicting generalization. Perhaps linguistic and phonological theory have been explored in this way most often, because generalization is a primary component in these theories (McReynolds and Bennett, 1972; Elbert and Gierut, 1986). The theories have been found to be partially successful in predicting generalization. However, what is more customarily tested in generalization, regardless of the theoretical underpinning, is production of the sound in untrained contexts and perhaps production of other sounds that are thought to be related to the target sound in some way, usually, topographically. In other words, there is not much room for variation in constructing generalization probes.

Thus, targets chosen on the basis of a theory may differ considerably, but usually the same behaviors are trained to reach those various targets. Theories may be effective instruments for predicting generalization, but thus far the data for this effectiveness are scarce. Primarily, though, the issue is not necessarily which behaviors should be trained and tested, but rather what these behaviors, when tested, represent, e.g., generalization, rules, innate mechanisms, or environmental variables.

In sampling client behaviors in the natural environment, the clinician may not employ formal norms obtained from normative studies, but undoubtedly uses informal norms. The informal norm may be derived primarily from observations of the way those without communication problems speak in everyday situations: language forms produced frequently, topics discussed, individuals addressed. The observations may include casual notations of the communication interactions in which the client eventually participates. Such observations give the clinician targets for treatment that help the client to sound "normal." Therefore, although formally obtained normative data are not used to identify behaviors for remediation, informal "norms" often provide useful information for intervention planning.

CLIENT-SPECIFIC TARGETS

Another question often raised is whether the targets for treatment should be chosen directly from each client's behavioral inadequacies or from some general and external base, such as normative data discussed earlier (Hegde, 1985). The question in this case is not one of similarities in patterns during development and intervention, but rather whether group, averaged, or externally derived data should be used to select targets for individuals with disorders that vary from one person to another. One objection to use of group data is that such data are averages and no individual conforms to an average because there are no average clients. In fact, the variability within and across clients makes standards derived from normative studies or any group studies reporting mean data unrealistic for selecting target behaviors for treatment. Clinicians are cautioned not to adhere too closely to norms, not only because they are averages, but also because the norms and sequences are derived from descriptive, not experimental, studies. Thus, there is no evidence that certain behaviors cannot be learned until other behaviors have been acquired. Data do not show that some behaviors are prerequisite to acquisition of behaviors that appear later in the developmental sequence. Therefore, it may be more useful to observe the behaviors in need of treatment and to select the sequence in which they are to be trained on the basis of behavior needed by the client in order to function better, than to follow developmental sequences based on norms.

Another concern is that there are no data suggesting that acquisition or generalization is enhanced if normal developmental sequences are used for selecting targets. In addition, even if data had been obtained, it would be impossible to follow a fixed sequence simply because the studies identifying the sequence have not been conducted. Therefore, such information is not available for all possible target behaviors. Even if it is and if it can be demonstrated that there are some developmental sequences, there is no evidence to indicate that everything is learned in a specific sequential order.

A better rationale for selecting targets and sequences for training may be based on each client's specific problems and needs. For this purpose, standardized tests may be used, but observation of the client's behavior in natural circumstances is preferred. Such observations supply information about the specific behaviors that are impaired in each client and about how much of a detriment the impairment presents in daily exchanges and activities in which the behaviors occur. The point is that spontaneously produced behaviors in natural situations are more representative of the communication behavior of the client in everyday interactions at home, at play, at school, or at work. It is particularly important to obtain measures of the client's behaviors in the settings and situations in which generalization is expected to occur. The more the behaviors trained are the behaviors produced in everyday situations, the greater the probability that generalization will be facilitated in training. To identify these behaviors, standardized tests are inadequate. It is necessary to sample the client's behaviors in the natural environment, or in a situation closely simulating the natural environment, and in situations in which the behaviors occur. Sometimes the suggestions for obtaining measures of all relevant behaviors and in all environmental situations in which generalization is expected to occur are grossly unrealistic from a clinical viewpoint. Such extended observations cannot be practically implemented. Instead, as in planning treatment, it is wholly reasonable to make measurements in just a representative sample of situations to obtain a picture of how well the targeted behavior generalizes. That is to say, in treatment the behavior is trained in a small number of exemplars, not in all possible contexts. Similarly, we should not have to sample all contexts in which generalization is expected in order to confirm that it has occurred in those contexts.

INTERVENTION ENVIRONMENT

The second issue regarding a relationship between the normal, natural environment and the clinical situation in which target behaviors are to be taught centers on how different the two situations should be, both in terms of the target behaviors selected and in terms of the treatment situation if generalization is desired. The questions are whether to choose target behaviors on the basis of those most often appropriate in the natural environment or on some other basis, and whether training should be carefully structured or more broadly conceived to reflect the natural environment. This last question is discussed next.

A criticism of the conventional interventions offered is their dissimilarity to the natural environment to which the target behaviors are expected to be extended after treatment is completed (Spradlin and Siegel, 1982). Many differences have been pointed out. For example, the target behavior is elicited through such events as imitation or visual stimuli such as pictures, and the responses to these stimuli are often followed by consequent events that are not used or present in the natural environment (e.g., tokens or candy). They are not often related in a direct way to the response. Rather, they are arbitrary and artificial. For instance, if a child names a picture of a rabbit correctly, the clinician may administer praise and a piece of candy. Neither has a direct or functional relationship to the picture named. In the natural environment the response may be one that is more appropriate to the situation and so is followed by appropriate consequences. For example, if the child requests "milk," it is highly probable that he obtains a glass of milk. Another dissimilarity might be the response trained. For instance, learning to name colors is relevant, but probably there are other behaviors that are more functional and should therefore be trained before colors. When the differences are great between the clinical intervention situation and the natural environment, it is easy to understand why generalization does not occur from one to the other.

To solve this problem of little generalization, suggestions have been made to increase somehow the similarity between the two situations. Suggestions range from introducing stimuli and individuals from the natural environment after the response has been established firmly in the client's repertoire to introducing stimuli from the natural environment at the beginning of treatment, thus planning for generalization at the initiation of treatment. There has also been a suggestion that training should be shifted to the home environment from the clinical environment so that it occurs in the natural environment from the beginning. The suggestions come from a belief that the closer the training environment is to the natural environment, the greater the probability that generalization will occur.

Although it is readily recognized that generalization is not as extensive as hoped when training is restricted to the clinic, there is some unease in moving training to the home environment with parents as trainers. Some of the problems that have been raised are as follows: first, the situation at home has been shown to be ineffective for language learning, as evidenced by the fact that the child has a language problem; second, research has not identified what variables in the home environment and the parent behaviors are responsible for language acquisition; third, we have not yet identified the variables in the environment or within the child that are responsible for the language problems, so we do not know what aspects of the environment need to be modified; and fourth, the complexity of training in the natural environment, particularly speech and language responses that require perceptual skills to identify correct and incorrect responses, may result in a less efficient, more time-consuming effort.

Thus, we may be increasing the complexity and decreasing the efficiency of our treatment programs if we move treatment to the natural environment or attempt to train in all the stimulus conditions in which the behavior occurs outside the clinic. Given that impaired individuals have not learned the behavior in their natural environment, is it efficient to try to simulate, in intervention, the environment in which they failed to learn in the first place? Secondly, it is possible that the training program could be extended considerably if the clinician introduced in treatment all the stimuli, settings, individuals, and situations in which the behavior is expected to occur. One of the premises on which we operate is that all forms of a response in all situations do not have to be trained because generalization does occur. If it did not, our task would be impossible.

Thus, the issue is whether generalization is best facilitated by conducting training in a structured situation that quickly establishes the behavior in the child's repertoire and then shifts to concerns about generalization, or by modifying the natural environment so that treatment can be conducted there. In between are all the other possibilities that bring the natural environment into a closer relationship with the clinic (Baer, 1981). The trend appears to be in the direction of planning for generalization from the initial steps of treatment and introducing stimuli and events from the natural environment into the clinic from the beginning of treatment. However, the data to support any of the proposed procedures are lacking.

A related issue is the context in which treatment should be administered. That is, should it be in a clinic therapy room with minimal distractions and structured procedures or in the natural environment with little structure, in order to enhance occurrence of generalization? The same concerns apply to this issue as apply to the issue of selecting target behaviors that are frequently produced in the natural environment in contrast to behaviors that are developmentally sequenced or lacking in the client's repertoire. We must consider and weigh the advantages and disadvantages of each setting. For example, would the natural environment contain too many distracting stimuli, making treatment a difficult task? Would the treatment have to be so powerful that it could override all the extraneous variables present in the natural environment?

TARGETS FROM CLINICAL RESEARCH

Another alternative to selecting targets on the basis of developmental milestones, or client needs, is choosing targets that have experimentally obtained data for support (Hegde, 1985). That is, selection of targets can be based not only on behaviors that are important for the client in relation to the environment in which he operates, but also on behaviors that have been experimentally identified as relevant, manipulable, and facilitative to generalization.

The clinical research that has identified targets for

selection has been behavioral in orientation. The variables that have been explored experimentally have been derived from several sources, including theoretical ones. Thus, if theory indicates that a number of behaviors are related, the research is designed to evaluate the nature of that relationship. Primarily, the research has been directed at attempting to identify behaviors that are grouped together as members of a larger category usually known as a response class. A good portion of the research in language and phonology was designed to evaluate the validity of structural classes as defined by linguistic theory. For example, linguistic theory (structural) suggests that copula *is* and auxiliary *is* are separate behaviors and that copula *is* develops earlier than auxiliary *is*. Based on the theoretical formulation, then, the clinician would plan to train copula *is* first and auxiliary *is* second and each one separately because they are individual behaviors, and generalization from one to the other would not be expected. However, clinical research indicates that the two may not form separate classes, because if the copula is trained, clients also begin to produce the auxiliary, an indication that the two are members of the same response class. If one is trained, generalization to the other occurs, so it does not have to receive individual training, or only requires minimal training before generalization occurs (Kearns and Salmon, 1984; Hegde, 1980; Hegde and McConn, 1981). Although the research in response classes is still in the early stages, enough data are available to make some choices in language targets on a scientific basis and on the basis of targets that have been shown to have facilitative effects for generalization. However, language is a complex behavior in which many structures are involved. Only a few have been experimentally evaluated, and strong relationships among the structures that have been explored have not always been found. Such research is sorely needed and is continuing.

The notion of response classes, although useful, has thus far not been extended across all communication disorders. In fact, as mentioned, even the research on grammatical structures has been directed primarily at examining responses that have structural (i.e., topographical) similarities, to determine if those similarities function to evoke the same or related responses. That is, we have depended on physical similarities to establish the relationship for defining response classes. (Although, see Costello Ingham's chapter on stuttering in this volume for an example of two topographically *dis*similar responses that covary in treatment.) The dependence on topographical similarity may limit the kinds of variables that are examined. It is possible that researchers are missing more potentially powerful variables because they are not the most obvious ones.

Response classes have also been demonstrated on the basis of functional similarities. For example, if a child was taught to categorize a knife, fork, and teaspoon as tableware, he or she, when presented with a soup spoon or gravy ladle, would label each with the class label although the specific items have never been trained directly. The items have a similar use and therefore can be categorized as members of one class.

The concept of response classes sometimes is elusive. For example, it is possible to develop response classes arbitrarily if functional and topographical similarities have not been identified either theoretically or empirically. One definition of a response class is that it is a group of responses that share antecedent and consequent events and are created by the presentation of the same contingencies. Therein may lie a problem. By programming arbitrarily selected stimuli and by reinforcing particular responses in the presence of the stimuli, an investigator may develop several responses that appear to be members within a class. Testing for generalization to other stimuli, also arbitrarily selected, may reveal that responses are not produced to them because there are no aspects or parameters they share. That is, the response class was arbitrarily formed. On the other hand, the stimuli controlling responses are not always obvious ones. Some research indicates that when such training is administered, the subjects may be responding to stimulus similarities that have not been identified by the experimenter. In that case, generalization may be expected and shaped to stimuli that appear to be topographically or functionally dissimilar. (See Spradlin's discussion of stimulus equivalence in this volume.)

The notion of response classes is discussed in several of the subsequent chapters in this book. Generally it is defined in the same way by the various authors. However, Spradlin presents a somewhat different view of response classes in his chapter, and the discussion is directed partly to the issue presented in the previous paragraph.

GENERALIZATION AS A TERMINAL GOAL

Although generalization is desirable during and after treatment, generalization as the terminal goal in treatment has been questioned (Hegde, 1985). Hegde points out that the generalization obtained in the laboratory and as defined by the procedures used to test it in the laboratory is unsuitable as a treatment goal in the clinic. As described earlier, in the laboratory the subject is taught a discrimination through differential reinforcement. After the response to the training stimulus has been established, generalization to other stimuli is tested, some very similar to the training stimulus and some less similar to it. Responses in the presence of these test stimuli are not reinforced. The farther the test stimulus is from the characteristics of the training stimulus, the fewer the responses. As the test stimuli become less and less similar to the training stimulus, responding ceases entirely; it has not been reinforced and it disappears.

According to Hegde, our goal should be maintenance of the trained response. This goal requires that the behavior continue to be reinforced when it is produced outside of the clinic. Thus, if the laboratory procedural definition of generalization is applied to clinical activities, it is no wonder that the behavior is extinguished, and that little or no generalization is obtained. Or if it is obtained it soon disappears. One possibility for handling the problem is to think of the procedural definition of generalization as a powerful demonstration of generalization, recognizing that the definition is only one of several available. One way to circumvent the problem is to implement procedures proposed for facilitating generalization (Stokes and Baer, 1977; Costello, 1983; Spradlin and Siegel, 1982). Most of the procedures include some form of reinforcement for the target behavior as it is produced in contexts that gradually shift from restricted clinical environments to the client's natural environment. Because reinforcement is a part of the procedures and generalization in a literal sense has involved extinction, it is contended that the procedures are more accurately described as maintenance procedures, not as generalization procedures (Hegde, 1985; Hughes, 1985). Thus, the terminal goal in treatment should not be generalization; it should be maintenance. Because maintenance requires selective reinforcement of the target behavior in some manner, clinicians may test for generalization and use it to initiate maintenance procedures, but the terminal goal in treatment should be maintenance. This is not a denial of generalization; in fact, generalization should be probed and recorded throughout treatment. Responses on the probes would inform the clinician about which responses should be placed on maintenance. Treatment plans, therefore, should include procedures for maintaining the behavior outside the clinical environment by gradually introducing antecedent and consequent events that are present in the natural environment so that the behavior is not extinguished.

The issue poses a number of questions for planning interventions and for theoretical constructs that form the foundation for different approaches to treatment of communication disorders. The most crucial, of course, is whether clinicians should relinquish generalization as the terminal goal and devote more effort to planning contingencies for maintaining the target behavior after it has been acquired in the clinic. If so, several options are available.

Clinicians can formulate treatments that include plans for generalization early in the treatment sequence (Hughes, 1985). For instance, from the beginning of training, the clinician might use contexts in training that resemble contexts from the client's natural environment, or use a variety of exemplars for teaching a target response rather than using a restricted set of training items. In planning for generalization from the start of treatment, the clinician makes plans to introduce gradually into training variables that are present in the client's natural environment. At the completion of training, all relevant variables would have been introduced into the clinic, the target behavior has been produced in the presence of those variables. The shortcomings of that approach have been presented above.

Clinicians can choose other options which have been discussed earlier. For one, they can depend on topographical similarity between the training items and generalization items to evoke the target response if generalization is the goal. For example, in articulation training, it has been shown that children who learn the voicing distinction in pairs such as /s/ and /z/ can produce other voiced pairs such as /t/ and /d/, or /p/ and /b/ correctly without additional direct training on those pairs (McReynolds and Bennett, 1972). Another example would be the articulation generalization that has been obtained from nonsense syllables to words and phrases (Powell and McReynolds, 1969; Elbert and McReynolds, 1978). However, reliance on topographical similarity has limitations. Seldom is generalization as extensive as the topographical similarity would lead one to expect, and sometimes the similarity is not a characteristic that functions to evoke the response. In addition, subjects exhibit considerable individual variability, so it is difficult to predict who will generalize or to what extent. Finally, the topographical similarity may not be powerful enough to facilitate generalization to other environmental settings or to individuals other than the clinician providing the training. Topographical similarity can be one parameter to use for facilitating generalization, but when used alone, it is limited.

If topographical similarity is nonexistent, another parameter that can be used to promote generalization is the notion of response classes (explained earlier). For example, research has established that if children are trained to produce subject noun phrases, they will begin to produce object noun phrases without direct training on that construction (McReynolds and Engmann, 1974). Response classes have been experimentally demonstrated for a number of language constructions, but not all. As previously cautioned, using membership in a response class to predict generalization is sometimes useful, but it can present the same limitations as total reliance on topographical similarity. Generalization is not complete, not always replicable, and considerable across- and within-subject variability is evident.

Another option that can be chosen in planning treatment is not to rely on any of the parameters or procedures described above, but rather to continue training until the target behavior is produced correctly in all clinic and extraclinic contexts. If the clinician views generalization as an irrelevant notion because rules are acquired during training, the assumption is that no particular parameters need to be manipulated. With sufficient exposure and practice, the rule is acquired, and once acquired, is applied in all contexts. Thus, generalization is not an issue within this approach to treatment. Whatever his or her theoretical approach, the clinician is still constrained to select exemplars for exposure and practice in training that promise to provide the most effective opportunity for rule induction. In that selection, parameters need to be considered, whether topographical, physical, functional, or other.

Before rejecting generalization as the terminal goal, it is advantageous to consider two other options. One could, like Hegde (1985), assume that reinforcement is the only stimulus controlling a response. But it is possible that other stimuli are present that evoke the response and control it. Alternatively, one could define generalization less rigidly. Possibly the definition of generalization should not and cannot be limited to the procedural one Hegde offers. As a matter of fact, Hughes (1985) proposes that we distinguish among three different types of generalization. The first is *spontaneous generalization*, which occurs without special planning or additional training. The second type entails a special generalization phase of treatment after an establishment phase, when a probe indicates that the target behavior has not generalized to all the contexts tested. She calls this *posthoc programmed generalization*. The third kind is *preplanned generalization*. In this type, procedures and variables that are thought to facilitate generalization are initiated as soon as treatment starts.

The option chosen by each clinician is partly dependent on the theoretical viewpoint. It also depends on which parameters, if any, are considered important for promoting generalization. Primarily, the issue for the clinician is her or his definition of generalization. If generalization can include some form of reinforcement, then it can be trained during or after clinical activities. If generalization does not include reinforcement, then maintenance may be a better treatment goal. Both generalization and maintenance are included in the terminal goal.

PRACTICAL CONSIDERATIONS

Some of the issues that need to be addressed in research are more mundane than the ones discussed thus far. They are concerned primarily with criteria used to demonstrate that generalization has occurred, and how to use generalization data for deciding to terminate treatment. The issues are presented in the following section, but answers to the issues can only be offered for a few, mainly because research has not been directed to them. In other cases, the answers depend on the behaviors trained.

Number and Variety of Contexts

Often generalization is probed to a select, but hopefully representative, sample of untrained contexts during training. For example, if a language structure such as a locative "in the ______" is trained in a small set of exemplars (e.g., car, room, basket), generalization to another set of exemplars in untrained contexts such as "in the box," "in the bag," and others, is tested. Not all possible contexts are tested for generalization. The question is, how many untrained contexts should be tested in order to allow statements about generalization? Is it sufficient to test production to visual stimuli in the form of pictures, or should the subject produce the form spontaneously in conversation before the behavior can be said to have generalized? Or, in stuttering, should the client perform fluently in public situations as well as in private conditions with friends to be pronounced ready to enter his or her natural environment? Thus, it is necessary to decide not only how many contexts need to be tested, but also, how to select contexts that can be considered representative of the contexts in which the behavior is to occur in the natural environment. In this regard, data suggest that clients often generalize to items and contexts in the restricted environment of the clinic, but they evidence no generalization to spontaneous conversation or in the natural environment (Hughes, 1985). In articulation, for example, a hierarchy has emerged. Children generalize first, and most, to imitated items, then to spontaneously produced words in naming pictures, then to reading, and least, and last, to conversational speech (Rigor, 1980; Elbert, Shelton, and Arndt, 1967; Shelton, Elbert and Arndt, 1967). Therefore, if generalization to picture naming only had been tested, the clinician would not know whether the target response was ever produced in conversational speech. To obtain a realistic assessment of generalization, the appropriate contexts should be included in the testing. No data have been offered to suggest explicitly the number and variety of contexts to be tested, and there probably will not or cannot be a hard and fast rule within or across disorders. However, clinicians need to keep such considerations in mind when planning intervention programs and tests for generalization.

Another decision that has to be made concerns how many settings and which settings have to be used in generalization testing to obtain an accurate picture of the client's generalization. If the client is a child, for example, should generalization be tested in the home, in every room in the home, in the classroom, the playground, and so forth? Should generalization testing be conducted in stores, in the library, at the movies, and at a friend's home? The number of settings in which the target behavior may be required to be produced are too numerous to be included in the generalization testing. What the clinician would like to do is to make predictions about the strength of the generalization across settings. To do that, it is necessary to identify when a sufficient number of representative settings have been used to ensure, with a high probability, that the behavior will be produced in other settings. However, in all instances the clinician has to use practical considerations for selecting contexts in which generalization should be sampled. Every possibility need not be included in the schedule.

Measures of Generalization

Stability and consistency of the target behavior after it has generalized is important for determining that generalization has been attained and that behavior will be maintained. There are experimental data showing that if subjects are probed on the same items from one training session to another (Powell and McReynolds, 1969), generalization performance may change from one probe to another, at least in the early stages of intervention. So, if a subject produces the target response in test items on one occasion, it does not necessarily guarantee that the item will be correctly produced on the next generalization probe. For example, a client with aphasia may be enrolled in treatment to learn to produce noun phrases such as "the big cat" and may be tested on items such as "the big car" and "the big box." It is possible that on the first probe the client would produce "the big car" correctly. The clinician may be tempted to conclude that generalization has been obtained and that the response is stable. However, the clinician should not make such an assumption. It is equally likely that on the next probe the client will not produce "the big car" correctly. The variability within individuals has been discussed in an earlier section in this chapter. The response may be stable, but the clinician needs to test the consistency of the response before concluding that generalization is stable. To avoid misleading conclusions, it is necessary to establish a consistency criterion for demonstrating stability of generalization performance. In other words, each context in which generalization is tested needs to be tested more than once to establish consistency. Therefore, a minimum of two probes is necessary, but several probes are even better.

Clinical Significance

The decision concerning when generalization is clinically significant is tied to all of the issues discussed in this chapter. Another way to state the issue is to ask, "When is the client's speech and language similar enough to the speech and language of others in the community not to draw attention to itself?" The concern is with social validation, i.e., when others in the community judge the speech to be normal. Therefore, clinical significance is determined by the perceptions of others who are speaking normally. Thus, testing for clinically significant changes would require testing the behavior in nonclinic environments.

Another factor that needs to be taken into consideration is the specific target behavior that is trained and tested. Criteria may need to be different for different behaviors. The amount and kind of generalization needed to establish clinical significance vary across behaviors. Some behaviors occur, or have an opportunity to occur, frequently in a daily situation, whereas other behaviors do not. For example, active constructions in language are more frequently produced than passive constructions in daily communicative situations. Thus, if a 50 percent criterion is imposed on both structures, the criterion may provide misleading information, particularly if the probes consist of spontaneous conversation. How often would one expect to use a passive construction in daily conversation? How often would the criterion be met? Not often, but a zero percent correct does not always mean the subject cannot produce the structure; it may just mean there were no opportunities to do so. Thus, in determining the clinical significance of a behavior change as it transfers to untrained contexts, the factors of frequency and opportunity for occurrence need to be kept in mind.

SUMMARY

A number of philosophical, theoretical, and practical issues have been identified by clinicians and researchers interested in generalization. Most of them are directed at selection of behaviors to be trained and the situation in which the training should take place for optimum facilitation of generalization in treatment of communication disorders. Some answers, or at least plausible suggestions, have emerged from experimental research, but many issues remain to be studied. Nevertheless, a start has been made in identification of relevant variables across most communication disorders. The remaining chapters discuss these variables, particularly in relation to planning effective treatments.

REFERENCES

Baer DM. How to plan for generalization. Austin, TX: Pro-Ed, 1981.

Blough DS. The study of animal sensory processes by operant methods. In: Honig WK, ed. Operant behavior: areas of research and application. New York: Appleton-Century-Crofts, 1966:345.

Coggins TE, Olswang LB. The pragmatics of generalization. In: Ingham R, ed. Seminars in speech and language. Vol. 8. New York: Thieme Medical Publishers, 1987:283.

Costello J. Generalization across settings: language intervention with children. In: Miller J, Yoder D, Schiefelbusch R, eds. Contemporary issues in language intervention (ASHA Reports No. 12). Rockville, MD: American Speech-Language-Hearing Association, 1983.

Elbert M, Dinnsen D, Weismer G, eds. Phonological theory and the misarticulating child (ASHA Monograph No. 22). Rockville, MD: American Speech-Language-Hearing Association, 1984.

Elbert M, Gierut J. Handbook of clinical phonology. San Diego: College-Hill Press, 1986.

Elbert M, McReynolds LV. An experimental analysis of misarticulating children's generalization. J Speech Hear Res 1978; 21:136–150.

Elbert M, Shelton RL Jr, Arndt WB Jr. A task for evaluation of articulation change: I. Development of methodology. J Speech Hear Res 1967; 10:281–288.

Ferguson CA. Learning to pronounce: the earliest stages of phonological development in the child. In: Minifie FD, Lloyd LL, eds. Communicative competence and cognitive abilities. Baltimore: University Park Press, 1978:237.

Ferguson CA, Farwell CB. Words and sounds in early language acquisition: English initial consonants in the first fifty words. Language 1975; 51:419–439.

Ferguson CA, Macken MA. The role of play in phonological development. In: Nelson KE, ed. Children's language. Vol. 4. Hillsdale, NJ: Erlbaum, 1983:231.

Guess D, Sailor W, Baer DM. Children with limited language. In: Schiefelbusch RL, ed. Language intervention strategies. Baltimore: University Park Press, 1978:101.

Hegde MN. An experimental-clinical analysis of grammatical and behavioral distinctions between verbal auxiliary and copula. J Speech Hear Res 1980; 23:864–877.

Hegde MN. Treatment procedures in communicative disorders. San Diego: College-Hill Press, 1985.

Hegde MN, McConn J. Language training: some data on response classes and generalization to an occupational setting. J Speech Hear Disord 1981; 46:353–358.

Hughes DL. Language treatment and generalization. San Diego: College-Hill Press, 1985.

Johnston J. Discussion: Part I: What is language intervention? The role of theory. In: Miller J, Yoder D, Schiefelbusch R, eds. Contemporary issues in language intervention (ASHA Reports No. 12). Rockville, MD: American Speech-Language-Hearing Association, 1983.

Kearns KP, Salmon S. An experimental analysis of auxiliary and copula verb generalization in aphasia. J Speech Hear Disord 1984; 49:152–163.

Leonard L. Early language development and language disorders. In: Shames G, Wiig E, eds. Human communication disorders. Columbus, OH: Charles Merrill, 1982:221.

McLean J. Extending stimulus control of phoneme articulation by operant techniques. In: Girardeau FL, Spradlin JE, eds. A functional approach to speech and language (ASHA Monograph No. 14). Rockville, MD: American Speech-Language-Hearing Association, 1970.

McReynolds LV. Generalization in articulation training. Analysis and Intervention in Developmental Disabilities 1981; 1:245–248.

McReynolds L. A perspective on articulation generalization. In: Ingham RJ, ed. Seminars in speech and language: generalization and maintenance of therapy benefits with children. Vol. 8. New York: Thieme Medical Publishers, 1987:217.

McReynolds LV, Bennett S. Distinctive feature generalization in articulation training. J Speech Hear Disord 1972; 37:462–470.

McReynolds LV, Engmann DL. An experimental analysis of subject and object noun phrases. In: McReynolds LV, ed. Developing systematic procedures for training children's language (ASHA Monograph No. 18). Rockville, MD: American Speech-Language-Hearing Association, 1974.

Powell J, McReynolds LV. A procedure for testing position generalization from articulation training. J Speech Hear Res 1969; 12:629–645.

Rigor S. An experimental analysis of articulation generalization as a function of elicitation method and sampling context during articulation training. Master's thesis, University of Kansas, Lawrence, KA:1980.

Shelton RL Jr, Elbert M, Arndt WB Jr. A task for evaluation of articulation change: II. Comparison of task scores during baseline and lesson series testing. J Speech Hear Res 1967; 10:578–585.

Spradlin JE, Siegel GM. Language training in natural and clinical environments. J Speech Hear Disord 1982; 47:2–6.

Stokes TF, Baer DM. An implicit technology of generalization. J Appl Behav Anal 1977; 10:349–367.

Templin MC. Certain language skills in children (Institute of Child Welfare Monograph No. 26). Minneapolis, MN: University of Minnesota Press, 1957.

Vihman M, Macken M, Miller R, et al. From babbling to speech: a reassessment of the continuity issue. Language 1985; 61:397–445.

Chapter Two

METHODOLOGIES FOR STUDYING GENERALIZATION

KEVIN P. KEARNS, Ph.D.

A fundamental challenge facing speech-language pathologists is the call for clinical accountability. Hospital and school administrators and third-party payers are demanding that clinicians provide objective documentation that supports the effectiveness of their interventions, and this trend is likely to continue as the competition for health care dollars escalates. Speech-language pathologists must, therefore, acquire an increasingly sophisticated knowledge of methods and procedures that measure treatment effectiveness. However, clinicians and researchers alike now recognize generalization as the terminal goal of therapy, and the measurement of treatment effectiveness is rapidly becoming synonymous with attempts to measure and control factors that facilitate or inhibit generalized responding. Clinical accountability cannot, in fact, be fully achieved without documentation that communication skills that were trained in the clinic generalize to, and are maintained in, everyday functional settings and situations.

The purpose of this chapter is to consider practical methodologies that can be used for measuring and facilitating generalization of treatment effects for communicatively impaired individuals. Throughout the chapter I explore questions such as: What is a "generalization plan," and how does it differ from the traditional treatment plan? What measurement considerations are needed to monitor a client's performance and to determine if, and when, generalization occurs? Are some treatment techniques more likely to facilitate improvements that will generalize to the natural environment? Is it necessary to establish criteria to determine whether generalization has occurred? And, what can be done when generalization does not occur, despite our best efforts?

Our discussion begins with a consideration of recent terminological controversies in the generalization literature. This discussion is a necessary prerequisite to our exploration of factors that enter into the process of generalization planning.

TERMINOLOGY

The presence of terminological confusion, whereby multiple terms are used to describe the same phenomenon and new terms are proposed for known processes, indicates that a discipline has not fully matured as a clinical science. This lack of maturity exists in speech-language pathology and related fields, in which some researchers have borrowed terms from early experimental studies of generalization (Guess, Keogh, and Sailor, 1973; Hughes, 1985; Warren and Rogers-Warren, 1985), others have proposed new terms to describe generalization phenomena (Goldstein, 1985; Hegde, 1985), and many individuals have adopted definitions of generalization that were molded by clinical considerations (Stokes and Baer, 1977).

Problems often arise when technical terms are borrowed from the laboratory and applied to the clinic setting. As McReynolds noted in the previous chapter, the terms *stimulus generalization* and *response generalization* refer to specific behavioral processes that have been studied under tightly controlled laboratory conditions (Keller and Schonfeld, 1950; Skinner, 1953). However, when applied clinically the term generalization seldom meets the stringent requirements established for the experimental setting. Consequently, some authors have objected to the clinical use of the term on the grounds that many treatment procedures used to obtain responding in nontraining conditions are not consistent with laboratory definitions of generalization (Hedge, 1985; Johnston, 1979; Scott, Himandi, and Keane, 1983). From this perspective, use of the term generalization in the clinical setting is an unnecessary departure from definitional purity that may confuse clinicians and researchers alike. For example, Hedge (1985) points out that the conceptual and methodological distortion of the definition in clinical settings may lead clinicians to invest considerable time and effort obtaining generalized responding, without giving due consideration to maintenance. Hegde argues that *maintenance*, rather than generalization, should be the terminal goal of intervention (Kazdin and Esveldt-Dawson, 1981).

Despite such objections, clinicians' notions about generalization are purely pragmatic, and the term is firmly entrenched in their professional vocabulary. Clinicians are keenly interested in methods and procedures that enhance their ability to measure and obtain generalization clinically, but they have relatively little interest in, or knowledge of, the technical, laboratory use of the term.

Stokes and Baer (1977) recognized the need for a clinically viable approach to the study of generalization. They defined generalization as "the occurrence of relevant behaviors under different, nontraining conditions (i.e., across ... settings, people, behaviors and/or time) without the scheduling of the same events in those conditions as had been scheduled in the training conditions." While acknowledging that their definition is imprecise from a scientific standpoint, Stokes and Baer note that this definition captures the myriad of processes that may be present when clinical generalization occurs. As such, they view the definition as a legitimate compromise that is necessitated by clinical reality (Baer, 1981; Stokes and Baer, 1977).

The clinical usefulness of the Stokes and Baer definition arises, in part, from the fact that it emphasizes the need to plan actively for and "program" generalization. Although generalization has traditionally been viewed as a phenomenon that occurs in the absence of reinforcement, their definition stipulates that generalization occurs when the amount of training present in nontreatment conditions is somewhat less than the amount provided in treatment conditions. The definition also highlights the need for additional training or environmental manipulations when generalization does not occur, or when improvements are not maintained over time. In the final analysis, the Stokes and Baer (1977) definition is well suited to the clinical setting.

It has been 20 years since Baer, Wolf and Risley (1968) admonished that "generalization should be programmed rather than expected." Since that time numerous reviewers of the generalization literature have concluded that the amount and extent of generalization that occurs following treatment is often limited, unless specific steps are taken to promote generalized responding (Drabman, Hammer, and Rosenbaum, 1979; Garcia and DeHaven, 1974; Guess, Keogh, and Sailor, 1978; Marholin, Seigel, and Phillips, 1976; Stokes and Baer, 1977; Wahler, Berland, and Coe, 1979; Wildman and Wildman, 1975). As the chapters in this volume demonstrate, considerable progress has been made toward discovering treatment procedures and factors that influence whether generalization is likely to occur following intervention. However, the fact remains that we are not yet at the point of knowing, with any degree of certainty, which treatment procedures are most likely to facilitate generalized responding for the individual clients that we treat. As Baer, Wolf, and Risley (1987) recently noted, "... we still have no system for matching the most suitable generalization-promotion method to the behavior change at hand, and no certainty that there is such a system to be found." Clinicians can expect guidance from applied researchers, but concrete, data-based answers to the question of which treatment is most likely to facilitate generalization for a particular client are not forthcoming. However, clinicians can improve their ability to monitor and, hopefully, to obtain generalization in the clinical setting.

TRADITIONAL TREATMENT PLAN

Ideally the clinical process involves a complex series of logically related decisions that lead to principled assessment and data-based interventions (Yoder and Kent, 1988). Unfortunately, clinicians seldom practice exactly what is preached by those who write about the clinical process. Speech-language pathologists have been weaned on the notion that there are four distinct, sequential phases of the clinical process: evaluation, treatment, generalization, and maintenance (Fig. 2–1). The evaluation phase generally takes place in the hospital, school, or clinic setting, and it may involve as little as a single diagnostic session. The evaluation often includes the administration of a standardized test battery and, perhaps, informal observation of communicative abilities within the clinical setting. Based on the results of the evaluation, target behaviors

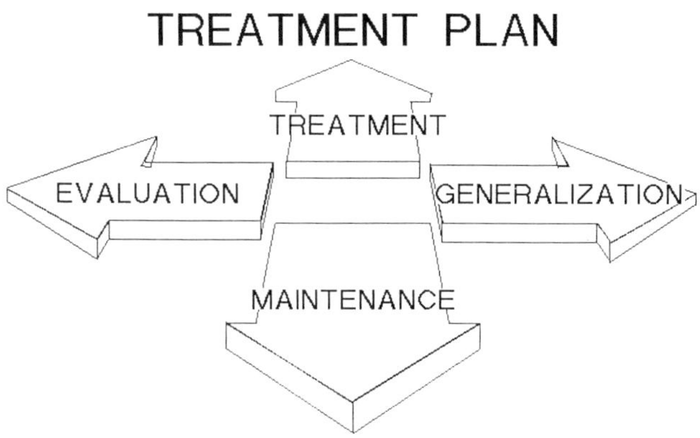

Figure 2–1 Four distinct phases of a traditional treatment plan: evaluation, treatment, generalization, and maintenance.

are selected for training, and a treatment plan is formulated. However, all too often, behaviors that are selected for training are never actually assessed during the traditional evaluation. That is, clinicians frequently administer standardized tests to select specific treatment behaviors. Yet, because of their broad format, these tests rarely provide information about the specific behaviors that are targeted in treatment. Moreover, when the behaviors of interest are included in formal test batteries, they are seldom sampled extensively.

Once target behaviors are selected for training, criteria for successful completion of treatment are often based on normative data or periodic readministration of the standardized tests used during the initial assessment. The schedule for retesting, when it occurs, is frequently based on nonclinical factors such as the end of a school year or the end of an academic or fiscal quarter.

Within the traditional treatment plan, clinicians often consider generalization *after* criteria are met on clinical treatment tasks, if they consider it at all. When they do examine it, they tend to assess carry-over informally and anecdotally. For example, clinicians may measure performance during group treatment sessions to evaluate generalization from individualized therapy; they may accompany the client to a cafeteria and subjectively assess generalization; or they may simply ask parents, teachers, or spouses about their clients' communication skills in nonclinical settings. However, specific procedures for assessing or facilitating generalized responding are rarely undertaken.

Similarly, post-treatment assessment of generalization over time (i.e., maintenance) is also the exception rather than the rule. Follow-up testing may consist of readministering standardized tests given prior to therapy; these, as noted previously, seldom measure behaviors or skills that are directly treated. Consequently, standardized tests often provide little or no information about generalization over time (maintenance). Furthermore, although clinicians sometimes counsel clients and families about the need to use and reinforce newly acquired behaviors in the home and other natural settings, steps are rarely taken to maintain treatment gains.

DEVELOPING A GENERALIZATION PLAN

On the surface, there are many similarities between traditional treatment planning and generalization planning. For example, many of the same clinical intervention activities and processes relating to evaluation, treatment, and generalization are considered with both approaches. However, the clinical process model involved in generalization planning is markedly distinct from the traditional intervention approach in terms of goals, methods, and procedures. In contrast to the traditional approach, the goal of generalization planning is to obtain generalized responding across behaviors, settings, people, and time. The methodology used to accomplish this goal is also at variance with the treatment planning methods, in that there are no discrete, sequentially ordered phases associated with generalization planning. On the contrary, each component of the generalization plan is dependent on, or overlaps with, all other components (Fig. 2–2). Thus, evaluation procedures are repeated periodically throughout intervention, treatment strategies are chosen because they may facilitate generalization, follow-up testing is routinely scheduled, and the results of such tests are used to continue, modify, or terminate intervention.

When intervention is conceptualized from a generalization planning perspective, it involves a number of unique considerations. We begin our discussion of generalization planning by considering factors relevant to evaluation procedures.

Evaluation

The evaluation component of generalization planning differs from the evaluation phase of treatment planning in that it requires that clinicians examine a broad range of behaviors and conditions that influence treatment outcome and generalization. In his monograph, *How to Plan for Generalization*, Baer (1981) suggests beginning the planning process by making four comprehensive lists: first, all behaviors that need to be changed; second, all situations (i.e., both setting and stimulus conditions change), settings, and places where changes are needed; third, all individuals with whom the improvements are desired; and fourth, all behaviors of significant others in the environment that affect production of the target behaviors. To these four lists I add a fifth: all environmental factors that might affect production of the communication behaviors.

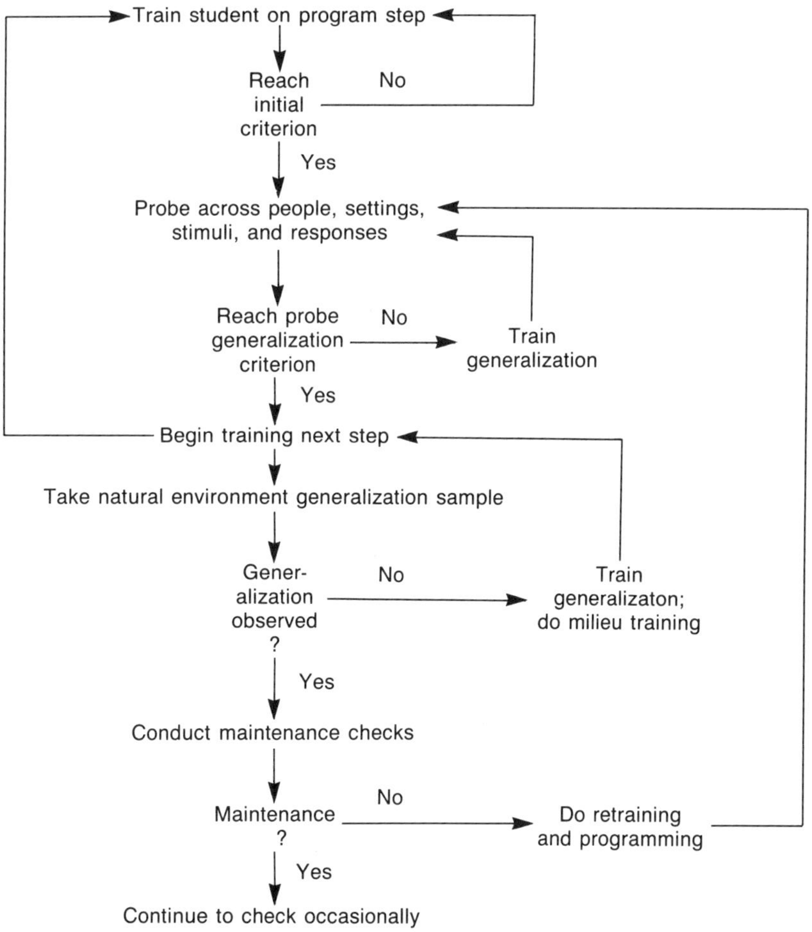

Figure 2–2 Integrated components of a generalization plan. (Reprinted by permission from Warren SF. Clinical strategies for the measurement of language. In: Warren SF, Rogers-Warren AK. Teaching functional language. Austin, TX: Pro-Ed, 1985.)

These particular lists were proposed because they are presumed to include the range of information needed for developing a comprehensive generalization plan. By listing all of the behaviors that need to be changed, the clinician is in a better position to decide which behaviors to treat and which behaviors simply to test periodically to determine whether generalization has occurred. Similarly, the list of relevant settings could be used as a resource for planning treatment goals and generalization test procedures; and the lists of individuals and environmental factors that affect patient responding could be used to determine whether indirect treatment approaches, such as family intervention or environmental manipulations, should be incorporated into the generalization plan. Finally, the lists might also prove useful for modifying treatment approaches following an unsuccessful generalization programming attempt.

A major task facing clinicians, therefore, is the process of narrowing the lists of behaviors, situations, individuals, and so forth, that are relevant for developing a generalization plan for a given patient. The necessity of gathering extensive information in so many areas and of selecting factors that are most relevant to programming generalization may, at first, appear overwhelming. However, as clinicians gain experience with generalization planning, they gradually become more organized and efficient, and the process of generalization planning becomes less time-consuming.

The process of gathering evaluative information on a broad range of behaviors and conditions and then using this information to aid generalization planning is analogous to learning how to operate a computer. Both activities require an initial time investment, and both tasks may initially seem overwhelming, frustrating, and even unmanageable at times. However, as one learns basic computer functions and acquires the ability to operate various programs, the initial frustration recedes and the benefits of the new skill become apparent. Likewise, as clinicians acquire the skills necessary to develop a generalization plan, time requirements diminish and the benefits become apparent. The initial time investment necessary to learn how to plan for generalization is rewarded when the time that it takes to establish an intervention strategy results in efficient and effective clinical management.

There are no absolute rules or infallible paths that lead to competent clinical management, and it is impossible to prescribe which behaviors, settings, people, and situations should be examined during the evaluation component of generalization planning. These types of decisions can only be made by the clinician responsible for managing a particular patient. Choosing among the possible options is frequently complicated by the fact that there is a wide variety of categories of generalization that could be examined clinically (Drabman, Hammer, and Rosenbaum, 1979). However, there are several logical and clinically proven guidelines that can be offered to help clinicians select the appropriate methods and procedures needed to develop a viable generalization plan.

First, after compiling the previously discussed lists of information, it is helpful to prioritize them with regard to generalization planning. That is, using all available objective data, clinical observations, and reports, select the communicative behaviors that most urgently need to be trained, and identify the people, settings, and situations in which these skills need to be produced. After ranking the lists and establishing priorities, select a minimum of two behaviors, one person and one setting or situation, that will be periodically evaluated or treated once intervention begins. By limiting the generalization plan to these priorities initially, the time constraints imposed by generalization testing become manageable, and a plan can be realistically devised and implemented.

Whenever practical, it is useful to evaluate systematically the influence of each generalization parameter in relative isolation from other parameters. We should, for example, initially attempt to hold setting and situation parameters constant if we are primarily interested in generalization across people. For example, we could measure carry-over by training a parent, spouse, or significant other to administer generalization probes (see below) within the clinical setting. Data collected under these restricted circumstances would serve as a measure of generalization across people (e.g., spouse), that would not be contaminated by other parameters.

It is, of course, possible and ultimately desirable to combine two or more generalization parameters for the purpose of testing. For example, it may be feasible to assess production of turn-taking skills of a patient with a closed head injury while he is interacting with his wife (generalization person), after dinner (generalization situation), at home (generalization setting).

Probes such as these, in which several important parameters differ from treatment conditions, provide an important means of assessing generalization to naturalistic conditions. However, by changing and measuring the effect of each parameter individually, the clinician is in a better position to make adjustments in treatment strategies that may promote generalized responding.

Compilation of comprehensive lists of factors relevant to generalization programming is a time-consuming and arduous task, but the advantages of thoroughness are considerable. As Baer (1981) notes, the listing of relevant considerations for generalization planning allows one to see problems in their entirety, so the complexity of the planned intervention becomes apparent. With the aid of the lists, clinicans can knowledgeably devise appropriate intervention programs that have the best chance of facilitating generalized responding.

Formal testing and within-clinic observations alone cannot provide the range of information needed to develop a comprehensive generalization plan. Therefore, it is usually necessary to gather additional information from parents, spouses, teachers, and other professionals. Industrious clinicians use any means at their disposal to obtain the information, including, for example, nonstandard preassessment questionnaires and family interviews (Lund and

Duncan, 1988). We now turn our attention to clinical probes, the most direct and common means of gathering generalization data.

Generalization Probes

Probes are tests of performance that provide information about acquisition, generalization, or maintenance. Any periodic test of performance that is used to measure the results of intervention can be considered a probe. However, more often than not, probes are nonstandard measures specifically designed by the clinician or experimenter as a measure of performance of target behaviors for which there exists no standardized test. Although probes are often structured to have a client respond in discrete stimulus—response situations (Warren, 1985), less structured assessments, and even in-vivo evaluations of spontaneous performance, have been used to assess generalization. Three representative types of generalization probes are briefly reviewed in this section: discrete-trial probes, environmental simulation probes, and spontaneous probes in natural environments. (These probe categories are neither all-inclusive nor mutually exclusive. They are presented for organizational convenience and clarity.)

Discrete-Trial Probes

Structured probes of performance on discrete-trial tasks that require patients to respond each time an examiner presents a stimulus are considered *discrete-trial probes*. Quite often, these assessments utilize the same or similar stimulus materials that are presented during treatment tasks, and they are designed to elicit responses on treated and untreated target behaviors.

Typically, discrete-trial probes include stimuli to elicit responses that are currently being trained, untrained exemplars of trained responses, and responses that are topographically or functionally similar to trained responses. These last items are included to assess generalization to similar, but untrained, behaviors.

For example, Kearns and Salmon (1984) conducted a study of the acquisition and generalization of auxiliary and copula verbs in aphasia. The criteria for successful completion of steps in the training program and the criteria for successful generalization of responding from trained to untrained auxiliary and copula verbs were based on periodic administration of structured probes. The procedure that was used to probe verb production consisted of individually presenting a stimulus picture that depicted trained and untrained auxiliary and copula verbs, in an attempt to elicit the subjects' verbal production of the target verbs. For example, the investigator presented a picture of a "boy running" and asked the aphasic patients to describe the picture. In all, thirty stimulus pictures were used to probe patients' responses to various classes of auxiliary and copula verbs. Performance on pictures that had not been used during training sessions provided information about the generalization of training effects. Data were also collected on items that were in the process of being trained, so that treatment effectiveness could be evaluated. Finally, performance on previously trained items allowed the experimenters to examine generalization across time (maintenance) for previous levels of performance on those items.

Two methods of probing that are commonly used to measure treatment gains and generalization were periodically administered throughout the Kearns and Salmon (1984) study. One method involved interspersing test items within the actual treatment sessions; the second method involved administration of the probes prior to the treatment sessions.

Because generalization probes are used as an assessment tool, an essential aspect of probes is that they measure performance in the absence of any reinforcement and feedback. Consequently, when the investigators interspersed probe items within sets of treatment items, feedback and reinforcement were never provided after the subjects responsed to probe items. This was accomplished by interspersing probe items within sets of treatment items during treatment sessions in which the clinician reinforced correct responding on an intermittent basis. That is, contingent feedback and praise were available after every three correct responses. This lean schedule of reinforcement allowed the investigators to intermix three probe items with seven treatment items to form ten-item sets of verb stimuli. The interspersed probe items were from verb categories that were not currently being trained. When one of the seven training items (e.g., copula *is*) was presented, modeling, feedback, and reinforcement were provided when an accurate response was produced. However when one of the three probe items (e.g., auxiliary is) was presented contingent praise or feedback was not provided. By proceeding in this manner, information was gathered on patients' ability to produce untrained verbs, previously trained verbs, and verb forms that were in the process of being trained.

One obvious advantage of the interspersing method of probing is that valuable information can be obtained about generalization and maintenance on untrained or previously trained behaviors during the actual training of a second behavior. However, this procedure takes careful planning and organization of treatment sessions. In addition, because a restricted number of probe items can be interspersed within a set of training items, it may take several treatment sessions to administer a complete set of untrained and previously trained items.

The second probe method used in the Kearns and Salmon (1984) study involved periodically presenting the entire set of thirty stimulus pictures prior to treatment sessions. After randomizing the stimuli, items were individually presented, and subjects were asked to describe the pictures. Again, contingent praise or feedback was not available to the subjects during the method of probing.

By randomly presenting the entire set of stimulus pictures on a periodic basis, the experimenters obtained information about the acquisition, generalization, and maintenance of the verb forms examined in this study.

Thus far, common forms of discrete trial probes have

been considered: those interspersed within training sessions, and those administered in their entirety prior to or after training sessions. It has also been noted that a common function of these probe techniques is to examine performance on items receiving training, on untrained exemplars of training items, or on related untrained (i.e., generalization) items, and on previously trained (maintenance) items. Another important function of discrete-trial generalization probes is to examine performance on untrained steps in a treatment program. Oftentimes, our treatment goals are hierarchically arranged in terms of sequential, presumably more difficult performance goals. Treatment programs typically proceed from least complex to progressively more complex behaviors. For a child with an articulation disorder we might, for example, initially train phonemes or phoneme contrasts in relatively simple consonant-vowel-consonant contexts until a predetermined performance criterion is reached. During subsequent steps in a program, we might require that performance criteria be reached in progressively more complex contexts, such as phrases, sentences, and conversational speech. In this example, and in other treatment approaches that include several intermediate steps prior to reaching a termination criterion level, it is important to measure performance periodically, prior to and throughout training. Using our previous example, this would mean that our discrete-trial generalization probes would include items that elicited responses at the single word, phrase, and sentence level. In addition, a separate probe of articulatory performance during spontaneous speech would also be of value.

The importance of systematically probing all steps in a treatment program cannot be overemphasized, because we rarely know the most efficient sequence of training steps to achieve our generalization goals. That is, in some instances, training at early steps in a treatment program may result in generalized improvements to subsequent training steps; it would then be unnecessary to train steps for which criterion level generalization has occurred.

Loverso, Prescott, and Selinger (1988), for example, found that generalization occurred to steps in a verb training hierarchy for aphasic patients, even though those steps in the program had not been directly trained. This information allowed these investigators to reduce the number of training steps in their protocol and to provide a more efficient treatment package. In addition, valuable generalization data were obtained from the probes of "higher" levels of the training procedure. Clinicians can also evaluate the efficiency of their training programs by probing untrained program steps to determine whether sufficient generalization has occurred and to establish the most efficient, cost-effective generalization plan.

For our purposes, "sufficient generalization" must be objectively defined before treatment begins. Thus, generalization criteria should be established for steps in a treatment sequence, and treatment can be withheld on untrained behaviors or training steps until generalization is met. Elbert and Gierut (1986) summarize this principle and provide an example for treatment of a phonologically disordered child. They state:

> Probes evaluate generalization following treatment on a specific program step, but can also be incorporated into the criterion for advancing to the next level of a program. For example, for a particular child probes are administered after the predetermined level of 90-percent accurate spontaneous production of a target sound has been reached on each step in the program. In addition, the child must also meet a predetermined level of probe (or generalization) performance. This may be 50-percent accurate spontaneous production of the target sound in untreated generalization (probe) items. If the child meets both the treatment criterion of 90-percent accuracy and the generalization criterion of 50-percent accuracy, then treatment is advanced to the next step in the program. If, however, the child meets the 90-percent treatment criterion but fails to meet the minimum 50-percent generalization, then additional treatment is provided. (p. 149).

By requiring clients to achieve both a treatment criterion and a generalization criterion, the clinician ensures that a minimum amount of generalization occurs prior to initiating training at subsequent steps in a treatment program. As we shall see in our discussion of treatment techniques that may facilitate generalization, decisions to terminate treatment should also be based on a generalization criterion for performance in the natural environment. The use of a generalization criterion to guide treatment decisions ensures the continuation of training until target behaviors are produced in the natural environment at sufficient levels so that they can make contact with naturally occurring reinforcers and, thereby, be maintained over time.

Discrete-trial probe procedures provide a relatively easy means of assessing generalization to untrained behaviors and program steps, and they can be adopted with minimal disruption of the clinic process. Once a set of probe items is compiled, it can be administered repeatedly over time without taking a great deal of time away from treatment activities. Because it is necessary to establish the stability of performance on treatment tasks prior to intervention, a set of probe items can be administered on three or more occasions, just prior to intervention to establish a patient's pretreatment level of performance or steps in a treatment program. Once treatment begins, the probe can be readministered periodically to assess progress. By comparing performance on the pretreatment (i.e., baseline) probes with performance during and after intervention, the clinician has an objective means of monitoring acquisition and generalization. At a minimum, discrete-trial probes should be readministered each time criterion is met at steps in a treatment program (Warren, 1985). However, it is desirable and often quite practical to administer probes on a more frequent basis, such as weekly or biweekly.

It is clinically advantageous if the results of probes are graphed immediately after they are collected. Discussions of procedures for graphing data are available (Barlow, Hayes, and Nelson, 1984; McReynolds and Kearns, 1983; Parsonson and Baer, 1978). The use of line graphs in which the rate or frequency of performance is plotted over time is particularly helpful for identifying trends in the data.

The ongoing monitoring of trends provides a degree of clinical flexibility that is not otherwise available (Connell and Thompson, 1986). That is, by immediately plotting and analyzing the results of generalization probes, the clinician can directly observe trends and determine when to alter intervention strategies. Graphic data presentation and analysis also provide an excellent form of feedback that can be made available to patients, families, quality assurance teams, and third-party payers.

As we have seen, the advantages of discrete-trial probe procedures are considerable. However, the structured information provided by this probe technique does not provide sufficient information for planning and monitoring generalization. As noted previously, a comprehensive generalization plan necessitates observing a client's performance in less structured conditions and in the natural environment. Our discussion of generalization probe procedures continues with a consideration of environmental simulation probes, because these assessment procedures approximate naturalistic observations.

Environmental Simulation

For our purposes, semistructured, clinician-controlled assessment conditions, which approximate elements of the natural environment and incorporate aspects of communicative interaction that occur in a patient's daily living, are referred to as *environmental simulation probes*. Although probes that simulate naturalistic conditions are regularly administered in clinical settings, they are not always planned or conducted in a manner that permits an objective assessment of communicative performance. As with all assessment procedures, clinicians should delineate goals, procedures, and measurement factors prior to initiating environmental simulation probes. Assessment procedures that approximate naturalistic conditions require careful planning, particularly with regard to making sure that the assessment situation can be accurately replicated over time, and that scoring procedures are a reliable and valid reflection of patient performance. Relevant measurement and scoring considerations are discussed later in this chapter (see "Natural Environments").

Lund and Duchan (1988) describe clinical examples of semistructured language elicitation techniques that fit our definition of environmental simulation probes. They suggest obtaining spontaneous language samples while observing the child interact with familiar and unfamiliar interactants. The stimulus conditions for the probes vary according to the child's interests and level of functioning. An attempt is made to select stimuli that the child may be curious about, and the interactant allows the child to direct the conversational flow to his interests. A typical spontaneous language probe would include observation of a parent teaching a task to his child and then interacting with the child while he played with a variety of toys. The clinician can serve as the unfamiliar interactant by gradually taking over the role previously served by the parent.

Lund and Duchan also describe several procedures for eliciting specific linguistic structures and communicative behaviors. For example, "set-ups" can be used to elicit commenting or requesting. A set-up involves arranging a naturally occurring event, such as an unexpected or unpredictable occurrence, to elicit desired structures. The clinician might introduce a broken toy or a logical absurdity, such as "blue milk," into the interaction.

In addition to set-ups, Lund and Duchan also describe the use of patterning, retelling or reenactment, pretending, and game playing as other semistructured techniques that can be used to probe a child's language and communicative behaviors. These environmental simulation probe procedures could be used to expand the clinician's personal repertoire of elicitation techniques.

Simmons, Kearns, and Potechin (1987) provide an example of a probe procedure that simulated known interactions that occurred in an aphasic patient–spouse dyad. The purpose of this study was to examine the effectiveness and generality of a spouse recognition training procedure. The procedure was designed to train spouses to recognize and modify behaviors that interfered with dyadic communication with their aphasic partner. For the couple in this study, target behaviors included the response classes of spouse interruptions, negative teaching behaviors, and use of convergent questions. Generalization of improvement in spouse interactive skills was evaluated by having the couple watch and discuss television shows, including news segments and a television talk show. These observations were designed to evaluate interactions under stimulus conditions that occur naturally in the couple's home environment. In addition to being convenient, this probe procedure had the added advantage of allowing the experimenters to control the length, content, and interest level of the videotape stimuli. Consequently, the researchers could consistently (i.e., reliably) repeat the probes over time. Environmental simulation probes include observation and analysis of situations and interactions that are similar to naturally occurring events taking place in everyday settings. An attempt should be made to incorporate significant others, to use stimulus materials from the natural environment, and to establish a realistic context or topic for the assessment. Environmental simulation probes should also be unobtrusive, and, whenever possible, these assessments should be recorded on audio equipment or videotape for analysis.

Audio- or videotaping provides a "hard copy" of the assessment that can be analyzed and subsequently compared with other evaluation sessions. Another advantage of taping interactions is that the tapes can also be used to check the reliability of clinicians' scoring of the communicative behaviors of interest.

Whenever possible, environmental simulation probes should supplement rather than replace observations obtained in natural contexts. The use of test conditions that simulate naturalistic settings or conditions provides an intermediate assessment step between discrete-trial probes and in-vivo testing. Consequently, creatively arranged controlled observations of simulated environmental conditions are an essential component of generalization planning.

Natural Environments

Naturalistic observations, like all other forms of assessment (Hawkins, 1979), can serve multiple functions, and the exact purpose of a probe in natural environments influences measurement decisions. For example, a pretreatment observation that is undertaken to help the clinician establish intervention priorities may be less focused than naturalistic probes that are administered to monitor generalization. Whereas in the former case, all significant communicative interactions or responses might be recorded, during naturalistic generalization probes a clinician might only record occurrences of specific target behaviors. Despite differences in measurement procedures, determined by the purpose of the probe, there are several broad issues that must be considered when the clinician wishes to conduct generalization probes in naturalistic environments. These issues are introduced next.

Oftentimes, the more difficult questions facing the clinician interested in naturalistic observations relate to the measurement and analysis of the assessments. Not the least of these questions is, "What variables exist in the natural environment that affect production of target and generalization behaviors?" Stated differently "What are the antecedent stimuli, responses, and consequences that either promote or inhibit communicative effectiveness?" An analysis of the "three term contingency" (Skinner, 1953; 1969) forces the clinician to attend to the functional relationships between environmental stimuli, responses, and the reinforcing or punishing consequences that increase or decrease the likelihood that target communication skills will be produced. Therefore, recording of observations in the natural environment should include the systematic description of these variables (Cooper, Heron, and Heward, 1987; Gelfand and Hartmann, 1984; Sulzer-Azaroff and Mayer, 1977).

In other words, clinicians should carefully observe and record the relationship between environmental factors that precede responding, the occurrence of the target response, and ways in which individuals in the natural setting reinforce the behavior of interest. For example, a laryngectomized individual who was more than 95-percent intelligible in sentences with his artificial larynx complained to his clinician that he wrote messages at home and seldom used his artifical larynx in that environment. This is somewhat perplexing given that he appeared satisfied with the artificial larynx and, in fact, relied on his instrument at work and while socializing with his friends. Interestingly, an analysis of periodic generalization probes of tape-recorded interactions between the laryngectomee and his wife at home revealed that attempts to use his artificial larynx were generally followed by comments from his wife such as, "What? I can't understand you with that thing." These derogatory remarks were found to be directly related to the frequency with which the patient attempted to use his artifical larynx at home. Thus, information from the generalization probe led to a treatment strategy that included training the spouse to attend to and reinforce the patient's successful attempts to communicate with his artificial larynx.

Measurement Issues. There are several factors to keep in mind when attempting to record the contingencies operating in the natural environment. First, a measurement procedure must be selected that is appropriate for the behavior of interest. Many communicative behaviors are discrete rather than continuous in nature, and a simple count of the number of discrete events that occur can be used for scoring these target behaviors. In the previous example, the number of times that the patient initiated a communicative interaction or responded to a question with his artificial larynx served as the basic measure of performance. This type of *event recording*, whereby a clinician records the number of responses produced, is commonly used during naturalistic observations. Of course, a more sensitive, multidimensional scoring procedure can also be employed to assess the quality of patients' responses. Thus, in the above example, a numerical score could have been recorded to reflect how efficiently and intelligibly he used his artificial larynx.

In addition to event recording, any number of time-based measurement procedures can also be useful for recording performance on probes obtained in natural environments. A clinician might, for example, choose to record target responses that were produced within a specified interval of time (i.e., interval recording). Relatedly, a clinician might wish to record the duration of a response, rather than the frequency of responding. Thus, a clinician could record the duration of responding for home observations of a patient who had suffered a right hemisphere stroke, because these individuals can be hyperverbal and fail to yield conversational turns during interactions. Whatever the behavior of interest, it may be necessary to select one or more types of less common measurement procedures to assess performance in natural environments. Clinicians interested in generalization planning should, therefore, familiarize themselves with the available alternatives (Cooper, Heron, and Heward, 1987; McReynolds and Kearns, 1983).

Once a clinician has selected a measurement procedure for naturalistic observations, it is necessary to develop a standard recording form that can be used for repeated observation. Ideally, the form should allow succinct recording of relevant stimuli, responses, and consequences that are observed. In this regard, observational recording is facilitated by the use of clinician-devised observational codes. For example, individuals in the probe environment could be appropriately identified as spouse (sp), brother (b), sister (s), and so on. A patient's responses could be recorded using a similar personalized code or an available multidimensional scoring system (Porch, 1971).

Besides being concise, the scoring form that is developed for naturalistic observations should attempt to capture the temporal relationships between environmental stimuli, patient responses, and consequences (Brookshire and associates, 1978.) By capturing the temporal relationship between events that occur in the observational setting, the clinician is in a better position to identify response patterns that may either facilitate or inhibit generalized responding.

It must be recognized that even the most well-intentioned and comprehensive evaluation of environmental contingencies still will not identify many variables that control or influence an individual's communicative abilities. The purpose of probes in natural environments is to observe and analyze directly the factors that affect patients' ability to respond. Yet, variables that affect responding may not be presented during observational sessions. Moreover, other variables that control responding are more complex than the restricted stimulus–response relationships that can be observed and recorded. Complex stimulus–response interactions that precede observation sessions and affect subsequent responding have been referred to as *setting events* (Wahler, Berland, and Coe, 1979).

Setting events are "complex...conditions, events, and stimulus–response interactions which may overlap or entirely precede subsequent behaviors that they affect" (Wahler and Fox, 1981, p. 329). Setting events are more complex environmental conditions or factors; they are specific to the patient or the patient's environment. Although we acknowledge that our clients' behaviors are influenced by the complexity of the home and school environments, by their attentional state, by sleeplessness, and by occurrences that are temporally and physically removed from the clinic, we rarely systematically evaluate these factors or consider them in treatment planning. However, we can record observations of environmental events and reports of significant events that precede naturalistic observations. By informally correlating notes on setting events with actual performance, we may identify factors that affect responding, and we can then attempt to control those environmental variables. For example, a dysarthric adult was found to perform more poorly than expected on probes of his intelligibility during spontaneous interactions in the nursing home where he resided. After observing that the patient's poor performance consistently occurred on the same day each week, the clinician asked the patient's primary nurse if there were any events preceding the probes that might be influencing performance. With some persistence and after several inquiries, the clinician discovered that the patient always had physical therapy just prior to the probes on which he did so poorly. Knowledge of this setting event allowed the clinician to adjust the schedules accordingly. As this example demonstrates, the ultimate success of a generalization plan may be determined by how well we identify and modify complex environmental factors above and beyond the simple contingencies observed during probes of performance in natural environments.

Finally, it should be noted that naturalistic observations are almost always costly, and some consideration should be given to the cost:benefit ratio of conducting probes outside the clinical setting. At times, the clinician's cost, in terms of time, salary, travel, and so on, far outweighs the benefits that are expected in terms of the clinician's ability to provide quality patient care. This is sometimes the case when a client's home or school is located a considerable distance from the clinic, school, or treatment setting. There are also times when naturalistic observations are clearly desirable, but an unusually heavy clinical caseload, transportation problems, and so forth, may prevent the clinician from observing the patient directly in his or her natural milieu. When practical problems such as these prevent or severely limit the clinician's ability to probe, then parents and other individuals can be trained to collect generalization probe data. (Some patients can, in fact, collect data on their own performance.) These confederates must be able to identify and score target responses reliably, and to administer probes consistently in the manner prescribed by the clinician. However, even after other individuals have demonstrated the ability to administer and score probes in natural environments, it cannot be assumed that they will remain reliable and unbiased. Therefore, it is occasionally necessary to tape-record naturalistic probes and reevaluate the reliability of the administration and scoring of these probes.

When other individuals are used it is, of course, necessary to provide these individuals with score sheets, tape recorders, or other items needed to complete the naturalistic observations. In addition, it is generally wise to keep observational sessions brief and on the same days and times. These tactics may improve compliance and ensure that the task is manageable. Finally, confederate observers may also be more cooperative if they are given feedback on their performance and if they are shown the value of their work. The clinician can, for example, graph a client's performance on the naturalistic observations, so that the data can be described and shown to the individuals who assisted with the probes.

A final note on probing concerns patient consent and confidentiality. It goes without saying that informed consent should always be obtained before patients are tape-recorded or observed, and the patient's confidentiality should never be violated. It is important that probes of performance in natural settings should be as unobtrusive as possible. However, every attempt must be made to keep patients informed of our intent to observe and record their communicative abilities.

FACILITATING GENERALIZATION

Inherent in the notion of developing a generalization plan is the belief that specific treatment techniques are available that promote generalized responding. Reviews of the applied behavioral literature (Stokes and Baer, 1977; Wildman and Wildman, 1975) and the language and communicative disorders literature (Garcia and Dehaven, 1974; Guess, Keogh, and Sailor, 1978; Harris, 1975; Risley, 1977; Spradlin and Siegel, 1982) provide concrete suggestions for facilitating generalized responding. Clinicians can also refer to recent texts that address the clinical management of communicatively impaired patients for further suggestions for programming and facilitating generalization (Elbert and Gierut, 1986; Hegde, 1985; Hughes, 1985;

Warren and Rogers-Warren, 1985). In this section I briefly review and demonstrate Baer's (1981; Stokes and Baer, 1977) list of tactics for facilitating generalization.

Aiming for a Natural Community of Reinforcement

The basis of this programming strategy is the belief that behavior is not maintained (i.e., generalized across time) in the natural environment if it is not sufficiently reinforced. In the absence of reinforcement, trained communicative behaviors are extinguished, and the rate of occurrence is gradually reduced to an insignificant level. Consequently, we should *only* train communication skills that will be maintained by reinforcement in the home or other natural setting. Baer (1981) states that this might be the most important tactic that can be employed for obtaining generalization: "A good rule is not to make any deliberate behavior changes that will not meet natural communities of reinforcement. Breaking this rule commits you to maintain and extend the behavior changes that you want by yourself, indefinitely...This is not just a good rule, but perhaps the best rule..." (p. 16).

How do we know when a behavior will be naturally reinforced in relevant contexts? Baer (1981) mentions two potential problems that, if avoided, may result in a better likelihood of a behavior's being maintained by natural communities of reinforcers. First, newly acquired behaviors may not be sufficiently taught to begin with, thereby limiting the number of times that the behavior can make contact with available reinforcers. One way to ensure that behaviors are sufficiently trained is to establish more stringent criteria for dismissing clients from therapy. As noted earlier, in addition to setting a terminal criterion based on, for example, percentage of correct production of a target behavior, it is useful to establish a stability criterion before proceeding to subsequent levels of a treatment program. Thus, instead of setting a criterion of 90 percent correct production of target phonemes in sentences on a discrete-trial probe, it might prove beneficial to extend training until 90 percent correct phoneme production is achieved on two or more consecutive weekly probes. Making sure that the trained behavior is firmly entrenched in the response repertoire may increase the likelihood that the targets are produced frequently enough to make contact with the natural community of reinforcers. However, the *only* way to be certain that responses are regularly produced in the natural environment is to base termination of therapy on actual performance in the home or other naturalistic setting. Thus, a clinician would establish a terminal criterion for a dysphonic voice patient as 90 percent correct voicing (+voice) on all items of a discrete-trial probe across two consecutive probes *and* 80 percent correct voicing during oral reading tasks at school. (If the terminal criteria were based solely on performance on the structured probes, the clinician could not know if treatment gains had generalized to the classroom situation, and he/she also would not know if the generalized improvements occurred frequently enough to elicit teacher praise.)

No data are presently available to aid clinicians in establishing naturalistic generalization criteria that would ensure that responses are produced frequently enough to come into contact with the natural community of reinforcers. It may be sufficient to use a 60-percent to 80-percent correct criterion level in the natural environment for termination of training on communication behaviors that are also consistently (80 to 99 percent) produced accurately on structured probes. These levels of responding may allow the behaviors of interest to make contact with naturally occurring reinforcers.

In any event, given how little we know about establishing dismissal criteria for performance in natural settings, it is imperative to schedule regular follow-up probes to be certain that desired levels of responding are maintained. A significant decline in performance on a single probe in the natural environment should not be cause for alarm, but excessive variability and/or performance decline should prompt the clinician to schedule additional probes within a relatively brief period of time. Closer monitoring of the target behaviors should reveal whether the decline in performance is a result of natural variability or if additional intervention is required.

The second mistake to avoid when following the natural contingency rule is to assume that there is no natural community of reinforcers available for a trained behavior. Baer (1981) points out that sometimes "the natural community is asleep and needs to be waked up and turned on." In other words, occasionally, no matter how well a communicative ability is taught and no matter how frequently an appropriate skill is produced in natural environments, reinforcement may not be forthcoming. Consequently, clinicians must train clients to recruit reinforcement in order to maintain the desired ability. For example, a dysarthric speaker who communicates successfully with the assistance of an augmentative communication device may not be reinforced for using this means of communication with his spouse. Such an individual could be trained, first, to cue the spouse that he wants to communicate, and then, to ask the spouse for feedback on the success of the communicative attempt. Baer warns that we can go too far in training individuals to recruit natural communities of reinforcers. Having a patient ask for feedback after every exchange could prove irritating to even the most patient and loving spouse.

In attempting to train individuals to recruit natural reinforcers, be sure that significant others support or at least will tolerate behaviors that are targeted for change. If difficulties arise when a client is trained to solicit reinforcement and feedback, family members, teachers, and peers can become actively involved in the generalization programming effort. That is, it may be necessary to provide direct training to significant others or to manipulate environmental factors so that social praise and feedback are readily available to the patient.

Teaching Enough Examples

Baer (1981) indicates that failure to teach sufficient examples of trained responses is the most frequent mistake made by teachers and clinicians interested in establishing a generalized behavior change. The cardinal rule here is to use multiple exemplars during treatment, because a single example is not likely to result in generalization. Thus, when attempting to teach a language-delayed child to use the singular–plural contrast, it would, in principle, be better to provide multiple contrasts that demonstrate the pluralization rule than to present a single or a few contrasts repeatedly. Unfortunately, applied researchers of generalization often train a small list of exemplars of a given behavior in an attempt to examine factors responsible for prompting generalization. Clinicians should avoid making this same mistake.

Choosing the Best Examples to Teach

What are the best examples to train in therapy, and how are they selected? We have far too little data to guide us with regard to selecting treatment hierarchies and determining the necessary sequential steps in a training sequence. However, we can use the notion of representative exemplars as one criterion for helping us select appropriate examples for training. By selecting those forms and considering the situations in which they are most needed, we may be able to select training examples that expose our clients to the dimensions that are relevant for obtaining generalization. The previous lists of relevant people, settings, behaviors, and situations are useful for selecting appropriate stimuli for training. When reviewing the lists for the purpose of selecting appropriate exemplars for training, the clinician should attempt to identify components of the generalization behaviors and conditions that could be incorporated into training. For example, if generalization to other people is desired, then two or more clinicians should be involved in training of that patient. Even though this type of intervention can be somewhat difficult to arrange in highly structured training settings, it is imperative that we break the mold of only training in therapy cubicles, with a single clinician, at the same time, on the same days, if we are truly interested in exposing our clients to many situations and examples that may be needed to facilitate generalized responding. Generalization is most likely to occur if, as a result of training, patients have sampled many relevant dimensions, conditions, and behaviors in which we desire transfer.

Teaching a Few Examples at the Same Time

In the early stages of treatment it is often necessary to establish an initial, restricted repertoire of responding by training only one or two examples of a behavior. That is, stimulus–response conditioning is often required when a skill is in the early stages of acquisition. However, Baer recommends simultaneous teaching of multiple examples of a rule or behavior as soon as possible. This generalization promoting strategy may result in slowing down the initial rate at which the target behavior is acquired, but the strategy may pay off in terms of enhanced generalization.

Loose Training

I noted previously that highly structured training that establishes discrimination between training and nontraining conditions may result in a limited degree of generalization. The reciprocal of this phenomenon is also true. That is, when we loosen the control over the stimuli and responses in therapy and expose the patient to a sufficient number and variety of relevant conditions, we enhance the probability of obtaining generalization. Baer (1981) summarizes this generalization prompting strategy this way, "If you cannot teach every aspect of what you want learned, you have to teach examples of every aspect that you want learned. You probably have to represent all the dimensions of the final generalized behavior change that you want. And you might as well try to represent a number of them at the same time. That might save time and is likely to further generalization..." (p. 24). Many of the previous suggestions are relevant to the notion of loose training, and the above strategies can be combined for use during a single training program so that the parameters of training are sufficiently loosened to facilitate generalized responding.

It is important to note that loose training should not be an excuse for uncontrolled or haphazard therapy. This treatment approach is a systematic attempt to vary the structure of stimuli and responses in treatment. The clinician must decide exactly what dimensions of training should be altered and how they should be altered. If anything, loose training approaches require additional planning and discipline beyond that required of many other treatment approaches. Numerous examples of "loose training" are available in the communication disorders literature (Hart and Risley, 1975; 1982; Kearns, 1986a; Kearns and Potechin, 1988; Thompson and Byrne, 1984).

Programming Common Stimuli

The assumption involved in programming common stimuli is that generalization is more likely to occur if there are common stimulus components in training and natural settings. Perhaps the best known examples of programming common stimuli are studies in which peers are used to bridge the gap between the training and generalization settings. Goldstein and Ferrell (1987) recently demonstrated the usefulness of having peers serve as common stimuli in training and generalization conditions in a study of intervention for language-delayed children. Clinical examples of the use of programming common stimuli demonstrate the feasibility of incorporating this generalization programming principle into clinical practice. One might, for example allocate time in the weekly treatment schedule for significant others to join the clinician and the patient in therapy and social activities. The primary advantage of having a peer or significant other act as a common stimulus is that people are mobile and can actually be present in both training and generalization settings. In addition, people can also monitor communicative behaviors and provide appropriate social reinforcement and feedback.

Adjusting Reinforcement Schedules

Stokes and Baer (1977) remind us that intermittent reinforcement schedules are particularly resistant to extinction. Thus, generalization over time (maintenance) is enhanced by schedules of reinforcement that are intermittent and less predictable. Contingencies can also be made less discriminable by delaying reinforcement once a target behavior has been established. Thus, immediate social reinforcement should be phased out once a client begins to master a therapy task. The use of delayed or intermittent feedback and reinforcement helps obscure distinctions between training and generalization, and this may facilitate generalization and maintenance.

Mediating Generalization

Patients who have relatively intact cognitive abilities can be taught to act as mediators of their own generalization. Self-monitoring and self-management programs provide an opportunity for patients to participate actively in assessing and programming their own carry-over. For example, it is also possible to have patients mediate their own generalization by teaching self-cuing and prompting strategies. The use of self-cuing strategies is fairly common in aphasia rehabilitation. Skelly (1979), for example, trained aphasic-apraxic patients to produce iconic gestures (Amer-Ind) as a means of facilitating verbal responding. The essence of self-cuing strategies is to train a behavior that a patient can produce and to pair it with an impaired function in an attempt to improve communication. By teaching patients to transport their own cuing strategies from the clinical setting to the natural environment, clinicians are teaching patients to mediate their own generalization.

CLINICAL EXAMPLE

At the beginning of our discussion of methodologies for studying generalization, the critical elements of a generalization plan were described and compared with traditional treatment planning. After that brief overview, procedures for measuring and facilitating generalization were also considered. In this concluding section, a clinical example is presented to highlight generalization planning as an integrated clinical process.

Yedor and Kearns (1987) reported a generalization training study involving a 63-year-old, left-handed Broca's aphasic-apraxic patient (R.G.) who was seen 8 months after the onset of a left hemisphere cerebrovascular accident. The patient's residual communicative abilites were severely impaired (Table 2–1). His verbal repertoire was restricted to stereotypic or "perseverative" (repeated) utterances, and his graphic output consisted of meaningless strings of single letters. His auditory comprehension abilities were adequate for following simple auditory commands and requests, but R.G. could not reliably read single words. After 8 months of individual and group therapy, R.G.'s auditory comprehension skills improved somewhat, but verbally he was still nonfunctional. He refused augmentative forms of communication that were introduced during treatment, and he did not have a functional means of communication. R.G. reached a plateau on formal language testing 3 months prior to being enrolled in this clinical study.

TABLE 2–1 Mean Percentile Scores for R.G. on the Boston Diagnostic Aphasia Examination (BDAE)*

Subtests	Percentile
Auditory comprehension	38
Naming	22
Repetition	30
Reading	35
Writing	30

Aphasia Severity Rating = 1
Classification = Broca's Aphasia
* Goodglass H, Kaplan E. The assessment of aphasia and related disorders. Philadelphia: Lea & Febiger, 1983.

During the course of therapy R.G.'s clinician noticed that his ability to draw common objects and simple actions remained relatively intact. However, he did not spontaneously use this skill in communicative exchanges, and he rarely communicated through drawing even when prompted by his clinician.

Purpose

To establish the goals for this study, the clinician obtained information from formal test results, probes of the patient's drawing ability, analysis of the results of previous therapy, discussions with nursing personnel, and observations of the patient in his nursing home environment. After reviewing this information a generalization plan was developed to pursue three questions. First, would a "loose training" procedure (Response Elaboration Training—Kearns, 1986a; Kearns and Potechin, 1988) facilitate an increase in the amount of information (number of content units) produced during a structured drawing task? Second, would an increased ability to communicate through drawing generalize to untrained stimuli and to another person (i.e., the clinician)? Finally, would improved communicative drawing ability generalize to spontaneous interactions in the clinic and in another setting (the dining room)?

Design Strategy

R.G. was somewhat unusual in that he was a left-handed aphasic individual who had suffered a left hemisphere cerebrovascular accident and had relatively intact drawing skills. Consequently, the design strategy used to study the patient was more formal and extensive than is typically found in many clinical settings. A multiple-baseline, across-behaviors design (Kearns, 1986b; McReynolds and Kearns, 1983) was used to document the effectiveness and generality of treatment. Experimental control is demonstrated with this design when improvement occurs only at times when treatment is applied, not at other times, such as during pretreatment baseline testing. The basic format of the multiple-baseline design is as follows. First, performance is evaluated on two or more behaviors during an initial baseline (testing) phase. Baseline test results establish pretreatment levels of responding and provide information about the stability of responding. Following baseline testing, treatment is administered to one behavior while testing continues on the remaining behaviors. Treatment is withheld from the second behavior until a termination criterion is met on the first behavior. Generalization probes are often administered throughout this type of study to examine generalized responding to behaviors, settings, and people.

The primary goal of the Yedor and Kearns (1987) study was to increase the amount of information (number of content units) communicated through drawing. Two sets of stimuli were chosen for training, and one set was withheld from training so that generalization could be assessed. In accordance with the requirements of the multiple-baseline design, baseline measurements were initially obtained on all three sets of stimuli, and response elaboration training was then sequentially applied to the two sets of training items.

Evaluation Components

During the course of this study three types of generalization probes—discrete-trial, environmental simulation, and natural environment probes—were administered to evaluate treatment effectiveness and generalization.

Discrete-Trial Probes

Fifteen black and white line drawings were used to evaluate performance on training and generalization stimuli. The two sets of training items consisted of five verb pictures arranged in categories of "activities of daily living" and "sports." The five-item generalization set contained related, untrained items from these same categories. All fifteen pictures were administered during discrete-trial probes.

These probes were administered during the pretreatment baseline phase, and they were also administered on a weekly basis during treatment. Discrete-trial probes were administered by presenting each picture individually and then asking R.G. to describe (draw) completely the pictures and whatever else they brought to mind. The number of content units drawn in response to each picture served as the primary performance measure (i.e., dependent variable). Generalization to a clinician not involved in training was assessed by having this clinician also administer discrete-trial probes periodically.

Environmental Simulation Probes

The patient's ability to use drawing as a means of communication during "conversational" exchanges was also probed. A natural communication situation was simulated by having the patient and clinician view and discuss 5-minute videotaped segments of a news broadcast. After viewing the tapes, the clinician presented a series of open-ended questions to prompt a communicative exchange. The drawing content units produced during these probes were tallied and analyzed. These environmental simulation probes were also periodically administered by the generalization clinician.

Natural Environment

R.G. was a resident in an extended care facility while he received speech-language therapy. As part of his daily routine, he ate lunch at a senior adult center. It was decided, therefore, to conduct naturalistic observations of spontaneous communicative drawing ability during lunchtime conversations. These probes were obtained by having the clinicians discuss daily activities with R.G. These naturalistic observations were again conducted by both treatment clinician and a generalization clinician.

By incorporating discrete-trial, environmental simulation, and natural environment probes into the generalization plan, the experimenters obtained information about generalization across behaviors (i.e., stimuli), across people (i.e., clinicians), across settings (a senior adult center), and over time (i.e., maintenance). The three types of probes were administered prior to treatment, periodically during treatment, and several weeks after therapy was terminated. The elements of the generalization plan pertaining to treatment are reviewed next.

Training to Generalize

One of the first treatment decisions faced by the experimenters was, "What generalization facilitator(s) would most likely result in generalized responding?" After careful consideration they decided to adopt a "loose training" strategy (Stokes and Baer, 1977) called *response elaboration training* or RET (Kearns, 1986a; Kearns and Potechin, 1988). RET is a loose training approach to facilitate increased elaboration of communicative abilities in nonfluent aphasic patients. The emphasis in RET is on shaping and chaining spontaneous patient-initiated responses rather than training clinician-selected responses. Using this technique, training was sequentially applied to the two sets of treatment stimuli. Generalization items were never trained.

The criterion for termination of training on each training level was successful drawing of four or more content units on at least four of the five training items (80 percent). The same criterion was also established for the generalization set. That is, if, after training the two training sets, four or more informational content units had not been produced on four or more generalization items, it would have been necessary to initiate training of these items. Fortunately, sufficient generalization occurred so that treatment on these items was not necessary.

Finally, the same criterion was also applied to the spontaneous (i.e., news) condition. That is, if probes conducted after completion of training did not demonstrate at least four drawing content units per communicative exchange for at least 80 percent of the turns, then additional training would be necessary in this spontaneous condition.

Before we scan the results of this study, it is worth mentioning the reliability of the scoring procedures used in this study. Assessment of reliability is an essential, albeit overlooked, aspect of clinical practice, and clinicians should routinely consider the reliability of their scoring procedures during generalization planning (Barlow, Hayes, and Nelson, 1984; Cooper, Heron, and Heward, 1987; Gelfand and Hartmann, 1984; McReynolds and Kearns, 1983; Sulzer-Azaroff and Mayer, 1977). Without an estimate of reliability, we can never be sure if our patients improve or (if the apparent is really a reflection of the subjective) if we are using biased or inadequate scoring procedures.

During each phase of this study, probe sessions were tape-recorded and independently rescored by another clinician. Scores of the treatment clinician and of the second clinician were compared on a response-by-response basis, and the percentage of overall interobserver agreement (i.e., reliability) was calculated for the number of drawing content units produced. The formula used to calculate overall reliability was: *Total number of agreements ÷ total number of agreements + total number of disagreements × 100.*

An 85 percent interobserver agreement level was obtained for the clinicians in this study. It appeared, therefore, that the scoring procedures used in this study were reliable and that they could be objectively used by the treatment clinician and other clinicians as well.

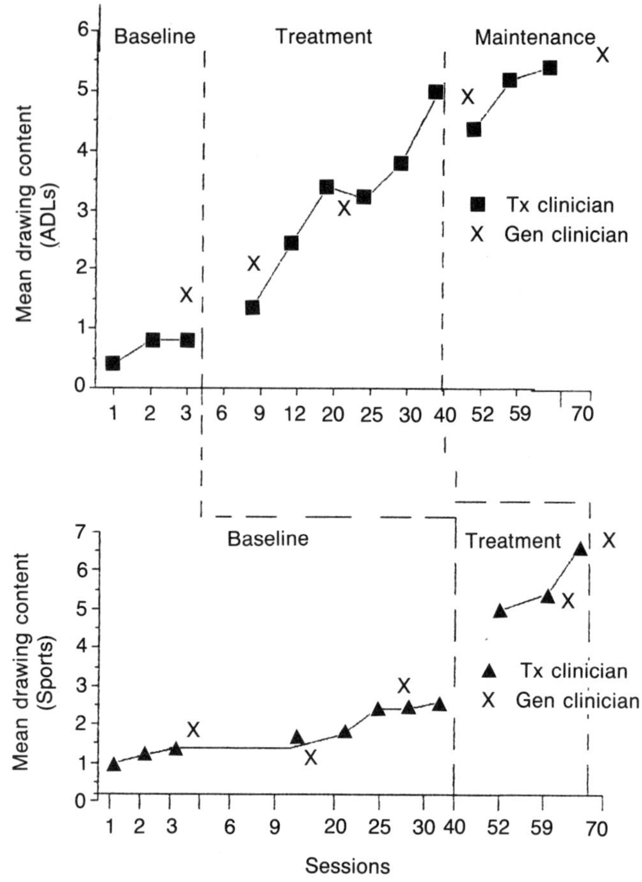

Figure 2–3 Treatment pictures (R.W.). Mean drawing content units produced on baseline (i.e., pretreatment), treatment (i.e., loose training), and maintenance probes. Data are shown for the treatment clinician (■) and a generalization clinician (*X*). (After Yedor K, Kearns KP. Establishing communicative drawing in severe aphasia through response elaboration training. Paper presented at American Speech Hearing Association, New Orleans, LA, 1987.)

RESULTS

The results of the generalization plan used in this study are depicted in Figures 2–3 to 2–5. Each graph displays the mean drawing units produced during probes over time (i.e., sessions). The results of the discrete-trial probes are displayed in Figures 2–3 and 2–4. The data in Figure 2–3 show that, prior to treatment (i.e., at baseline), R.G. produced very little communicative content in his drawings. However, rapid improvements were apparent on both sets of stimulus pictures after the RET was applied. The patient's improved drawing ability also generalized to the nontraining clinician (*X* in the figure). The data in Figure 2–4 demonstrate that improved drawing ability generalized to untrained picture stimuli that were similar to the training items. The amount of generalization obtained on the untrained pictures was virtually the same for the treatment clinician (■) and the generalization (*X*) clinician.

The data shown in Figure 2–5 represent follow-up training that occurred after the treatment was completed on the two sets of picture stimuli. These data are revealing in several respects. First, despite marked improvements in ability to draw for communicative purposes following training on the picture stimuli (see Figs. 2–3 and 2–4), the low level of baseline responding in Figure 2–5 indicates that there was little generalization in spontaneous interactions. Importantly, this was true despite the fact that generalization occurred across stimuli (see Fig. 2–4) and clinicians (see Figs. 2–3 and 2–4). It appeared that the loose training facilitator was successful, but only to a point. Thus, even in the face of a considerable degree of generalization following a treatment procedure that incorporated

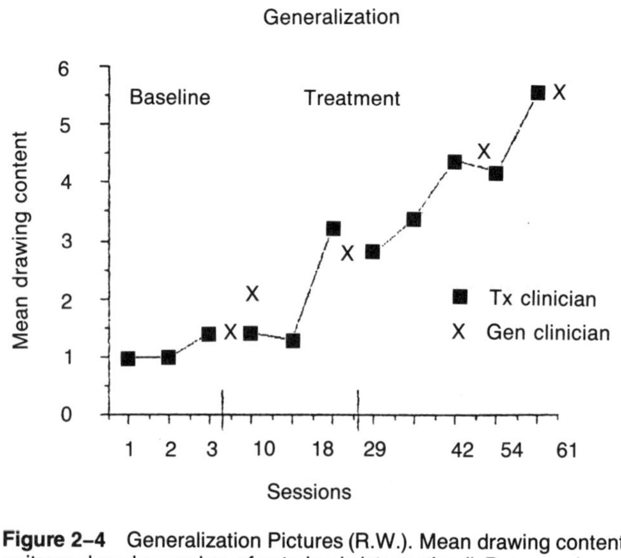

Figure 2–4 Generalization Pictures (R.W.). Mean drawing content units produced on probes of untrained picture stimuli. Data are shown for the treatment clinician (■) and a generalization clinician (*X*). (After Yedor K, Kearns KP. Establishing communicative drawing in severe aphasia through response elaboration training. Paper presented at American Speech Hearing Association, New Orleans, LA, 1987.)

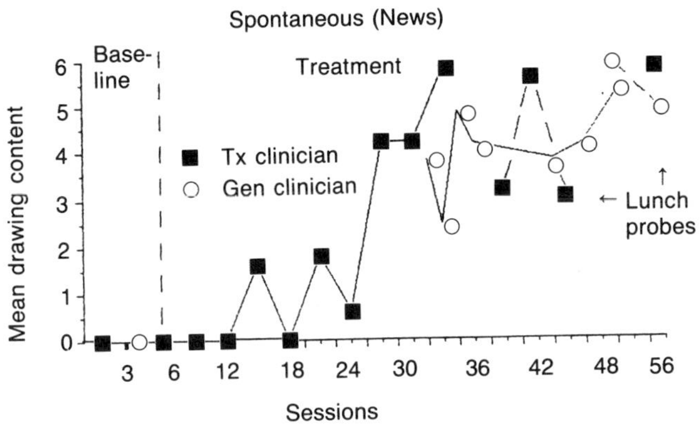

Figure 2–5 Spontaneous training (R.W.). Mean number of drawing content producing during pretreatment (i.e., baseline), and spontaneous treatment probes. Data are shown for the treatment clinician (■) and a generalization clinician (○). Arrows designate performance during spontaneous interactions during mealtime probes. (After Yedor K, Kearns KP. Establishing communicative drawing in severe aphasia through response elaboration training. Paper presented at American Speech Hearing Association, New Orleans, LA, 1987.)

a generalization facilitator, generalization to the spontaneous condition was not automatic.

A second important point relates to the fact that the generalization probe procedures and the graphic presentation of the data clearly revealed the need for additional training. Thus, had they not had an adequate generalization plan, which included environmental simulation and naturalistic probes, the experimenters might have been pleased with the amount of improvement and generalization found in the more structured conditions, and they might have decided to terminate therapy. However, given the low level of performance on baseline probes of spontaneous interactions, it was apparent that additional programming was necessary.

After baseline testing, the experimenters reinitiated treatment by continuing the RET during spontaneous interactions that occurred after the patient and clinician viewed the videotaped news segments. The results of the additional training are shown in Figure 2–5. It is apparent that the loose training procedure was again successful. Following session twenty-six, R.G. spontaneously produced four to six informational drawing units on each spontaneous probe. Importantly, probes of spontaneous interactions during lunch (see *arrows*) demonstrate that improvements in communicative drawing ability also generalized to lunchtime interactions. An equal amount of generalization occurred to these spontaneous interactions regardless of whether the treatment clinician or generalization clinician administered the probes.

The results of this study demonstrate a major assumption that underlies generalization planning. That is, generalization to natural environments is not an automatic process that occurs as a result of intervention. Generalization must be actively planned for and programmed rather than expected (Baer, Wolf, and Risley, 1968; Stokes and Baer, 1977). By clinging to the false assumption that generalization is an automatic by-product of intervention, speech-language pathologists may unwittingly sentence their patients to communicative inadequacy. Consequently, failure to consider generalization to the natural environment as the primary goal of therapy, and failure to incorporate methodologies that may achieve this goal, might be considered unethical clinical practice (Warren, 1985).

Besides demonstrating the need to plan for generalization, the previous example also highlights basic methodologies that can be used to study generalization. For example, the benefits of evaluating a broad range of behaviors and conditions and of periodically probing these variables were also demonstrated. By systematically incorporating generalization probe procedures, Yedor and Kearns (1987) evaluated generalized improvements in communicative drawing ability to various behaviors, people, settings, and situations. Also, by establishing generalization criteria prior to intervention, we were able to make objective clinical decisions about whether treatment should be continued or terminated, and about when generalization was sufficiently established. The graphic presentation of the data proved an invaluable interpretation aid to the decision-making process.

Moreover, this clinical example demonstrates both the value and the limitations of incorporating techniques into treatment that may facilitate generalized responding. The use of a "loose training" procedure facilitated acquisition of elaborate communicative drawing ability, and these skills generalized to untrained stimuli and people. However, this generalization programming attempt was not entirely successful until additional treatment was applied using the same procedure in a spontaneous, interactive condition. This sequential modification strategy (Stokes and Baer, 1977), in which training is applied sequentially to additional settings and conditions, ultimately proved successful. Thus, although the initial "loose training" facilitator was somewhat successful, a second generalization promoting technique (i.e., sequential modification) was required to achieve the goal of establishing a functional communication system in the natural environment.

SUMMARY

To summarize, clinical methodologies that can be used to measure generalization and facilitate generalized responding were described and demonstrated. Emphasis was placed on the need to adopt a generalization planning approach to clinical management, and the components of this approach were discussed. Our dicussion of the *evaluation* component of the generalization plan has been primarily concerned with generalization probe procedures and related measurement issues. It was noted that a broad range of factors can influence the success of a generalization plan and it was suggested that compiling comprehensive lists of these factors can facilitate generalization planning. Following Baer's (1981) lead, I have suggested that, within reason, an attempt should be made to gather information about behaviors, situations or settings, significant others, and environmental factors that can effect generalized responding. Ideally, if the lists contain all relevant information, and if clinicians prioritize the information from these lists, all the data necessary to develop a comprehensive generalization plan would be available. However, as with most "ecological assessments," obtaining such detailed lists is impractical, so I have suggested that clinicians use formal test results, observations of patients' behaviors, and parental interviews to narrow the focus of the generalization assessment. Based on clinical and research experience, it is feasible to select and periodically probe two behaviors, one naturalistic setting, and one significant other in the clinical setting.

Following discussion of the breadth of the evaluation component, measurement considerations relating to three types of *generalization probe procedures:* discrete-trial, environmental simulation, and probes of performance in the natural environment were reviewed. I described two methods of *discrete-trial generalization probes*, the interspersing method and presession or postsession probes. Both methods can be used to assess performance on training items, generalization items, and previously trained (maintenance) items. Discrete-trial probes are also used to evaluate generalization to steps in a treatment program, and generalization criteria should be established to determine when to proceed to subsequent steps in a treatment hierarchy. Similarly, discrete-trial probes should be administered several times prior to initiating treatment, and periodically during treatment, so that generalization can be monitored and adjustments can be made in intervention strategies. Graphically displaying the data obtained from generalization probes provides a judgment aid that is useful for making appropriate modifications to a generalization plan.

During the review of *simulated environmental probes,* I emphasized the need to incorporate significant others into the assessment process, by soliciting their views on the importance of treatment goals and by having them actively participate in generalization probes that approximate naturalistic conditions. Measurement considerations relevant to the use of environmental simulation probes were also discussed, and special emphasis was placed on the need to develop standard testing conditions that can be reliably repeated over time.

Finally, measurement issues pertaining to *probes in the natural environment* were reviewed. Emphasis was placed on the need to choose an appropriate measure of generalization carefully and to develop standardized recording forms. At a minimum, it is important to observe and record the antecedent stimuli, patient responses, and consequences that occur in the natural environment. In addition, the clinician should be alert to the possible influence that setting events—complex stimulus–response interactions that precede observations—may have on inhibiting generalization. When circumstances prevent the clinician from conducting naturalistic observations, individuals from the environment or even patients themselves can be trained to conduct probes in daily living settings.

Comprehensive generalization plans incorporate treatment procedures that may actually *facilitate generalization.* After all, without powerful treatment procedures that promote generalized responding, we would be faced with the nearly impossible task of intervening for every behavior, setting, and condition to which we desire generalization.

A number of techniques that may increase the probability of obtaining generalization were presented and discussed. These techniques are representative of generalization prompting techniques that can be incorporated into intervention strategies in an attempt to facilitate generalized responding. Although numerous strategies were considered, the strategy of making sure that generalized behaviors are exposed to a natural community of reinforcers is a generic technique that can be utilized in conjunction with more specific treatment approaches. Moreover, this strategy can be easily put into clinical practice by establishing termination criteria for generalization to natural environments. Continuing treatment until a generalization criterion is met in natural environments helps to ensure that target behaviors are produced in natural environments frequently enough to come into contact with natural communities of reinforcement. Unfortunately, generalization facilitating procedures have not been extensively studied in the communicative disorders literature, and one cannot be certain that a given technique will work for any individual client. Thus, clinicians have an ethical obligation to monitor the success of these and other intervention approaches so that treatment strategies can be appropriately modified when they do not provide the degree of generalized responding necessary to meet preestablished generalization criteria.

Because we can never be certain that a particular generalization facilitating technique will be effective, we should explore the use of combined procedures. Gelfand and Hartmann (1984) advocate such a "blockbuster approach," in which numerous generalization promoting aids are applied simultaneously. This suggestion appears to have merit, because naturalistic language training approaches, such as incidental teaching (Hart and Risley, 1975, 1982; Warren and Kaiser, 1986) and the delay technique (Charlop, Schreibman, and Thibodeau, 1985; Halle, Baer, and Spradlin, 1980), which surreptitiously incorporate several generalization facilitating techniques, have consistently resulted in generalized improvements in language ability. Clinicians should, therefore, consider in-vivo training when the opportunity presents itself (Siegel and Spradlin, 1982), because the easiest way to be sure that trained communication skills are being produced in a natural setting is to conduct training in that setting. However, this may not always be possible or even desirable.

Regardless, given the paucity of data regarding procedures for prompting generalized responding, a blockbuster approach that combines generalization facilitating techniques should be considered the rule rather than the exception for generalization planning.

The ultimate reward of clinical management comes from the realization that we contribute to our patient's quality of life by improving communicative abilities in naturalistic settings and situations. After all, it is rather meaningless if treatment gains do not generalize beyond our clinical walls. Achieving significant, generalized changes in our patients' communicative abilities may not be easy, but our attempts are likely to be rewarded to a degree that is commensurate with the amount of effort expended. Generalization planning requires additional time and effort beyond that required by the traditional treatment planning approach. However, for clinicians who are willing to invest the energy and resources, the potential reward in terms of stimulation, self-satisfaction, and patient benefits far outweigh the costs.

Acknowledgments The writing of this manuscript was supported, in part, by the Veterans Administration Rehabilitation Research and Development funds. The assistance of Kathy Yedor and Patricia Williams is gratefully acknowledged.

REFERENCES

Baer DM. How to plan for generalization. Austin, TX: Pro-ed, 1981.

Baer DM, Wolf MM, Risley TR. Some current dimensions of applied behavior analysis. J Appl Behav Anal 1968; 8:91–97.

Baer DM, Wolf MM, Risley TR. Some still-current dimensions of applied behavior analysis. J Appl Behav Anal 1987; 20:313–328.

Barlow DH, Hayes SC, Nelson RO. The scientist practitioner: research and accountability in clinical and educational settings. New York: Pergamon Press, 1984.

Brookshire RH, Nicholas LS, Kreuger KM, Redmond KJ. The clinical interaction analysis system: a system for observational recording of aphasia treatment. J Speech Hear Disord 1978; 43:437–447.

Charlop MH, Schreibman L, Thibodeau MG. Increasing spontaneous verbal responding in autistic children using a time delay procedure. J Appl Behav Anal 1985; 18:155–166.

Connell PJ, Thompson CK. Flexibility of single-subject experimental designs. Part III. Using flexibility to design or modify experiments. J Speech Hear Disord 1986; 51:214–225.

Cooper JO, Heron TE, Heward WL. Applied behavior analysis. Columbus, OH: Merrill Publishing, 1987.

Drabman R, Hammer P, Rosenbaum M. Assessing generalization in behavior modification with children: the generalization map. Behavioral Assessment 1979; 1:213–219.

Elbert M, Gierut J. Handbook of clinical phonology. Approaches to assessment and treatment. San Diego, CA: College-Hill Press, 1986.

Garcia EE, DeHaven ED. Use of operant techniques in the establishment and generalization of language: a review and analysis. Am J Men Defic 1974; 72:169–178.

Gelfand DM, Hartmann DP. Child behavior analysis and therapy. New York: Pergamon Press, 1984.

Goldstein H. Enhancing language generalization using matrix training and stimulus equivalence. In: Warren SF, ed. Teaching functional language: generalization and maintenance of language skills. Austin, TX: Pro-ed, 1985:225.

Goldstein H, Ferrell DR. Augmenting communicative interactions between handicapped and nonhandicapped preschool children. J Speech Hear Disord 1987; 52:200–211.

Guess D, Keogh W, Sailor W. Generalization of speech and language behavior. In: Schiefelfusch RL, ed. Bases of language intervention. Baltimore: University Park Press, 1978:374.

Halle JW, Baer DM, Spradlin JE. Teachers' generalized use of delay as a stimulus control procedure to increase language use in language handicapped children. J Appl Behav Anal 1981; 14:387–400.

Harris SL. Teaching language to nonverbal children—with emphasis on problems of generalization. Psych Bull 1975; 82:565–580.

Hart B, Risley T. Incidental teaching of language in the preschool. J Appl Behav Anal 1975; 8:411–420.

Hart B, Risley T. How to use incidental teaching for elaborating language. Austin, TX: Pro-ed, 1982.

Hawkins RP. The functions of assessment. J Appl Behav Anal 1979; 12:501–516.

Hegde MN. Treatment principles and procedures in communicative disorders. San Diego: College-Hill Press, 1985.

Hughes D. Language treatment and generalization. A clinician's handbook. San Diego: College-Hill Press, 1985.

Johnston JM. On the relation between generalization and generality. Behavior Analyst 1979; 2:1–6.

Kazdin AE, Esveldt-Dawson K. How to maintain behavior. Austin, TX: Pro-ed, 1981.

Kearns KP. Systematic programming of verbal elaboration skills in chronic Broca's aphasia. In: Marshall RC, ed. Case studies in aphasia rehabilitation: for clinicians by clinicians. Austin, TX: Pro-ed, 1986a:225.

Kearns, KP. Flexibility of single-subject experimental designs. Part II. Design selection and arrangement of experimental phases. J Speech Hear Disord 1986b; 51:204–214.

Kearns KP, Potechin G. The generalization of response elaboration training effects. In: Prescott TE, ed. Clinical aphasiology conference proceedings. Minneapolis, MN: College-Hill Press, 1988.

Kearns KP, Salmon SJ. An experimental analysis of auxiliary and copula verb generalization in aphasia. J Speech Hear Dis 1984; 49:152–163.

Keller FS, Schonfeld WN. Principles of psychology: a systematic text in the science of behavior. New York: Appleton-Century-Crofts, 1950.

Loverso FL, Prescott TE, Selinger M. Verbs: a treatment strategy for aphasic adults (CVT). J Rehab Research and Development 1988; 52:47–60.

Lund N, Duchan J. Assessing children's language in naturalistic contexts. Englewood Cliffs, NJ: Prentice-Hall, 1988.

Marholin D, Seigel LT, Phillips D. Treatment and transfer: a search for empirical procedures. In: Hersen M, Eisler RM, Miller PM. eds. Progress in behavior modifications. Vol III. New York: Academic Press, 1976:294.

McReynolds LV, Kearns KP. Single-case experimental designs in communicative disorders. Austin, TX: Pro-ed, 1983.

Parsonson BS, Baer DM. The analysis and presentation of graphic data. In: Kratochwill TR, ed. Single-subject research strategies for evaluating change. New York: Academic Press, 1978:101.

Parsonson BS, Baer DM. The graphic analysis of data. In: Poling A, Fuqua RW. Research methods in applied behavior analysis. New York: Plenum Press, 1986.

Porch BE. The Porch index of communicative abilities. Palo Alto, CA: Consulting Psychologists Press, 1971.

Risley TR. The development and maintenance of language: an operant model. In: Etzel BC, LeBlanc TM, Beger DM, eds. New developments in behavioral research: theory, method and application. Hillsdale, NJ: Lawrence Erlbaum Associates, 1977:81.

Scott RR, Himandi W, Keane T. A review of generalization in social skills training: suggestions for further research. In: Hersen M, Eisler RM, Miller PM, eds. Progress in behavior modification. New York: Academic Press, 1983:15, 114.

Siegel GM, Spradlin JE. Therapy and research. J Speech Hear Disord 1985; 50:226–230.

Simmons NN, Kearns KP, Potechin G. Treatment of aphasia through family member training. In: Brookshire RH, ed. Clin-

ical aphasiology conference proceedings. Minneapolis, MN: BRK Publishers, 1987:106.
Skelly M. Amer-Ind gestural code. New York: Elsevier, 1979.
Skinner BF. Science and human behavior. New York: MacMillan, 1953.
Skinner BF. Contingencies of reinforcement: a theoretical analysis. New York: Appleton-Century-Crofts, 1969.
Spradlin JE, Siegel GM. Language training in natural and clinical environments. J Speech Hear Disord 1982; 47:2–6.
Stokes TF, Baer DM. An implicit technology of generalization. J Appl Behav Anal 1977; 10:349–367.
Sulzer-Azaroff B, Mayer GR. Applying behavior-analysis procedures to children and youth. New York: Holt, Rinehart and Winston, 1977.
Thompson CK, Byrne ME. Across setting generalization of social conventions in aphasia: an experimental analysis of "loose training." In: Brookshire RH, ed. Clinical aphasiology conference proceedings. Minneapolis, MN: BRK Publishers, 1984:132.
Wahler RG, Berland RM, Coe TD. Generalization process in child behavior change. In: Lakey BB, Kazdin AA, eds. Advances in clinical psychology. Vol 2. New York: Plenum Press, 1979:35.
Wahler RG, Fox JJ. Setting events in applied behavior analysis: toward a conceptual and methodological expansion. J Appl Behav Anal 1981; 14:327–338.
Warren SF. Clinical strategies for the measurement of language generalization. In: Warren SF, Rogers-Warren AK. Teaching functional language. San Diego: College-Hill Press, 1985:197.
Warren SF, Kaiser AP. Incidental language teaching: a critical review. J Speech Hear Disord 1986; 51:291–299.
Warren S, Rogers-Warren A. Teaching functional language. Generalization and maintenance of language skills. Austin, TX: Pro-ed, 1985.
Wildman RW, Wildman RW. The generalization of behavior modification procedures: a review—with special emphasis on classroom application. Psychology in the Schools 1975; 12:432–448.
Yedor K, Kearns KP. Establishing communicative drawing in severe aphasia through response elaboration training. Paper presented at American Speech Hearing Association, New Orleans, LA 1987.
Yoder DE, Kent RD, Decision making in speech-language pathology. Toronto: BC Decker, 1988.

Chapter Three

GENERALIZATION IN THE TREATMENT OF PHONOLOGICAL DISORDERS

MARY ELBERT, Ph.D.

The occurrence of generalization is often viewed as rather wondrous. Take the case of the child who misarticulates fricatives. When we teach the child to produce and use one fricative and then observe that he or she is not only beginning to use that sound correctly but other fricatives as well, we are both pleased and somewhat amazed. And yet this happens. Even though we have observed the occurrence of generalization often in the clinic and documented it in numerous research investigations, we still do not entirely understand it. Nevertheless, we expect generalization to occur; otherwise, we would be faced with the overwhelming necessity of teaching every error sound in every possible word and context in which it occurs. We know this is an impossible situation, and we know also from experience that, at some point, generalization of information learned in one context or situation will occur in other untrained contexts and situations.

How or why it occurs has been the practical question asked by clinicians in the field. The same question has provided the impetus for the many research studies in the literature. In this chapter an attempt is made first to describe the problem faced in the clinical situation and then to present clinical cases to illustrate an approach to solving the problem. In the following sections evidence from experimental investigations is presented to provide support for the approach. The clinical population of concern in this chapter is the group of children that have been labeled "functional misarticulators," that is, children for whom no organic problems can be identified but who have disordered phonological systems from unknown causes. These children have normal hearing and are functioning within normal limits in the environment. Even though the cause of the problem is unknown, speech-language pathologists have the responsibility of providing the intervention that will help the children to learn the English phonological system and become proficient speakers of the language.

For the clinician faced with a child with a moderate to severe articulation or phonological disorder, the first problem is where to begin. What error sound or error pattern should be targeted first for treatment? Depending on the clinician's orientation, the question could be answered in a variety of ways. One could look at developmental norms and select the target sound that appears to be learned earliest by normally developing children and then proceed to teach each sound in a progressive sequence. Another approach would be to work on all of the error sounds at the same time. These two approaches represent the opposite ends of a continuum, and both have advantages and disadvantages. The biggest problem of these two approaches is that neither takes into consideration the process of generalization.

Perhaps the question should not be simply what speech sound or pattern should be the first target, but rather what target should be chosen first in order to promote the greatest generalization and thus the most efficient change in the child's phonological system. When the question is posed in this way, the focus is on the actual learning process.

The notion of planning for generalization prior to treatment has been discussed in current literature (e.g., Hughes, 1985; Rockman and Elbert, 1984; Stokes and Baer, 1977). The articulation generalization approach offered here is based on two important assumptions. The first assumption is that phonologically disordered children are similar to normally developing children in that both types are active, creative participants in the learning process. It is assumed that children have normal learning capacities and that they use these capacities as new information becomes available. Every child brings to the language learning situation general abilities that are used in all areas of acquiring new information and skills. Children can recognize new information and store new lexical items and, at the same time, categorize the information in terms of similarities. Children also are able to compare input from the adult to their own output. This comparison ability allows children to modify responses based on information from the environment.

The second assumption is that each child possesses, at any one point in time, a unique set of facts about the community phonological system. However, for the phonologically disordered child the system may differ substantially from the adult system. As new facts are learned, either about the production of particular sounds or the appropriate distribution of the sounds within the system, the child incorporates the new knowledge and integrates it with already established knowledge. It is at this point that generalization begins to occur. Because each child begins treatment with a unique system, it follows that individual differences in learning patterns also result.

When we accept the assumptions that children play an active role along with the clinician in the learning process and that phonologically disordered children possess unique phonological systems, then our approach can focus on utilizing the cognitive abilities and knowledge that the child brings to the clinical situation to assist the child in the learning process. Even though phonologically disordered children have incomplete sound systems compared to adults, their systems are not haphazard or random but are orderly and regular. All children are faced with the problem of sorting out from the multitude of speech input some segments and units for communication purposes. They are forced to organize the input into some sort of sound system. The fact that each child organizes the input data somewhat differently should not be a surprise; the fact that some children are more efficient in this process is also not surprising.

CASE STUDIES

Two children are discussed here in order to illustrate how two factors—the unique knowledge of the sound system that a child possesses prior to treatment and the particular phonemes selected for treatment—interact to cause changes throughout a child's phonological system. These two female children (M, age 4 years 3 months, and K, age 3 years 8 months) were selected from a larger pool of 40 subjects in a current research study. The two children are representative of other children in the group. Both children had normal hearing and no observable organic problems. Their receptive language abilities, as measured by the Peabody Picture Vocabulary Test—Revised (Dunn, 1986); were within normal limits. Their only presenting problem was unintelligible speech.

A standard generative phonological analysis (Dinnsen, 1984; Elbert and Gierut, 1986) was used to analyze the data. Generative phonology is a theoretical linguistic framework for describing sound systems. The analysis procedures have been used to describe sound systems of many languages. In this analysis procedure, the primary focus is on a description of a child's system as a unique phonology. That is, the child's sound system is described independently of the target, or adult, sound system. In a sense, the child is viewed as a speaker of an exotic language. After the child's system is described, it is compared with the adult sound system. This comparison helps to determine the similarities and differences between the child's phonological system and the adult system.

Data on the children's speech were obtained from spontaneous speech samples and responses to a specially designed 306-item word list, which elicited sounds showing contrastive use and morphophonemic alternations. *Contrastive use* of sounds is determined by providing the child with the opportunity to produce potential minimal pairs such as *key* and *tea*. If the child uses the two sounds to contrast meaning, then there is evidence that the sounds operate as separate phonemes in the child's phonological system. *Morphophonemic alternations* refer to pairs such as *dog* and *doggie* or *run* and *running*. Elicitation of these forms provides evidence of the child's underlying representations (lexical representation) for particular words and the sounds in the words. If a child produces [da] for *dog* but also produces [dagi], this evidence from the child's own production suggests that the underlying representation of the morpheme *dog* contains all three phonemes and that a phonological rule of neutralization is being used to delete the final sound in the word. If, on the other hand, the child did not produce the /g / in either form, there is no evidence to suggest that the child has the complete (adultlike) form in the underlying representation. This distinction is important in distinguishing different types of sound usage. More detailed explanations of phonological rules and procedures for determining underlying representations can be found in Dinnsen (1984) and Elbert and Gierut (1986).

The results of the analysis were used to determine the productive phonological knowledge unique to each child. Productive phonological knowledge includes a characterization of both the competence (underlying representations) and the performance of the child. Performance includes the specification of the sounds that a child uses whether correctly or incorrectly (phonetic inventory) and the sounds that are used to contrast meaning (phonemic inventory). In addition to establishing the phonetic and phonemic inventories, the distribution of the sounds in the system is determined (i.e., whether the sounds are used in all word positions or only in some positions).

From this analysis a profile of productive phonological knowledge was constructed for each child. At one extreme of the profile were the sounds that the child used accurately, as in the ambient (standard English) language. The child was presumed to have complete productive phonological knowledge of these sounds, because they were produced accurately in all contexts. At the other extreme were sounds that were never produced, and thus were accounted for by inventory constraints. Inventory constraints imply no phonological knowledge, because these sounds were never produced in any context. At midpoints on the profile were sounds that differed in usage from the ambient system in various ways, for example, positional constraints or phonological rules. In these cases, the child was credited with partial productive phonological knowledge, because the sounds were produced correctly in at least some well-defined contexts. This characterization of phonological knowledge is limited to productive aspects of the sound system without any necessary appeal to perceptual knowledge; however, both children had auditory discrimination scores within normal limits on the Goldman-Fristoe-Woodcock Test of Auditory Discrimination (1970), which would suggest that their discrimination abilities were intact.

The profiles showing the two children's phonological systems pretreatment and posttreatment are presented in Figures 3–1 and 3–2. The first child, M, had three sounds that only occurred in specified positions and that are shown in the box labeled "positional constraints." The /t / did not occur postvocalically, and /tʃ/ and /l/ never occurred word-initially. The two sounds /θ/ and /ð/ were never produced and were characterized by inventory constraints. All other sounds were produced in adultlike fashion and were thus not listed in the profile.

The second child, K, also had three sounds that were described as positional constraints. The sound /ð/ never occurred postvocalically; /r / and / l / never occurred prevocalically. Two sounds, /θ/ and /ʃ/, were never produced and were thus described by inventory constraints. All other sounds were produced accurately.

The two children were similar in several respects; they both had five sounds in error and the errors were in the

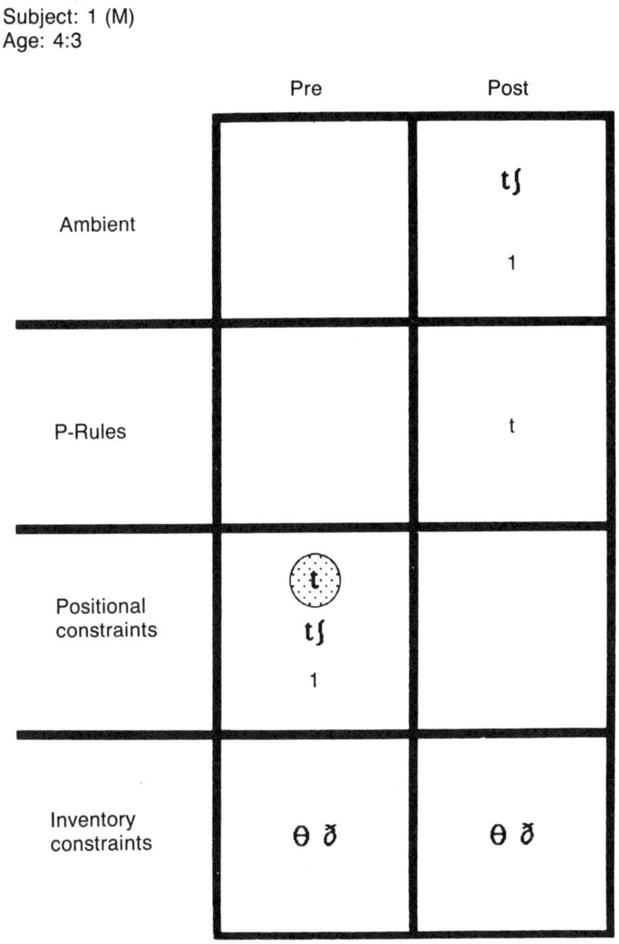

Figure 3–1 Phonological profile pretreatment and posttreatment for child M.

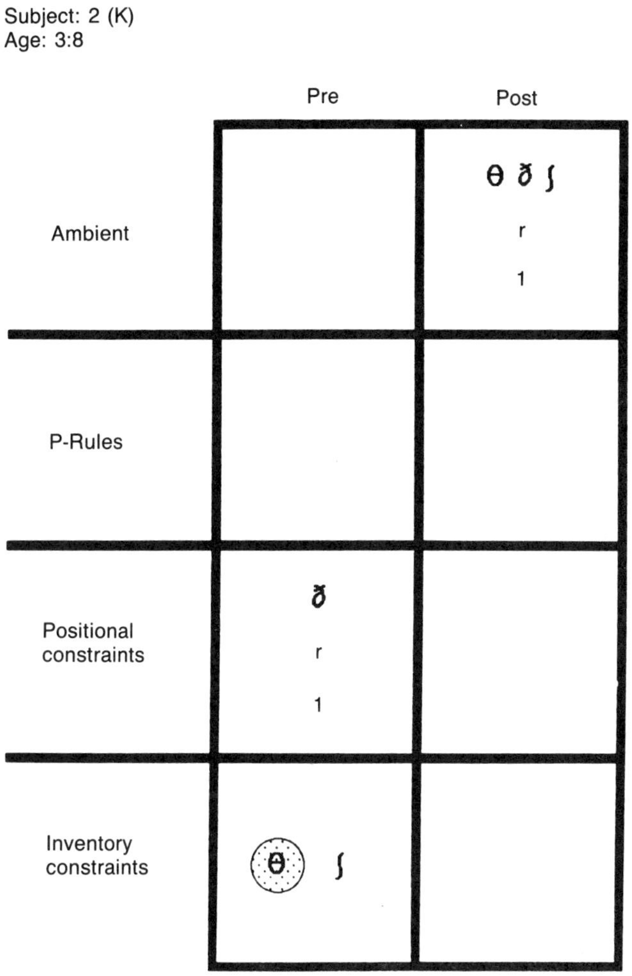

Figure 3–2 Phonological profile pretreatment and posttreatment for child K.

category of either positional or inventory constraints. However, the sounds selected for treatment were different for the two children. The treatment targets are shown within circles on the two figures. The treatment target for M was /t/ and for K was /θ/.

Treatment procedures employed minimal pairs contrasting the target phoneme with the error substitution, the omission or both. This type of treatment focuses on both the phonetic and phonemic aspects of phonology. The child is taught the phonetic aspect by the repeated production of the target sound until the sound is produced correctly and effortlessly. The phonemic aspect is learned through the contrasting of the minimal pairs illustrating the difference in meaning. For M, the contrast taught was /t/ versus null in postvocalic position in word pairs such as *boat–bow*. For K, the contrast taught was /θ/ versus /f/ in prevocalic position in word pairs, such as *thin–fin*. No more than five minimal pairs were taught. Criterion levels were established so that each child correctly produced the target sound spontaneously in words by the end of treatment. The criterion level was reached by M after 15 treatment sessions and by K after 19 sessions.

The target sound was tested imitatively in 20 untrained items during treatment to determine whether generalization had occurred. Production of all error sounds, both treated and untreated, was tested (probed) on a longer 306-item test before and after treatment in order to show change in the phonological system.

The changes in each child's phonological system as a result of treatment are shown in Figures 3–1 and 3–2. For M, treatment on the one target /t/ resulted in change in all three of the sounds characterized as positional constraints. The treated sound /t/ improved as a result of treatment and was listed as an optional phonological rule, because it was not produced correctly in all instances. The two sounds, /θ/ and /ð/, for which the child had no productive phonological knowledge and which the child had never produced, did not change. The two sounds in the category of positional constraints (/tʃ/ and /l/) changed spontaneously: this change can be attributed to the fact that the child possessed productive knowledge of those sounds in postvocalic position and generalized the production to the prevocalic position.

The results for M can be compared with the results for K, who received treatment for the sound /θ/, an inventory constraint. The taught sound, /θ/, improved because of treatment, but the other targeted sounds in error all changed spontaneously. The change in /ð/ could be accounted for because it is the cognate of /θ/ and might be expected to change; also, the child had knowledge of the sound in some positions. The change in the liquids also could be accounted for on the basis of the child's productive phonological knowledge of the sounds in other positions. The change in production of /ʃ/ is more problematic. The change may have occurred because of the child's knowledge of the stridency contrast. That is, the child did use /z/ and /ð/ contrastively in prevocalic position, and this knowledge may have contributed to the change in production (Rockman, 1983).

Comparison of the results from the two children shows that K made the greatest improvement in response to treatment. M continued to need treatment on the two sounds characterized as inventory constraints. We could speculate that if M had received treatment on one of the sounds listed as an inventory constraint, the other sounds might have improved without treatment as they did in K's case. The notion of productive phonological knowledge offers a possible explanation of why some sounds that were not directly taught or phonetically related to taught sounds often change. When children demonstrate at least partial productive phonological knowledge of specific sounds and these sounds are produced in some contexts, even though restricted by a phonological rule in others, there is a strong likelihood that these sounds will be extended without direct treatment.

These findings have implications for treatment of phonologically disordered children. In planning intervention strategies, it seems important to look at the entire phonological system for any given child. That is, one needs to determine the phonetic and phonemic inventories, the way the sounds are distributed in the system, the underlying representations of morphemes, and the phonological rules being used. Although many of these concepts are currently being used in research, they are not as well known to clinicians. The practicing clinician who is unfamiliar with some of the linguistic concepts might simply classify sounds in three major categories: sounds that a child uses correctly, sounds that are never produced, and sounds for which the child has at least partial productive phonological knowledge. In order to maximize generalization, it seems preferable to choose sounds for treatment for which the child shows no productive phonological knowledge (those sounds that are never produced), with the expectation that these sounds will not readily change without treatment (Gierut, 1985).

EVIDENCE FROM RESEARCH

In 1981 McReynolds stated, "Review of the research in articulation generalization is problematical. Research has not been systematic and the data do not fall neatly into place" (p. 246). The research to date has not been, perhaps, as systematic as one might wish. Individual researchers seem compelled to follow their own particular paths, pursuing their own favorite hypotheses and intuitions, rather than working through each problem in a programmatic sequence. However, even though the investigations are somewhat scattered, they have yielded a rich data base from which certain facts have emerged.

One type of generalization that has been demonstrated is that in which a target sound in taught words is extended to untaught words containing the same sound (Arndt, Elbert, and Shelton, 1971; Elbert and McReynolds, 1975, 1978, 1985; Elbert, Shelton, and Arndt, 1967; Hoffman, 1983; McReynolds, 1972; McReynolds and Elbert, 1981; Mowrer, 1971; Powell and Elbert, 1984; Shelton, Elbert, and Arndt, 1967). This basic finding has been replicated many times. It seems clear that children are able to extend their correct use of a sound taught in only a few exemplars to a larger set of untrained items containing the same sound.

Generalization also has been observed across word positions (Elbert and McReynolds, 1975, 1978; McReynolds, 1972; Powell and McReynolds, 1969; Rockman, 1983). When a sound is taught in one position of a word, correct production frequently is extended to other positions.

Another type of generalization is the use of untreated sounds in more complex linguistic units (Gierut, 1985; McLean, 1970; McReynolds, 1972; Wright, Shelton, and Arndt, 1969). If a sound is taught in syllables, generalization has been shown to occur to words, sentences, or conversation. A gradient of correct production has been demonstrated from imitative tasks, to reading, to spontaneous speech.

The generalization patterns described so far have primarily dealt with the generalization that occurs within a particular sound. A more complex type of generalization is across-sound generalization. One finding is well established. Generalization is influenced by the relationship that exists among sounds. The research investigations of the late 1960s and 1970s have demonstrated this relationship, and the results have been replicated many times, so we can have confidence in the findings. In fact, there is an element of predictability about the fact that if you train certain sounds, some generalization will occur to other sounds that share common features. For instance, if you teach correct production of one member of a cognate sound pair, the child will begin to produce the other sound correctly without direct teaching (Elbert, Shelton, and Arndt, 1967; Mowrer, 1971; Shelton, Elbert, and Arndt, 1967). If you teach one allophone, production of other related allophones will improve (Elbert and McReynolds, 1975; Hoffman, 1983). If you teach a distinctive feature, untreated sounds sharing a common feature will also improve (McReynolds and Bennett, 1972; Costello and Onstine, 1976).

What do these findings mean? It appears from this research that sounds are organized into natural groups and these groups are described by features, either broad features such as place, voice, and manner or more discrete features, such as distinctive features. These features have been formulated by linguists and speech scientists based on the acoustic, perceptual, and physiological characteristics of the speech sounds. The fact that children seem to generalize across sounds that share common features is an indication that these groupings have a psychological validity and that children as well as linguists recognize the similarities among sounds.

So, at least one facet of generalization has been made clearer. This information concerning features appears to explain some of the generalization patterns obtained. And yet, there is still individual variability among subjects. There are examples in the literature of children who present puzzling variations. Consider the following examples. One child, after being taught the feature of (+) stridency in the sound /f /, generalized to other fricatives, such as /v /, /s /, and /z /, but not to each of the sounds equally. There was less generalization to the sounds /v / and /z / and only to certain word positions (McReynolds and Bennett, 1972). In another study investigating the effect of context on generalization, three subjects out of five generalized across all contexts, but two subjects generalized to all contexts except clusters (Elbert and McReynolds, 1978, 1979). In yet another study, children who omitted final consonants generalized from training on a few final sounds to other final sounds, but each subject differed in the type and amount of generalization. That is, one child produced more final stops than final fricatives, and another child produced more fricatives than stops (Elbert and McReynolds, 1985). What kind of explanation can we offer to clarify these variations?

There are, no doubt, many variables that together help to explain some of these individual differences. Recent investigations at Indiana University have focused on one variable that appears promising in providing some further explanations of individual differences (Dinnsen and Elbert, 1984; Elbert, Dinnsen, and Powell, 1984; Gierut, Elbert, and Dinnsen, 1987; Weismer, Dinnsen, and Elbert, 1981). That variable is a subject variable, specifically, the individual child's unique productive phonological knowledge about the phonological system at the point in time before he or she begins treatment. This knowledge base that the child brings to the learning situation very likely influences the amount and kind of generalization patterns that occur. The case studies presented earlier were used to illustrate this notion.

Even though the concept of productive phonological knowledge is the focus of our most recent and our current research, this concept of differential knowledge affecting learning has been a persistent, albeit understudied, variable for many years. The beginnings of this concept can be traced back to the first study that mentioned stimulability. Diedrich (1983), in his comprehensive review of studies of stimulability, points out the variety of definitions for the concept and the somewhat conflicting results obtained in various studies. Nevertheless, the concept has survived and appears robust despite the confusion concerning exactly what stimulability is and how it affects learning. *Stimulability*, or the ability to imitate error sounds correctly in syllables or words, may be conceptualized as one level of phonological knowledge.

Another level of knowledge that has been shown to differentiate misarticulating children concerns feature usage. A clear demonstration of the differences among children on the basis of feature use was presented in the 1971 study by McReynolds and Huston. They studied a group of ten children who had multiple articulation errors. Figure 3–3 is taken from this study and shows the percentage of error on the different sounds for two subjects who were representative of the other subjects.

As can be seen in Figure 3–3, the children had many different sounds in error at high percentages. These children would be considered to be a somewhat homogeneous group in that they each had moderate to severe articulation problems. McReynolds and Huston analyzed these children's errors using a distinctive feature analysis (Chomsky and Halle, 1968) and discovered that the children's errors could be described according to specific features. However, there were two different patterns of feature errors. These patterns are shown in Figure 3–4. For some children most of the sound errors could be attributed to errors on a few features, such as stridency, continuancy, or voicing. This proved to be a very economical way of characterizing the errors. Other children displayed a different pattern. They had many features in error but all at low percentages. Pattern 1 was described by the authors as a phonetic problem; the children either could not produce the sounds or could produce the sounds but did not because they considered the sounds nonfunctional. These are the children who either omit the sounds or use a few sounds as substitutions for most other sounds. In pattern 2, where there were low feature errors, the children could produce the sounds, that is, they had a more complete phonetic inventory, but they used the sounds inappropriately. These children were described as having a phonemic problem. Although McReynolds and Huston did not speak directly to a difference in knowledge between the two groups of children, these data provide clear evidence that the children knew different aspects of the phonological system. However, the authors did state, "According to our results, articulation problems cannot be regarded solely as problems in motor productions; they also consist of inappropriate phonemic rules. Consider that children lacking features in their repertoires also evidence inappropriate rule behavior. Inappropriate use of features contributes considerably to the articulation problems of these children. To a large extent, therefore, we would agree with individuals who contend that articulation problems should be considered within the framework of a phonological system, as systems at variance with adult phonemic systems" (McReynolds and Huston, 1971, p. 165). The authors further suggested that different treatment procedures should be used with children in the two groups.

The children in pattern 1 were studied further by McReynolds and Bennett (1972) and were provided treatment on sounds containing the highest feature error. Their findings indicated that training a feature in one sound resulted in increased correct production of other sounds that also contained that feature. Children like these have been studied often in generalization studies. They are the children who begin treatment with very low baseline scores, who simply do not produce a sound correctly. When they are trained to produce the sound correctly in a few contexts, they generalize across many untrained items containing the sound and across some other pho-

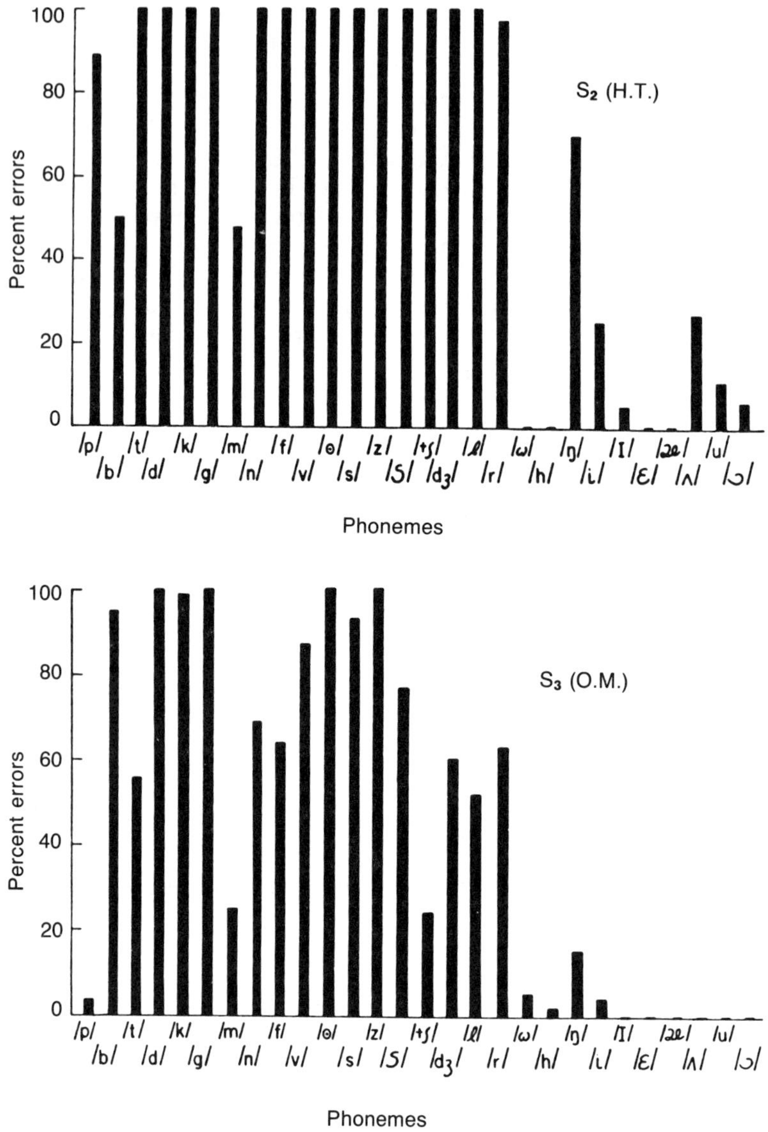

Figure 3–3 Percentage of incorrect articulation of phonemes measured on the McDonald Deep Test of Articulation for subjects 2 and 3. (McReynolds LV, Huston K. A distinctive feature analysis of children's misarticulations. J Speech Hear Disord 1971; 36:155–166).

netically similar sounds. Generalization patterns like this lead to the conclusion that their problem was primarily a phonetic problem, that is, once they have learned the motor skill required to produce the sound, they are able to use that sound appropriately.

But what about the children in pattern 2? They appear to have the motor skill available but do not distribute the sound within the phonological system in an appropriate manner. Children with phonemic problems are not easy to identify in the research literature, so it is not possible to describe the generalization patterns for this group. Generalization patterns may be different depending on whether a child has a phonetic problem, a phonemic problem, or some combination of the two. In other words, what a child "knows" about the phonological system when he begins remediation may influence the generalization pattern.

PHONOLOGICAL KNOWLEDGE

The term "knowledge" has been operationally defined in several studies as the child's actual productions of speech sounds and the use of the sounds in the phonological system. Thus, productive phonological knowledge becomes a measurable entity. In one study concerned with consonant clusters (Elbert, Dinnsen, and Powell, 1984), productive phonological knowledge was operationally defined as a score of 10 percent or greater on a baseline test. In another study concerned with final consonant omis-

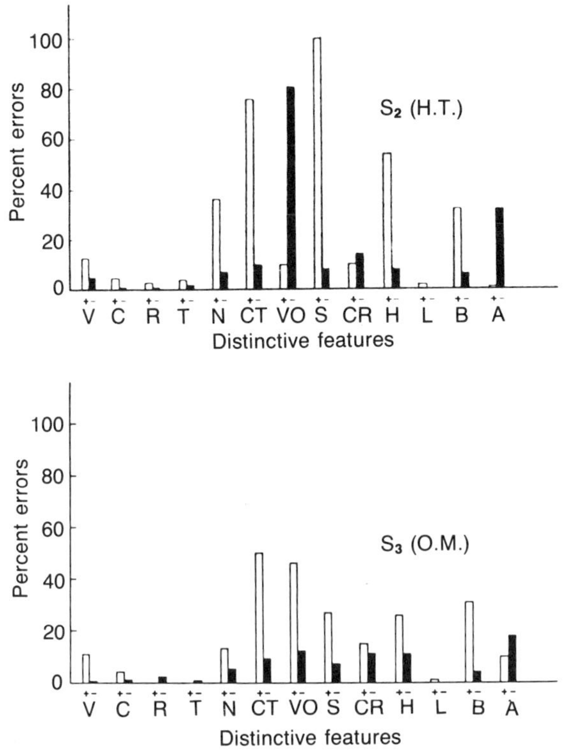

Figure 3–4 The percentage of incorrect usage of features in the phonological systems of subjects 2 and 3. (McReynolds LV, Huston K. A distinctive feature analysis of children's misarticulations. J Speech Hear Disord 1971; 36:155–166).

sion (Dinnsen and Elbert, 1984), knowledge was based either on a subject's inconsistent production of a final sound or on production of a sound in a related diminutive form. For instance, one subject might say [pi] one time and [pig] another time, for target "pig," or another subject might say [pi] but also say "piggy." In both of these cases the subjects actually produced the sound in the morpheme and thus they were credited with productive phonological knowledge of the final /g /. In this definition there is no need to infer what the child has stored mentally; the child is given credit for knowing those sounds that he produces and uses. The term *knowledge* as used in this context refers only to productive phonological knowledge; it implies nothing about speech perception. Speech perception and subphonemic distinctions may, indeed, represent other levels of knowledge. The use of the word "knowledge" should be understood to be restricted to evidence from speech production alone. The terms "knowledge" and "productive phonological knowledge" are used interchangeably here.

What is it that children need to know in order to master the phonological system of the English language? In the first place children need to be able to produce the speech sounds of the language. They need not only to produce the sounds but also to use the sounds contrastively to distinguish meanings. For instance, minimal pairs such as "fat" and "bat" differ in meaning, and thus the sounds are said to be used contrastively. Additionally, children must understand which sounds can occur in different positions in words; for instance, / ŋ / can occur intervocalically and postvocalically but not at the beginning of a word. Linguists refer to these distributional properties of the language as *phonotactics*. Many normally developing children learn most of these aspects by the age of 3. However, the children that we see in the clinic differ from their normal peers and present patterns that show varying amounts of knowledge about the sound system.

FEATURE GENERALIZATION

There are some examples in the research literature that illustrate different generalization patterns that may have been affected by the productive phonological knowledge the child possessed prior to treatment. Two studies deal with feature usage. Referring again to the McReynolds and Bennett (1972) study, three subjects from the pattern 1 group were trained on three different features—(+) stridency, (+) voicing, and (+) continuancy. All three subjects showed changes in phoneme usage after the training. The subjects generalized not only to untrained items of the sound being trained but also to some untrained items in some other sounds containing the trained feature. This study showed clearly the influence of features on generalization patterns; however, the authors noted individual differences. One subject generalized mostly to sounds in the releasing position of words, and another, mostly to voiceless sounds. Although the authors did not present a complete phonological analysis for each subject, we can speculate that the children's restrictions in generalizing to different sounds may have been related to their initial ability to use the voicing feature contrastively and to a problem in producing sounds in final position.

A more detailed example of feature use and generalization patterns was presented in a study by Rockman (1983). In this study six subjects who never produced /s / and /z / prior to treatment were taught /s / in identical treatment procedures. Given this situation, we might expect to see very similar generalization patterns, but actually there were three different patterns. Close examination of the data revealed three distinct patterns of productive phonological knowledge at the feature level, which corresponded with three different generalization patterns. In this study, the status of the stridency contrast in the child's phonological system appeared to be related to generalization. The two subjects who generalized most extensively had a phonemic stridency contrast in their systems prior to treatment. Specifically, although they never produced /s / or /z /, they did produce / θ / and / ð / and /f / and /v / contrastively. Thus, they showed contrastive production of both strident and nonstrident phonemes in their systems.

Two subjects who generalized at a slower rate and in a limited fashion had a stridency contrast at the phonetic level but not at the phonemic level, that is, one subject produced / ǰ / (a plus strident sound) and / ð / (a minus strident sound), and the other subject produced / ʃ / and / ð /, but these sounds were not used contrastively. The last two subjects, who generalized very minimally, lacked the stridency contrast at any level. They produced either strident or nonstrident segments, but not both. Specifically, one subject only produced /f / and /v / and the other subject produced only / θ / and / ð /. Thus, it appears that the knowledge that these subjects possessed about strident and nonstrident phonemes influenced the learning of the specific strident sound /s /.

PATTERN GENERALIZATION

Several studies dealing with clusters also reveal differences in learning patterns related to error patterns at the beginning of treatment. Elbert and McReynolds (1979) reported on five children who misarticulated /s / and were subsequently taught correct production of /s / as a singleton in three nonsense syllables. Two patterns emerged from the children's performance on consonant cluster generalization. In one pattern three subjects substituted / θ / for /s / in all clusters at the beginning of the study. These children who marked the cluster with / θ / began to use /s / correctly in probe items. The other two subjects omitted /s / in clusters at baseline. These subjects progressed through a series of stages before producing /s / correctly in clusters. First they went from omitting /s / to inserting / θ / in the cluster and then finally to replacing the / θ / with /s /. It appears that two pieces of information are important in learning cluster production. The first is the phonotactic rule that two consecutive consonants can occur in sequence. The second is the actual production of the correct segment. Three subjects appeared to know the phonotactic rule at the onset. They only had to learn correct production of /s / in order to produce clusters correctly. The other two subjects, who had less knowledge at the beginning of treatment, had to learn not only correct production of /s / but also the rule that two consonants could occur sequentially.

Two other studies specifically investigated generalization to clusters when clusters were trained. In one study (McReynolds and Elbert, 1981), six children were trained to produce /s / and either /r / or / l / clusters. The baseline scores for these children showed that the subjects never produced the clusters in more than 10 percent of the probe items. The results showed that with one exception, children generalized only within class clusters, not across class clusters. That is, when the children were trained on /s / clusters, generalization occurred to untrained /s / clusters, but not to /r / or /l / clusters, and vice versa.

In a separate study (Powell and Elbert, 1984), six subjects who misarticulated stop plus liquid (e.g., /tr/) and fricative plus liquid (e.g., /sl/) clusters were trained on either one or the other type of cluster. In this study, generalization occurred to both the treated and the untreated categories. This finding differs from the McReynolds and Elbert (1981) study. An explanation for this difference seemed to be related to the baseline performance of the subjects. In the Powell and Elbert study, the subjects were able to produce all of the phonemes as singletons prior to the onset of treatment; in contrast, subjects in the McReynolds and Elbert study did not produce the sounds as singletons. It appears that the productive phonological knowledge that the subjects possessed prior to treatment may have been a factor influencing their generalization patterns.

ROLE OF KNOWLEDGE

The data from the Powell and Elbert study were examined more closely in a separate investigation (Elbert, Dinnesen, and Powell, 1984), in order to clarify the role of knowledge at the onset of treatment and its relationship to generalized learning. In this study an operational definition of a child's productive phonological knowledge of a particular cluster class was determined according to two criteria. The first requirement was that a subject must achieve an average score of 10 percent or greater over the three baseline tests; the second requirement was that a subject must score at least three or more correct responses in either cluster category in any one baseline session. From these criteria each subject was characterized either as having knowledge of a cluster category or as having little or no knowledge of a cluster category. This factor of productive phonological knowledge combined with the treatment factor (i.e., which category was taught) appeared to be predictive of generalization patterns. For instance, if a subject had productive phonological knowledge of the category stop plus liquid and was trained on fricative plus liquid, he or she generalized to both cluster categories almost equally. Conversely, if a subject had knowledge of fricative plus liquid clusters and was trained on stop plus liquids, generalization occurred to both categories. Only two subjects of the six studied did not demonstrate knowledge of either of the two cluster categories.

The results from this study seem to have some implications for clinical decisions. That is, if children have some minimal knowledge of sound usage, they are able to increase this knowledge without direct training. Specifically, if a child can produce a sound in some contexts before treatment starts, he or she may begin to extend this ability to correct production of the sound in other contexts (e.g., different positions in words) without direct treatment. Sounds for which children have no knowledge do need direct training.

Another series of studies investigating the error pattern of omission of final consonants contains further information concerning children's individual knowledge. Elbert and McReynolds (1985) provided treatment to four subjects who consistently omitted final consonants. These subjects were taught to produce a limited number of exemplars of either final stops or final fricatives. The results indicated that the children generalized only to the class of sounds being taught, not across sound categories. Once again, individual differences in generalization were noted; for instance, the children did not generalize to all stops or fricatives equally. Rather, more generalization occurred to some stops and fricatives than to others, and this varied among subjects.

The individual differences noted among the children led to further investigations. Extensive additional data had been gathered from these children prior to treatment. Complete phonological analyses were performed from these pretreatment data (Dinnsen and Maxwell, 1981), and acoustic analyses were also completed to study subphonemic characteristics (Weismer, Dinnsen, and Elbert, 1981). The phonological and acoustic analyses were performed independently from the treatment study, and the results are reported in separate studies.

The acoustic study by Weismer, Dinnsen, and Elbert (1981) investigated the vowel duration of three of the four experimental subjects who omitted final consonants. The purpose of this study was to explore the possibility that children who omit final stops mark the voicing of the "missing" consonant with differential vowel durations. In English, adults and normally articulating children as young as 3 years produce greater vowel durations before voiced, as compared to voiceless, stops. The results of this study indicated that two of the children evidenced systematic differences in vowel durations depending on the voicing of the omitted final consonant. In other words, vowel durations were longer for targets that should have contained final voiced sounds but shorter when the target should have contained final voiceless sounds. One child did not produce a systematic difference. Therefore, even though the children had the same surface error pattern of omission of final consonants, at a subphonemic level there were indications of individual differences.

These differences were supported by the phonological analyses on the same children. The child who showed no voicing distinction also showed no productive knowledge of final stops or fricatives. The other subjects did show varying amounts of knowledge for specific sounds. The evidence for productive knowledge was obtained from subject responses to word final sounds and morphophonemic alternations. For instance, in some cases a child might produce variable responses to final sounds, so that "dog" might be realized at times as [da], but produced [dagi] when the word was inflected as a diminutive. These two types of evidence were the basis for deciding that a child had the correct underlying representation for a particular sound and thus showed productive phonological knowledge of that sound.

Based on evidence from the acoustic and phonological analyses, it was possible to describe each child's unique knowledge about final consonants. This knowledge was reflected in the individual generalization patterns. Three factors seemed related to the patterns: the class of sounds being trained, the knowledge of underlying representations, and the order of training. None of these factors was sufficient by itself to explain all of the variations in individual learning patterns. However, when taken together they do account for a great deal of the variation observed.

These findings have been extended in a recent study (Gierut, Elbert, and Dinnesen, 1987), in which no particular error pattern was selected for study. Rather, the entire phonological system was analyzed for six misarticulating children. Based upon these analyses, each child's productive phonological knowledge was determined and ranked on a continuum from "most" to "least" knowledge relative to the adult target. Each child received treatment for sounds selected from different points on the continuum. The results indicated that a child's knowledge at the onset of treatment influenced the overall amount of generalization, and also that generalization learning was associated with the point on the knowledge continuum at which treatment was initiated.

An example of a continuum for one child is shown in Figure 3–5. At the top of the continuum are the sounds that were produced accurately and were never in error relative to the adult target; next were the sounds [t,d] which were optionally (sometimes, but not always) deleted in postvocalic position. The sounds /ʃ/ and the voiced affricate were inconsistently produced in different word positions. At the bottom of the continuum are sounds that were never produced correctly relative to the adult system and that never occurred in the child's phonetic or phonemic inventories.

In general, the findings indicated that when children were trained on sounds from the bottom of the continuum,

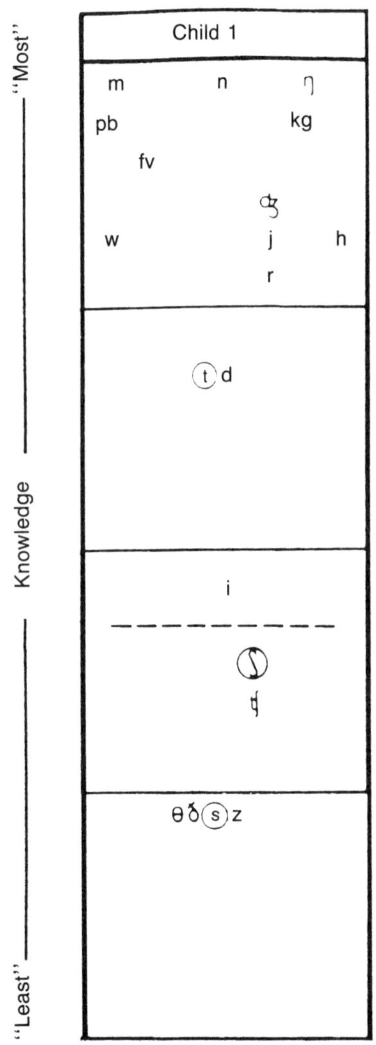

Figure 3–5 Continuum of productive phonological knowledge for child 1.

they showed increased correct production not only on the sounds directly treated but also on sounds higher on the continuum for which they already had some knowledge. However, when a child was trained on sounds at the other end of the continuum, the changes were restricted to the sounds being trained. Sounds at the bottom of the continuum did not change.

Information from studies concerned with phonological knowledge and learning patterns is in the early stages. The results seem promising, but continued research is needed before these relationships can be more fully understood. Other factors must be investigated, such as the type of training provided and other subject variables including the motor and perceptual abilities of individual children.

STRATEGIES FOR FACILITATION OF GENERALIZATION

In addition to the research findings presented in this paper, many suggestions have been made over the years about ways in which generalization can be facilitated. The following suggestions have been culled from suggestions in the literature and are taken from material presented by Elbert and Gierut (1986).

Characterize the child's phonological system. Obtain a representative speech sample. Determine stimulability. Determine intelligibility. Analyze to determine phonetic inventory, phonemic inventory, pattern of errors, and productive phonological knowledge.

Select targets that will provide new information to the child. After analyzing the child's phonological system, it should be possible to determine which sounds are being used correctly in all cases, which are used correctly on an inconsistent basis, and which are never produced correctly. When you select a target from the category of sounds that are never produced correctly, you will be teaching the child new information about how a sound is produced and how it is used in the phonological system. You are also assuming that the child will continue to learn those sounds he can already produce and will increase correct production of these sounds without direct treatment.

Select treatment items that are relevant to the child and that serve a communicative function. The clinician needs to consider the individual and his or her environment. Consider, for instance, the child's favorite activities, names of family and friends, and common communication needs at home or in school. Choosing meaningful items for treatment increases the likelihood that the words will be used outside of the clinic in daily communication.

Present different and diverse treatment items. Diversity in the treatment items allows the child to discover the underlying pattern being taught and the range of application of that pattern. When a child is presented with words like *bus, soup, tricycle, stop, scissors, skipping,* he or she must learn to identify the common element across the items and notice the differences. The child is given the opportunity to discover that the sound /s / is common to all of the items and that the sound occurs in many different types of words (nouns and verbs), in many different positions, and in different syllable shapes.

Structure the treatment plan loosely. Provide many and varied activities in treatment, encouraging sound use in different communicative tasks. Although drill work on a particular sound in a limited set of words may be an important part of the treatment plan, it is also useful to extend the use of the words into other domains. Examples would include games, such as concentration, "go fish," conversations on play telephones, or role playing with puppets. By varying the task activity, the clinician gives the child an opportunity to manipulate sounds actively and to recognize that sounds can and should be used in different communicative situations.

Monitor daily progress as well as progress in learning over time. Regularly record accuracy of performance and periodically probe for generalization. *Learning performance* refers to how accurately the child is producing target sounds in the clinical treatment tasks; *generalization performance* refers to how accurately the child is producing target sounds in new treatment items and tasks. Daily progress can be evaluated by recording the percentage of correct response of the target sound on a set of trials; generalization performance can be evaluated by administering a probe, testing related but untreated items. Both are important measures. If a child does not transfer accurate sound production after a series of treatment sessions, it may be that the child needs additional practice in learning to produce the sound in a more effortless manner or that a more diverse set of items needs to be introduced. In any case, failure to generalize indicates a need to reconsider the treatment plan.

Keep the attentional demands on the child to a minimum. Early in treatment, when the emphasis is on correct production of a sound, the attentional demands of the task should be few. Once the production is known but the production is not yet automatic, the demands of the task can be increased.

Engage the child in problem-solving tasks. The use of minimal pair training is one example of a problem-solving task. In this type of task the child learns that sounds are associated with a change in meaning. When a child is presented with pairs, such as *pin–fin, pat–fat,* and *Pete–feet* and is required to use the words appropriately, the child learns something about the contrastive elements of sounds. Another problem-solving task might involve sorting and matching. For example, in a sorting task the child may be asked to name treatment items and then to sort items into respective piles representing target sounds. In this task the child learns that there is some similar property among the items in each pile, that is, they all contain a specific sound. In a matching task, the child may select an item from a group of pictures, name the item, and then match the item with other pictures in the group that have the same sound.

A PUZZLING CONCLUSION

The complexities of the data and the number of unexplained variables in articulation generalization make it difficult to arrive at a final summary statement. However, the following analogy may help to summarize some of the points presented in this chapter.

In this analogy, the phonological system is viewed as a giant puzzle that has to be solved by the child. The child begins with a few pieces of the puzzle, a few sounds that he began to use in babbling that have been adopted into words, and he moves forward from there adding new pieces to fit into the puzzle. From what is known about normal phonological acquisition, most children proceed to solve the puzzle in quite individual ways, selecting different pieces in the beginning but managing to reach a fairly complete solution by age 3 years.

Children who come into the clinic seem to have reached a temporary impasse. They arrive with many assorted pieces but need some help in finding other pieces. If you visualize this puzzle as containing in a two–dimensional form all of the English consonant sounds in three positions (pre-, inter- and postvocalic) as a simplified version of the puzzle, children's knowledge of the phonological system can be characterized by how many pieces of the puzzle they possess (Fig. 3–6).

Figure 3–7 illustrates a child who has a very restricted phonetic inventory and thus very few puzzle pieces. When he learns a new sound he gains one more piece but has very few clues about where the sound fits into the puzzle. This is a very severe type of problem.

Figure 3–8 shows a child who has a larger phonetic inventory but who presents problems with phonetic production of some sounds in some positions. This child has more information about the puzzle and more clues about how new pieces fit into the picture.

Another type of child is seen in the school-age population. This child misarticulates /s / and /z / only (Fig. 3–9). So, the child has an almost complete phonetic and phonemic inventory and is only missing small pieces of the puzzle. Once the child learns correct /s / and /z / production, he can fill in the blanks and have the full picture.

CONCLUSION

Although much information has been obtained over the years in research concerning articulation generalization, there are still many intriguing questions to be answered. Both clinicians and researchers need to be concerned with these questions and with providing answers. Even though we are generally successful in effecting change in the

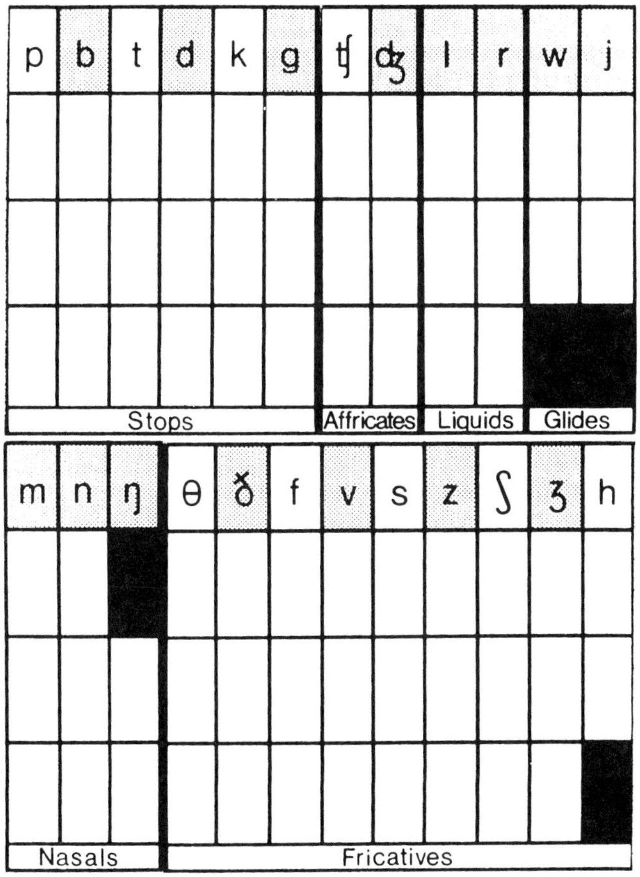

Figure 3–6 English consonant sounds in three positions.

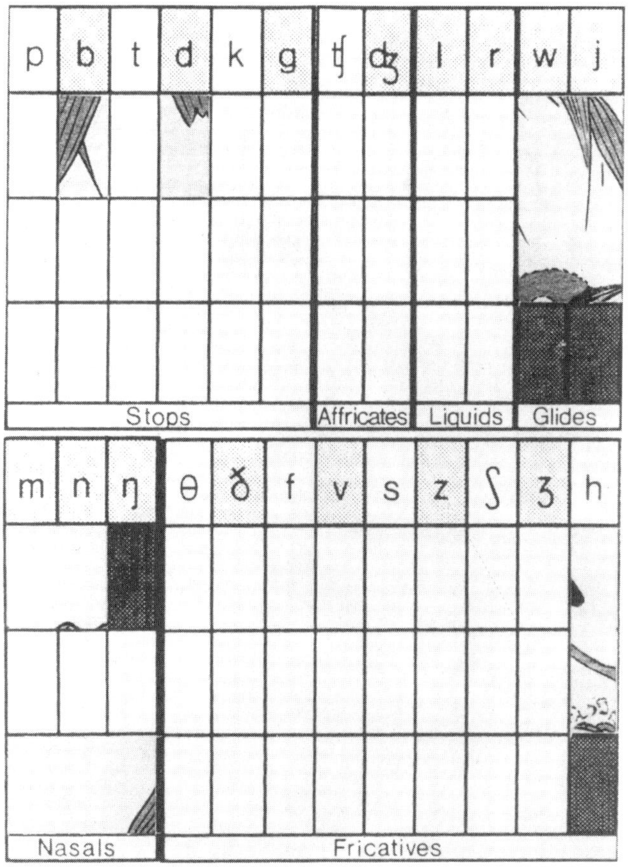

Figure 3–7 Puzzle analogy for child with restricted phonetic inventory.

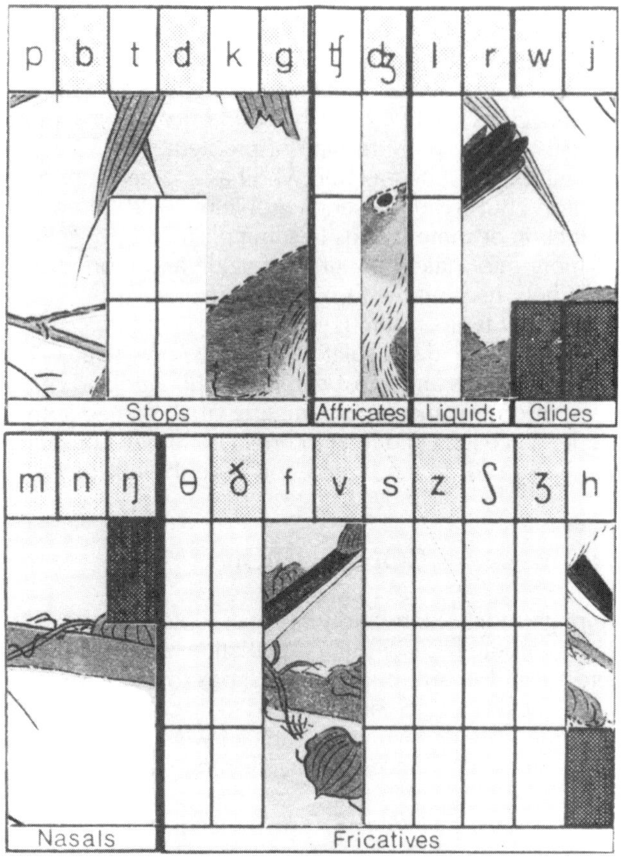

Figure 3–8 Puzzle analogy for child with larger phonetic inventory.

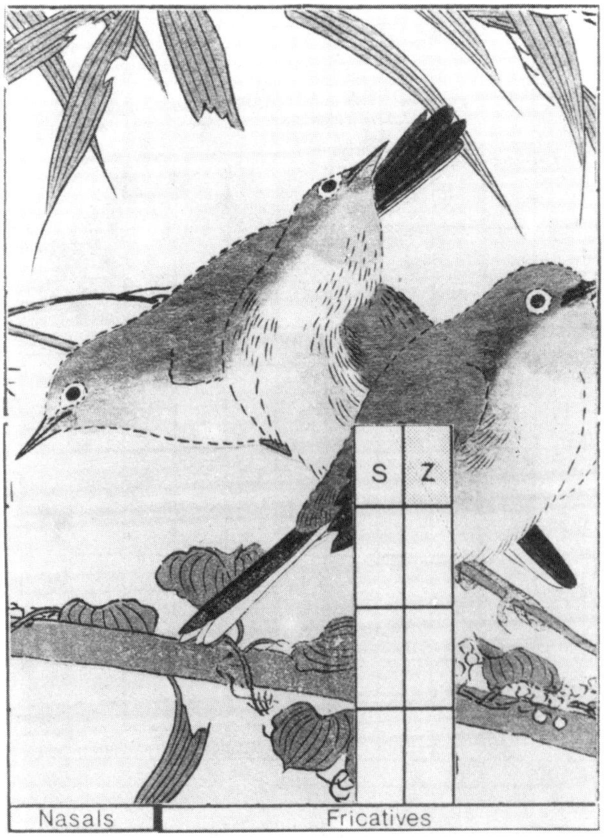

Figure 3–9 Puzzle analogy for child with misarticulations of /s / and /z /.

speech of functionally misarticulating children, we must continue to explore the reasons for our success or lack of success. Efforts to do so help to build a much-needed empirical base for our clinical work.

This research was supported in part by a grant from the Department of Health and Human Services, Public Health Service, NIH grant number R01 NS 20976.

REFERENCES

Arndt WB, Elbert M, Shelton RL. Prediction of articulation improvement with therapy from early lesson sound production task scores. J Speech Hear Res 1971; 14:149–153.

Chomsky N, Halle M. The sound pattern of English. New York: Harper & Row, 1968.

Costello J, Onstine JM. The modification of multiple articulation errors based on distinctive feature theory. J Speech Hear Disord 1976; 41:199–215.

Diedrich WM. Stimulability and articulation disorders. Seminars in Speech and Language 1983; 4:297–312.

Dinnsen DA. Methods and empirical issues in analyzing functional misarticulations. In: Elbert M, Dinnsen DA, Weismer G, eds. Phonological theory and the misarticulating child (ASHA Monograph No. 22). Rockville, MD: ASHA, 1984:5.

Dinnsen DA, Elbert M. On the relationship between phonology and learning. In: Elbert M, Dinnsen DA, Weismer G, eds. Phonological theory and the misarticulating child (ASHA Monograph No. 22). Rockville, MD: ASHA, 1984:59.

Dinnsen DA, Maxwell EM. Some phonology problems from functional speech disorders. Innovations in Linguistics Education 1981; 2:79–98.

Dunn L. Peabody Picture Vocabulary Test—Revised. Circle Pines, MN: American Guidance Service, 1986.

Elbert M, Dinnsen DA, Powell TW. On the prediction of phonologic generalization learning patterns. J Speech Hear Disord 1984; 49:309–317.

Elbert M, Gierut JA. Handbook of clinical phonology: approaches to assessment and treatment. San Diego: College-Hill Press, 1986.

Elbert M, McReynolds LV. Transfer of /r / across contexts. J Speech Hear Disord 1975; 40:380–387.

Elbert M, McReynolds LV. An experimental analysis of misarticulating children's generalization. J Speech Hear Res 1978; 21:136–150.

Elbert M, McReynolds LV. Aspects of phonological acquisition during articulation training. J Speech Hear Disord 1979; 44:459–471.

Elbert M, McReynolds LV. The generalization hypothesis: final consonant deletion. Lang Speech 1985; 28:281–294.

Elbert M, Shelton RL Jr, Arndt WB Jr. A task for evaluation of articulation change: 1. Development of methodology. J Speech Hear Res 1967; 10:281–288.

Gierut JA. On the relationship between phonological knowledge and generalization learning in misarticulating children. Doctoral dissertation, Indiana University, Bloomington, IN, 1985.

Gierut JA, Elbert M, Dinnsen DA. A functional analysis of phonological knowledge and generalization learning in misarticulating children. J Speech Hear Res 1987; 30:462–480.

Goldman R, Fristoe M, Woodcock R. The Goldman-Fristoe-Woodcock Test of Auditory Discrimination. Circle Pines, MN: American Guidance Service, 1970.

Hoffman PR. Interallophonic generalization of /r/ training. J Speech Hear Disord 1983; 48:215–221.

Hughes D. Language treatment and generalization. San Diego: College-Hill Press, 1985.

McLean JE. Extending stimulus control of phoneme articulation by operant techniques. In: Girardeau FL, Spradlin JE, eds. A functional approach to speech and language (ASHA Monograph No. 14). Rockville, MD: ASHA, 1970:24.

McReynolds LV. Articulation generalization during articulation training. Lang Speech 1972; 15:149–155.

McReynolds LV. Generalization in articulation training. Analysis and Intervention in Development Disabilities 1981; 1:245–248.

McReynolds LV, Bennett S. Distinctive feature generalization in articulation training. J Speech Hear Disord 1972; 37:462–470.

McReynolds LV, Elbert M. Generalization of correct articulation in clusters. Appl Psycholing 1981; 2:119–132.

McReynolds LV, Huston K. A distinctive feature analysis of children's misarticulations. J Speech Hear Disord 1971; 36:155–166.

Mowrer DE. Developing precision in recording speech behaviors. Salt Lake City, UT: Word Making Productions, 1971.

Powell J, McReynolds LV. A procedure for testing position generalization from articulation training. J Speech Hear Res 1969; 12:629–645.

Powell TW, Elbert M. Generalization following the remediation of early and later-developing consonant clusters. J Speech Hear Disord 1984; 49:211–218.

Rockman BK. An experimental investigation of generalization and individual differences in phonological training. Doctoral dissertation, Indiana University, Bloomington, IN, 1983.

Rockman BK, Elbert M. Generalization in articulation training. In: Winitz H, ed. Treating articulation disorders: for clinicians by clinicians. Baltimore: University Park Press, 1984:131.

Shelton RL, Elbert M, Arndt WB. A task for evaluation of articulation change: II. Comparison of task scores during baseline and lesson series testing. J Speech Hear Res 1967; 10:578–585.

Stokes TF, Baer DM. An implicit technology of generalization. J Appl Behav Anal 1977; 10:349–367.

Weismer G, Dinnsen D, Elbert M. A study of the voicing distinction associated with omitted, word-final stops. J Speech Hear Disord 1981; 46:97–103.

Wright V, Shelton R, Arndt W. A task for evaluation of articulation change. III. Imitative task scores compared with scores for more spontaneous tasks. J Speech Hear Res 1969; 12:875–884.

Chapter Four

FACILITATING GENERALIZATION THROUGH INDUCTION TEACHING

PHIL J. CONNELL, Ph.D.

This chapter presents a description of a particular approach to teaching language that is called here *induction teaching*. The focus of the description is on factors that make the approach as effective as possible, that is, on factors that contribute to the generalization of the effects of induction teaching. The kinds of procedures contained within the approach have been designed to teach language to children who have demonstrated a difficulty in learning language naturally from nurturing and interacting caregivers. Because of the detrimental effects that delayed language development can have on academic progress and psychological and social adjustment (Aram, Ekelman, and Nation, 1984), these children need the assistance of skilled language teachers if they are to succeed in a highly competitive society. A basic assumption made within the approach that is described here is that teachers of language need to have several areas of expertise to be effective, some of which are as follows: (1) a knowledge of the structure and function of language that can be translated into teaching content, (2) a knowledge of the process by which structure and function are learned, (3) a knowledge of the nature of language learning impairment from which to create a working hypothesis about the cause of a client's failure to learn language, and (4) a knowledge of the process of language teaching from which to create a working hypothesis about how the client's learning difficulty can be overcome through instruction. These four areas of expertise form the structure of the chapter that follows.

The four areas of knowledge fit into four sections of the chapter: the nature of language structure and function, the process of language acquisition, the nature of language learning impairment and a description of induction teaching. Each section presents positions taken related to major issues of debate in the field. The positions taken here are justified as much as possible by comparison to alternative approaches and by reference to the findings of theoretical, developmental, and clinical research. It is assumed that all approaches to language teaching, by practical necessity, take definitive positions on the central questions of the field, questions such as: what is language? how is it learned? and how can it be taught? Some approaches, in their description, convey their positions only implicitly through the procedures advocated.

As will soon be obvious to the reader of this chapter, I assume that one of the major responsibilities of those advocating any teaching approach (besides providing empirical evidence for the effectiveness of the procedures within the approach) is to defend explicitly the theoretical validity of the approach with regard to competing approaches. This requirement is especially important in a field such as clinical language teaching (and equally so in other clinical teaching fields such as stuttering, aphasia and articulation disorders, and others), because there are different and opposing approaches that have submitted evidence of effectiveness. At the present time, the field is far too ignorant of the factors that should be controlled and of the methods by which language teaching should be evaluated to select a teaching approach solely on the results of the few research studies that have evaluated teaching effectiveness. In the present state of its development as a science, clinical language teaching is groping for a promising research direction that will uncover the nature of the language learning problem itself. Until progress is made in this direction, the results of teaching research must be viewed with caution. One of the most promising directions seems to be the development of models of disorder that fit into larger models of cognitive organization, models that view language learning as part of the overall cognitive process of learning. Whatever the direction taken during this preliminary stage of the science, an overemphasis on comparisons of the effects of different teaching approaches may have the unfortunate effect of selecting the best procedure from a group of relatively bad teaching methods. In the long term, it may impede our search for models that are much better suited for our clinical population.

The following two sections are devoted to a brief explanation of the theoretical background of induction teaching and to a brief comparison between it and the operant approach that has been thoroughly described in the other chapters of this book. Following this, a discussion of the possible causes of language learning problems is offered. The causes proposed are predictable for the conclusions reached in the theoretical discussion. The next section details the methods by which the approach is being implemented. It also summarizes the applied research that supports the approach. In this section, the principles that guided the creation and implementation of the procedures are summarized, and suggestions for the future direction of the clinical research program from which the approach was developed are discussed.

LANGUAGE STRUCTURE AND FUNCTION

Language is defined within the approach as a system of mental representation, that is, one of the several systems of knowledge that compose human cognition. This particular system relates language meanings to language utterances by means of a set of rules that permit generation of sentences by specifying the sounds and meanings of each. One part of the knowledge of this system of rules, the syntactic part, has been described as an algebraic type of knowledge (Lightfoot, 1982). For example, one's knowledge of a rule specifying that sentences contain the grammatical categories NP (noun phrase), AUX (auxiliary), and VP (verb phrase) (S→NP AUX VP) is similar in some respects to one's knowledge of a mathematical formula such as $y = 3x^2 + 3xz + 4z$.

To claim that one knows formal rules such as these means that one assumes two types of knowledge. The first type is knowledge of the nature of the elements that compose the statement, and the second is knowledge of the relationships among the elements or the process of computation described by the statement. In the mathematical case, to have the first kind of knowledge means that one knows that the numerical variables (x, y, and z) can be replaced by numerical values (e.g., $x = 5$, $y = 3$, and $z = 2$) and that each of these values represents a discrete point on an abstract number line. To have the second type of knowledge means that one knows the operational basis for mathematical operations (e.g., multiplication, division, and addition) that are performed on these values as specified by the formula. In the grammatical case, to have the first kind of knowledge means that one knows that the grammatical variables (NP, AUX, and VP) are replaced by linguistic values (e.g., The dog, PRESENT TENSE, and bite) in the process of sentence formation. This means that one knows, for example, what an NP is and how it differs from other abstract grammatical categories that compose language. To have the second type of knowledge means that one knows the linguistic operations that are performed on these values specified by the statement (e.g., ordering and affixing placement).

The knowledge of mathematical and grammatical rules can be separated, at least in a descriptive sense, from their application. The use of language rules generates behaviors such as spoken sentences. Although rules are used when encoding and decoding spoken sentences, the actual occurrence of a behavior of language (i.e., the speaking or comprehending of a spoken sentence) is not compulsory for asserting that certain grammatical rules are known. Just as the absence of the act of mathematical computation does not necessarily mean that one does not know a mathematical rule, the absence of the behaviors of language cannot be interpreted as lack of the knowledge of language rules. The act or behavior of adding, subtracting, or saying sentences is transitory; it has a beginning and an end. In contrast, the knowledge of adding, subtracting, and formulating sentences has a more permanent mental existence. Thus, data that indicate that a rule has been used, such as a person's production or comprehension of a sentence in a certain communication context, could support the assertion that the person had knowledge of the rule, but the lack of such data would not, by itself, support the assertion that the person did not know the rule in question.

This model of language differs drastically from the operant model that underlies a considerable amount of the teaching research reported in the literature and the teaching programs that are available for purchase. Behavioral explanations of language make no appeal to cognitive mechanisms underlying behavior (Baer and Guess, 1973; Skinner, 1957; Warren, 1985). They refer only to the occurrence and physical attributes of verbal behavior and their relation to the occurrence and functional attributes of environmental events. What is conceived as language structure and use to a cognitivist is labeled as a speaker's verbal behavior (*expressive language*) and a listener's response (*receptive language*) by a behaviorist. Within this latter view of language, the structure of the verbal behaviors of a speaker is entirely a function of its effect on listeners. Behaviors that have similar effects are classed together and the resulting "response classes" constitute the only internal structure of the behavioral system of language.

This difference between the behavioral level of organization advocated by the operant theory and the cognitive level advocated by the other major theories of language is critical to the difference between the present approach and that underlying the teaching practices advocated in the other chapters of this book. It is assumed here that language is more than the behaviors that emanate from its rules. It is assumed that to learn language, one has to learn the rules, and thus that to teach language, one has to teach rules. The behaviors of language are given a priority secondary to the rules that generate them. Thus, it is assumed that the structure of language is far more complicated than a system of behaviors and that to think otherwise seriously misrepresents the system of language. Consequently, to teach language as if these rules do not exist is tantamount to teaching the wrong content and should, in principle, inevitably fail.

Although it is argued that behaviors and knowledge must be separated when discussing the nature of language, there are other domains of learning in which the distinction is not as necessary or clear. Surely it would seem unnecessary to postulate a system of mental representations for learning a golf swing. A system for explaining how a learner slowly increases the precision and strength of certain body movements would seem to be all that would be necessary, and operant theory would seem to be as good a candidate as any for teaching this. Operant theory stresses the need for repetition and feedback, two prominent aspects in a golf teacher's arsenal. Of course, there is more to the game of golf than the physical aspects, and these aspects might require a more abstract descriptive apparatus. But at least the physical acts themselves need no such machinery. This is essentially the point that Chomsky made about Skinner's book *Verbal Behavior* in his famous 1959 review. He claimed that the logic of operant theory was not wrong, only that it is wrongly applied to systems of complex human cognition such as language.

LANGUAGE ACQUISITION

The induction teaching approach is modeled after the induction learning hypothesis of language acquisition. The induction learning mechanism is perhaps the most widely used general approach to explaining language learning in theories of natural language acquisition. It was the centerpiece of the language acquisition theory proposed by Bloomfield (1933), which was popular before the advent of transformational generative grammar (Chomsky, 1957). According to Bloomfield, a child begins the induction learning process by storing in memory relevant facts or data garnered from input sentences. The selection of only appropriate data and the nature of the processes subsequently performed on the data are considered to be the products of an innate induction ability that is not necessarily limited in its operation to language acquisition. When the stored data reach some critical mass, they are analyzed to uncover distributional patterns or similarities that might be used to classify them into linguistically relevant categories. The distribution of these categories, in turn, is analyzed to discover patterns of sentence structure. The learner is said to make inductive generalizations about the distribution of the raw data leading to the creation of grammatical categories such as noun, verb, and adjective, and to make generalizations about the distributions of these categories, leading to the creation of rules of sentence structure.

Even though the syntactic focus of Bloomfield's theory of language is not as popular as it once was (see Maratsos, 1982, for a more contemporary version), the induction learning mechanism is a component of most currently popular explanations of language learning. The social-interactional (Berko Gleason, 1977; Nelson, 1977) and the similar cognitive-interactional (Bates and MacWhinney, 1979, 1982) models of language acquisition describe the learning processes in inductive terms (Bohannon and Warren-Luebecker, 1985). The process of language learning is described in these theories in terms of inducing categories and rules from developmentally tailored input spoken about salient objects and events in an immediately available and interacting environment. As with Bloomfield's explanation, the cognitive mechanisms that a child brings to bear during the induction process are not thought to be limited to language learning but are available to other learning activities as well.

The cognitive emphasis of the theory of language acquisition that emanates from induction learning stands in stark contrast to explanations of language learning associated with operant theory. In operant theory, the term generalization covers many of the phenomena associated with what has been called rule learning. *Behavioral generalization* is defined as the extension of a behavior learned as a response to an environmental stimulus in a novel context (i.e., to a context that does not contain the stimuli or reinforcers that originally controlled it). Children are thought to learn language by learning specific responses that are later generalized to broader contexts and new situations (Warren, 1985). A second kind of generalization stems from the response class structure of language. In this type, learning a modification of some aspect of one response in a response class changes the other members of the class in the same way (Baer and Guess, 1973). Both of these types of generalization are concerned with the organization of behaviors and not with the organization of rules. The idea of *learning rules* that generate sentences is not possible within a theoretical framework that is predicated on the claim that language can be explained (as can any type of behavior) solely by the relation that is established between responses and environmental stimuli.

The critical differences of these opposing conceptions of the nature of language learning are, of necessity, reflected in the approach taken to teaching language. From even a cursory examination of the language teaching literature, it is clear that approaches taken to teaching are essentially an emulation of the process that is conceived for learning language in a natural situation. Thus, one of the responsibilities of an advocate of a teaching procedure is to explain how the approach emulates the particular model of acquisition selected. The next responsibility is to explain how the approach can overcome the obstacles to learning that the child experienced when failing to acquire language naturally. That is, the justification of an approach should demonstrate that it is as close as possible to the natural process of language learning (as the advocate perceives it), while being different enough from the natural process to overcome the learning difficulty the learner experienced in the natural learning situation.

THE NATURE OF LANGUAGE IMPAIRMENT

The children who are used here as examples to demonstrate and justify the induction teaching approach to language teaching are specific language-impaired (SLI) children (Rosenberg, 1984). These children are labeled as *specific*, because their language learning difficulty seems to be the only unusual thing about their cognitive development. Although recent studies seem to be uncovering subtle cognitive difficulties in other cognitive areas (e.g., Ellis Weismer, 1985), it is not yet clear whether these difficulties will prove to be the cause or the effect of their delay in language learning. These children generally have difficulties at all stages of language development: they are late in saying their first words, they are late in sequencing words to express meaningful propositions, and they are late in learning morphosyntactic elements and syntactic operations. At any stage, their language seems to be no different than that of normal children, only they learn it later and slower and apparently will never attain a normal language facility (Aram, Ekelman, and Nation, 1984).

One of the major language difficulties in the later stage of these children's development appears to be syntactic (Connell, 1986a; Johnston and Kamhi, 1984); this fact is significant for the kinds of teaching approaches that would be most effective. Those aspects of language that are most closely akin to the abstract grammatical code of language, such as subject–verb agreement and transformational operations (e.g., question inversion and complex sentence formation), are consistently missing from their sentences. This problem can be portrayed as a failure to acquire the syntactic mode of language (Givon, 1976), the mode in which sentences are structured by abstract grammatical features (e.g., S→NP AUX VP). This kind of structure develops relatively late in normal children (after 2 years [2;0] to 2 years 5 months [2;5 years] of age; Brown, 1973) and is relatively far removed from the meaning the sentences convey or the context in which they are used. This distinction between abstract syntax and meaning and context is amplified in the following discussion. The distinction has important implications for the composition of teaching procedures, as is explained below.

Examples of the sentences that these children use in the later part of their language learning progression are presented on the left side in Table 4–1. The sentences on the right side of Table 4–1 were produced by normal children much younger than the SLI children (2;0 to 2;5 compared to the 3;3 to 3;5 for the SLI children), and they demonstrate the similarity in the kinds of errors made by the two types of children. In (1) and (3) of the SLI sentences, the copular *be* that would be present in adult glosses of the sentence (*This is Tracy* and *It is mine*) is missing from the child's version. Copula is an element that is most related to the syntactic or abstract grammatical aspects of sentences, in that its sole function is to agree (accord) with the number (singular or plural) and the person (first, second, or third) of the subject of the sentence, in this case, the third person singular. The absence of the copula suggests a lack of understanding of the subject–verb agreement system of English which, in turn, suggests a lack of understanding of the syntactic structure of sentences and the operations (e.g., agreement) that the structure allows and requires. Of course, the lack of the behavior of saying the copula in this one sentence does not, by itself, preclude the possibility that the speaker has knowledge of the syntactic rules that govern the use of copula and the selection of one of its many forms (*am, are, was, were,* and *be*). Applying the same logic as was used in the earlier discussion of the distinction between the behaviors and the knowledge of language rules, the absence of copula can only be seen as a sign of the *possibility* that the speaker lacks knowledge of the rules that govern copula. The equally likely possibility that the speaker knows the rule but fails to use it in this sentence must also be entertained. If, for example, the speaker used copula in some other sentences and it was clear from the context that its use was not predicated on imitation of prior utterances or on the unanalyzed use of a memorized routine (e.g., the use of *that* and *where* by some children), then

TABLE 4–1 Excerpts of Language Samples From an SLI Child and a Normal Child

Specific language-impaired child (CA 3;3 to 3;5)	*Normal child (CA 2;0 to 2;5)*
1. This Tracy.	1. That mine.
2. This say Tracy.	2. Me see that.
3. It mine.	3. Adam see that (Adam = I).
4. Him looking out the window.	4. My get, mommy.
5. There toys in there.	5. No, my have it.
6. Why us not read that one?	6. What me think?

it would have to be assumed that the speaker knew the rules governing the copula. Thus, the behaviors of language must be used cautiously as evidence for or against hypotheses about a speaker's knowledge of the rules of language. The distinction between knowledge and use of a rule is discussed more later.

In (2) of the SLI sentences, the lack of syntactic structure is again made apparent by the missing third-person-singular verbal morpheme that would be contained in an adult gloss of the sentence (*This says Tracy*). Like the copula, the function of this morpheme is mainly to make the verb and the subject agree in person and number (third person, singular). Its absence is further evidence of a lack of knowledge of the syntactic nature of sentences.

Sentence (4) demonstrates another aspect of the syntactic problem the speaker has. The use of *him* where *he* would be used in the adult gloss suggests that the speaker does not distinguish among the syntactic roles that can be played by NPs in sentences. The distinction between the role of subject and the roles of direct and indirect object of the verb, object of the preposition, and modifier of a noun (possessive) forms the basis of the syntactic phrase structure rules alluded to earlier (S→NP AUX VP). Failure to mark this distinction by using different pronoun cases (e.g., *he, him, his*) suggests the speaker's system does not distinguish NPs on the basis of the syntactic role they play, providing further evidence that syntactic structure is not a part of the speaker's knowledge of language.

Putting the speaker's lack of syntactic knowledge into induction terminology, the speaker has failed to learn the kinds of rules that would generate sentences containing the syntactic elements alluded to above. The phrase structure rules that the speaker apparently knows generate sentences that are not abstractly syntactic in structure but that reflect the meaning relations among the words contained in the sentences and the context in which the sentences were spoken. For example, the sentence in (4) might have been structured according to a rule such as S→ Agent-Action-Location. This kind of rule would not require the use of a pronoun case that distinguishes subject NPs from other syntactic types, because only semantic distinctions between NPs (e.g., agent versus location) are coded. Nor would the speaker need to make the subject NP agree with the verb by means of the form of the auxiliary *be* (*is*, in this case), because there would be no subject designated in the sentence (nor any AUX).

Given the foregoing orientation to language, language acquisition, and language disorders, what this speaker needs is a teaching situation in which a set of abstract syntactic rules can be learned. As indicated previously, it is assumed that rules can be taught by emulating the natural induction learning process as closely as possible. By providing the kind of linguistic data that would lead one to discover patterns, the teaching approach detailed in the next section gives the learner the opportunity to hypothesize rules and implement them in language use. The rules are viewed as the learner's best solution to the problem of explaining patterns in the data, solutions that are motivated by a strong (and probably innate) tendency to search for order in the face of chaos.

IMPLEMENTING INDUCTION TEACHING

In order to describe induction teaching fully, it is necessary first to fill in certain gaps in the description of the normal induction learning process. The details that fill these gaps are a set of hypotheses about the process of learning language through induction. The details themselves are testable and undoubtedly should be tested, but their exact nature is not entirely crucial to the approach. That is, alternative ways of filling in the gaps would not change the approach in any substantial way. The level of detail that is used in this description is necessary, because a description of teaching requires more precision than a description of theoretical explanation. Aspects that are not fully understood cannot be glossed over in descriptions of teaching as they can in theoretical descriptions. A teacher has to fill in these fuzzy areas with a procedural description in order to use the description as a guide for teaching.

In the description of the induction process, it is assumed that learners enter into a language learning situation fully aware of how to induce. If the assumption of a predeveloped induction capability were not made, a complete description of the induction learning process of language acquisition would have to begin with the process of learning how to induce before describing the process of learning how to induce language. The mechanism for induction has been assumed to be innate in most developmental theories because of the difficulty that would be encountered in explaining its development. In accordance with these theories, the following description of induction teaching contains no method for teaching induction. It is assumed that children who have the capacity to learn language have the capacity to induce language rules.

The natural induction learning process is translated here into three steps that can be emulated by a procedure designed to teach a language rule. The induction learners' *first step* is to recognize that there is a pattern to some of the variation in the pronunciation and distribution of a certain set of language elements. Using a morphological example first, their induction learning mechanism allows them to recognize that a word for four-legged household pets is sometimes *dogs* and sometimes *dog*. They notice that this variation of pronunciation—sometimes pronounced with word-final frication and sometimes not—forms a pattern for many of the words that they hear spoken to them about objects and events. The process of recognizing a pattern is schematized in Figure 4–1. The pattern recognizer performs three related functions: pairs items so that they can be compared, finds the difference between the members of each of the pairs, and finds a pattern across all of the differences. Each of these operations has its own complexities, and each is assumed to be controlled by the predeveloped induction ability of the learner.

The purpose of the first step is to identify the pattern that exists in the data. The pattern recognizer accomplishes this goal by organizing the data into sets, comparing across these sets, and identifying a pattern. Words spoken to the learner are the raw data that are first examined by the pattern recognizer. It seems that the best way to organize these data is into pairs, with one member being one manner of pronunciation and the second member being the other, as indicated in Figure 4–1 by the dashed lines. This pairing could be accomplished by recognizing that two entries in the data pool make reference to the same object or event and that they are pronounced differently. These two criteria differentiate the data that will be critical for learning the rules from the data that have no bearing on the rule. By comparing across the identified pairs, it is possible to determine that the change in pronunciation is systematic, that is, that there is an identifiable pattern in the pronunciation change. In this case, that pattern is that the noun used to reference an object or event is sometimes pronounced with a word-final fricative and sometimes not.

The purpose of the *second step* in the process is to explain the pattern found in the first step. This is accomplished by searching the context for an element of meaning that coincides with the pronunciation pattern identified. One way to conceive of this process is that learners approach the pattern as if it were a mystery that needs solving. To solve this mystery, they know they have to determine what the speaker who utters *dogs* intends as a meaning that is different from when he utters *dog*. The search for a meaning solution to the problem would entail a systematic analysis of the context cues available when both elements were uttered. The data gathered in such a search might be something like the form and context information presented in Table 4–2. Such data would presumably lead a learner, after uncovering a number of similar situations in which the pairs of words identified by the pattern finder were used in similar contexts, to discover the fact that in one situation the speaker expresses the meaning *canine* and, in the other, a meaning in addition to canine, namely, *plurality*.

Once the pattern is explained by the context variation that is associated with it, learners can take the last step: they can hypothesize a rule that captures the nature of the correspondence between pronunciation and meaning in the observed pairs of words and for all related pairs that might be encountered in the language. The rule might be stated thus, "The meaning of more-than-one-item is expressed by appending a fricated sound to the name of the item." This rule could be tested by the learner listening to the words spoken by others and determining whether the use of the fricated suffix always corresponds to the

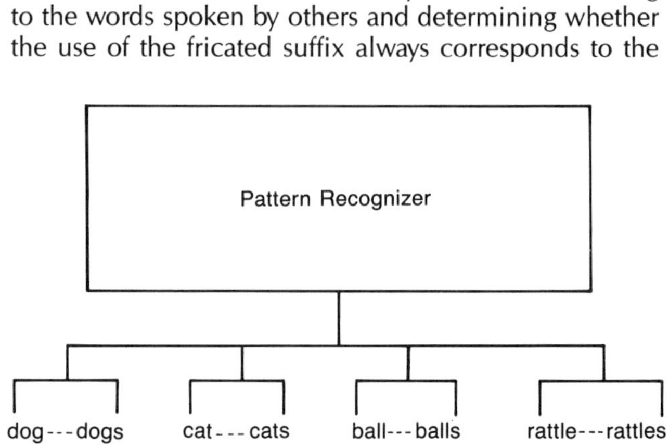

Figure 4–1 The pattern analyzing process in induction learning.

TABLE 4–2 The Process of Explaining Patterns in the Language Input

Form	*Context*
Dog	Parent and child are looking at a book. The parent says, "Look at the dog, it is a big dog." The topic of discussion is a picture of a large dog.
Dogs	Parent and child are walking on a sidewalk and two dogs come towards them. The parent says, "Here come two dogs. Let's pat the dogs."

meaning of more-than-one. Some of the data do not support the rule and this result eventually leads to changes in the rule, a sort of fine-tuning process. For one thing, the effect of phonetic context on the pronunciation of the appended morpheme would eventually have to be specified in more detail. That is, the pronunciation of the suffix depends on the voicing and place features of the final speech sound of the noun to which it attaches. Also, the fact that the rule is applicable only to count nouns (two dogs, two cats) and not mass nouns (flour, people) would have to be learned as a restriction to the rule's application. Perhaps most importantly, in view of the high proportion of irregular plurals in English, the *lack* of a pattern in the pronunciation of many plural nouns is to be accounted for in the rule. Thus, the application of the regular rule has to be limited to a set of regular nouns, and the pronunciation consequences of adding in a plural meaning have to be learned separately for the rest of the nouns in the lexicon. This means that the pronunciation of these pluralized nouns is not specified by the rule but has to be learned and stored separately for each irregular noun. The well-known fact that children overregularize plural, as in *mans*, and misapply the rule to mass nouns, as in *peoples*, during certain stages of their language development is evidence of the changing nature of the preliminary rule.

An example of learning a rule based on pragmatic factors illustrates other important aspects of induction teaching that are not readily apparent in the process of learning a morphological rule such as plural. In this example, children are learning a rule for pronominalizing NPs in sentences. The same three steps are described: recognizing a pattern, explaining the pattern, and hypothesizing a rule. The learners' first step in learning a pronominalization rule would be to recognize that there is a difference in the pronunciation and the distribution of terms referring to objects, ideas, and events. In this case, they might recognize that *she, he*, and *it*, are pronounced differently than *the girl, the boy*, and *the desk* even though they apparently refer to the same objects in some sentences in which the terms are used. Pairs would be constructed containing terms that refer to the same object, ideas, and events, such as *the boy–he, the dog–him, the desk–it*. By comparing across the pairs, the learners would recognize a pattern in the data. The pattern would be a bit more complicated than in the plural example where a single, general pronunciation difference—word-final frication—was identified. In this case, the change in pronunciation is more drastic, in that nothing of the pronunciation of two members of the pair necessarily matches, and further, there is no single pattern of pronunciation for either member of the pair: the lexical item or the pronoun. There is, though, some basis for a pattern to emerge. The lexical member of a pair comes from an open class of items, one in which there is no restriction on membership, whereas the pronominal member comes from a more closed class. After distinguishing between the members of all pairs in this way, the learner might restrict that pattern search to only those pairs that have as one member the pronoun *me*. This could make the pattern simpler and simpler to explain in the next step. An analysis of the context cues would reveal that the meaning intended by a speaker when using a pronoun and when using a NP would not be greatly different, that is, in both cases, the term would be used to make reference to an object, idea, or event. By disregarding this similarity and focusing on the conversational contexts in which the terms were used, learners should notice that the speaker who uses the lexical form describes information that is new to the conversation and the speaker who uses the pronoun form describes information that had previously been introduced into the conversation. Thus, they will come to discover that a difference or contrast in contextual situations (new versus shared information in a conversation) and the difference in utterance (NP versus pronoun) correspond to each other. Armed with this information, a learner can then hypothesize a rule that captures the nature of this correspondence in the observed pairs and for all related pairs that might be encountered in the language. The rule would be stated something like this: *"Replace a NP with a pronoun (PN) when reference is shared between the speaker and listener."*

Emulating the Induction Process

The details described in these highly idealized processes of rule learning can be translated into three teaching steps that correspond to the three steps introduced above. The steps of the process for teaching the plural rule are schematized in (1) and (2) of Table 4–3. In (1), a schematic version of the rule illustrates the instructional problem faced by the teacher: making the learner realize that the contrast in form (noun versus noun + suffix) corresponds to the contrast in meaning. The goal of teaching is to establish a network much like that depicted in (1). This network is the interrelation of the separate one-to-one correspondences established between two sets of forms and meanings. The network embodies the relation between the difference or contrast in form (noun versus noun + fricated suffix) and the difference in meaning (one versus more-than-one). This network is established through teaching by demonstrating that the contrast in form is associated with the contrast in meaning. The first two steps described for the model of induction learning are incorporated in

TABLE 4–3 A Teaching Interaction for the Pronominalization Rule

	Form	Meaning
1.	Noun	Single item
	Noun + fricative	More than one item
2.	"This is the cat."	Single item
	"These are the cats."	More than one item
	"The dog can run."	Single item
	"The dogs can run."	More than one item

induction teaching. In (2), a method for accomplishing this is presented in schematic form. Disregarding for the moment details that are attended to later, the pairs of sentences, each of which presents singular and plural manifestations of reference to the same object, present data both about the change in form that occurs and about the change in meaning that results. The data provided by these sentences, together with their associated contexts, constitute the input into the pattern recognition process. The pairs of sentences make the task of constructing the data pairs simpler. In the natural situation, the members of a pair would be unlikely to be said in two adjoining sentences. It is more likely that they are said at different times and in entirely different contexts. Thus, the natural learner must store each member in memory and make the pairing at some later time. The pairing process might involve scanning the lexical store for entries that have two pronunciations. For the learner who was being taught by being presented the paired sentences in (2), the pairs are preconstructed, thus reducing the need for the memory search and any related process. In addition, the contrast in the meaning associated with the pairs is presented to the learner at the same time, possibly simplifying the second step in learning, i.e., explaining the pairs. The natural learner would have to retrieve the contexts associated with each member of a pair when searching for an explanation. This retrieval process is not as necessary when the data are packaged as they are in (2).

The final step in the induction learning process has no counterpart in induction teaching, because inducing a rule is considered to be wholly within the learner's control. All the teaching can do is to provide the learner with data that are necessary and sufficient for inducing the rule and to provide the data in a manner that simplifies the induction process as much as possible.

The processes of teaching the pronominalization rule are presented in (1) and (2) of Table 4–4. In (1), a schematic version of the rule illustrates the kind of parameters that compose the rule: a distinction in form (lexical versus pronominal reference) and a distinction in context (new versus shared information). The method for establishing this kind of system is basically the same as before. The first two pairs of sentences presented in (2) represent one way to provide the information needed to teach the rule. The strategy for teaching is again to provide sufficient data within each pair of sentences to help accomplish the first two steps of induction learning: recognition of a pattern in the forms and discovery of an explanation for the pattern. An accumulation of such data is assumed to lead the learner to the last step: hypothesizing a rule.

Teaching Example 1

At this point, to bring the description of induction teaching to a more concrete level, the details of the teaching approach are given for a particular client who was a subject in a study recently performed on language teaching (Connell, 1986b). The client (LM) was 3;4 years old at the time of the study. He lived in a home in which English was the only language spoken. He was the second of three children of a mother who worked as a housewife and a father who worked as a stock broker. His birth history was unremarkable, and he met the milestones of motor development within normal limits. He appeared to have developed normally in all areas except language. LM was diagnosed as having SLI.

LM's language production was limited to one word at a time. He was never observed to utter a two- or three-word phrase either by his parents or by the clinicians who interacted with him prior to his enrollment in the study. He said the names of approximately 20 common objects, actions, locations (there, here), and states. The development of his receptive lexicon was measured by standardized means and was determined to be at the 3;0 level. Thus, he obviously knew many more words than he could or would say.

The evidence gathered appeared to place LM at the presyntactic level of language development, that is, a stage prior to Brown's stage I (Brown, 1973). This stage is signified by the lack of expression of relational meanings—meanings signified by the ordering of words in phrases. The meanings that LM expressed in his speech were only lexical in nature. He appeared to have no linguistic means for expressing meanings such as possession, agent-action, action-patient, or entity-location within a single phrase unit. He could communicate an entity-location meaning by pointing at an object and saying *there*, but

TABLE 4–4 Aspects of Pronoun and Semantic Relation Teaching

	Form	Meaning
1.	NP	New referent
	PN	Shared referent
2.	"This doll is Mary."	New referent
	"She is a nice doll."	Shared referent
	"The block is on the table."	New referent
	"It is yellow."	Shared referent
	Show a ball and bounce it.	
	"It can bounce high."	Shared referent
3.	Worm kiss frog.	Worm is agent, frog is patient.
	Frog kiss worm.	Frog is agent, worm is patient.

he could not express this meaning in a linguistic framework such as *ball there*.

In light of the previous discussion, the possibility that LM knew the linguistic framework for expressing such meanings but did not use them in his own speech had to be considered. That is, it is possible that a situation similar to that found in his lexical knowledge and use could have been present in his phrasal knowledge and use. This possibility was examined by testing LM on his ability to comprehend sentences expressing an agent-action-patient meaning. This meaning is expressed in English simple sentences by the order of the words referring to the entities and the objects involved in the relation. The entity before the action is the agent of that action, and the entity after the action is the patient. This is, of course, true only of active as opposed to passive sentences. The active sentence *the man pushed the dog* expresses the relational meaning in the manner described, but the passive sentence *the dog was pushed by the man* expresses the same relational meaning by other syntactic means. The active interpretation is used earlier by normal children, and it was the one used to test LM's knowledge of the linguistic expression of relational meanings.

The test was constructed around ten situations, each involving two entities. The situations were selected because they were reversible in terms of which entity took the agent and patient roles and they could be rendered in a line drawing by an artist. A pair of pictures presented the two opposite configurations of each situation. For example, one situation was depicted by two animated pictures of an interaction between a worm and a frog. One picture depicted the frog kissing the worm, and the other picture depicted the same worm kissing the same frog (see [3] in Table 4–4). Before using these pictures to test LM's knowledge of relational meaning, LM was tested to determine whether he could recognize the meanings of the words that would be used to describe the pictures. Thus, words like *frog, worm*, and *kissing* were tested in a comprehension format in which LM was asked to point to frog, worm, or kissing in an array of pictures of objects and actions.

In the relational meaning test itself, LM was presented with the pair of pictures and asked to point to either the worm kissing the frog or the frog kissing the worm. The order of these sentences and the position of the pictures were randomized. Some of the ten situations were presented to LM by means of three-dimensional objects in the form of a toy frog and worm. In this case, LM was told to make the worm kiss the frog or to make the frog kiss the worm. The result of both of these testing formats was the same: LM did not give any indication of understanding the relational meanings expressed by the serial order of the entities and actions. He randomly selected a picture or used either toy to act on the other. This result was interpreted to mean that LM was actually at the presyntactic stage of language development.

Given this stage of language development, a teaching strategy was created to facilitate the learning of relational meanings. The relational meaning selected for teaching was the agent-action-patient meaning tested in the diagnostic and evaluation sessions. Two teaching strategies were considered, but because LM was a subject in a study of the relative effect of the two treatment strategies, only one of them was selected. The two strategies were similar in that the approach taken to establish a relation between relational meanings and word order was based on the assumption that children acquire a language rule that specifies the relation. The rule could be formalized as S→ Agent-Action-Patient, which could be read as, "A sentence (of this type) is composed of three ordered meaning elements." The goal of both strategies was to facilitate LM's acquiring knowledge of this rule.

The approach taken to teaching this rule was to present LM with sufficient linguistic information in a format that allowed him to identify a pattern, to associate it with a meaning distinction, and to hypothesize a rule. The pattern that needed to be explained was the variation in the order of the words spoken by an adult. LM had undoubtedly experienced many occasions when people had spoken to him in sentences. Because he had no knowledge of a rule for relational meanings, he would have viewed sentences as lists or sets of words, some (major meaning words) having a meaning and others (functors) having none. He probably could have responded appropriately to some commands and questions spoken to him, because he was able to recognize certain words and, with them, to piece together a likely relational meaning (this scenario had been verified by parental report and from clinical observation). For example, he might respond to the command *help mommy close the door* by closing the door because he knew the meanings of each of the major words and he knew what relation is typical of this particular set of words. Thus, he would respond the same way if the sentence were said as *help the door close mommy*, because the set of words would not have changed.

The explanation for the word-order variation pattern is the change that results in meaning when word order is changed. Similar to the plural and pronominal rule-teaching examples, the goal of teaching a relational-meaning rule would be to establish a network of correspondence between pairs of forms and meanings, this time between one word order and the meaning it represents and the other word order and its meaning. The rule that would be hypothesized once this network is known can best be characterized as the phrase structure rule introduced previously: S→ Agent-Action-Patient. Hypothesizing this rule is apparently quite difficult for SLI children, as evidenced by LM's failure to solve the problem (and the failure of many other children in similar circumstances).

The method used to help LM develop the network of correspondences between form and meaning was to use paired forms and meaning as before. Constructing the network was made more probable by eliminating factors that might be distracting and by highlighting factors that are critically relevant. This process was implemented by presenting two opposing (reversed) meanings and two opposing (reversed) word orders together so that they could be analyzed as a unit. The pictures of a dog chasing a cat and of its opposite, a cat chasing a dog, were presented to LM in conjunction with sentences *dog chase cat* and *cat chase dog*. The information was presented as a unit by presenting the two pictures together and saying the sentences that correspond to each of them while pointing to the appropriate picture. LM was thus presented with two contrasts, the contrast between the meaning represented by the pictures and the contrast in the order of words in the list (from his perspective) spoken about each picture. Successfully relating the two contrasts and thereby forming a network relating meaning to word order would seem to be made more probable by the fact that the contrasts were presented as a unit.

The particular strategy used at first to teach LM was to have him imitate the two sentences as they were said by the teacher. After some practice, LM was expected to say the sentences while looking at the appropriate picture without having to hear the model sentence. An alternative approach, used with similar subjects but not with LM, was to have the child point to the picture representing a sentence spoken by the teacher, without imitating it. The result of this type of teaching is discussed in detail below, but suffice it to say at this point that imitating and later generating the sentence proved to be a far more effective procedure. The imitation–self-generation strategy was performed with LM in only three situations, that is, on three sets of reversible pictures and sentences. Again, the decision to limit the teaching situations to three was based on the needs of the study. In a more typical clinical situation, the number of pairs would have been greater. The comparison between the two teaching strategies was performed with regard to the amount of generalization resulting from learning the rule. Consequently, a minimal amount of exposure was given to situations in which the rule could be used so that generalization to these situations could be compared. If LM had not been a research subject, there would have been no reason to limit the situations so severely; on the other hand, there would have been no reason to have an overly large representation of situations. There is no reason to believe that children learn a rule only after substantial information from a vast range of similar situations is provided. Surely in normal acquisition, there are no data to suggest that a child needs a vast amount of redundant information across different situations to learn rules. It is assumed that, because children approach language learning with the predisposition to find patterns and form rules, they do not need to be convinced that there is a need for a rule in any given case, only that the rule must account for certain information, for example, information such as the contrast between meanings and word order.

LM was presented with 40 trials in each of six sessions held on separate days over a 2-week interval. The trials were presented as sets of two sentences in which LM imitated one sentence while looking at the relevant picture and then imitated the reversed sentence while looking at the reversed picture. LM was given feedback on how well he was repeating the sentences and looking at the pictures. Once he was relatively competent in his imitation of the sentences, he said the sentences in response to questions without an imitative model.

LM's performance on the pretest described previously was monitored on a daily basis throughout the teaching portion of the study. There was a steady increase in the percentage of picture sets about which LM could say a three-word sentence expressing the agent-action-patient relational meaning. In addition to these probes, conversational language samples were taken from LM on a daily basis. During the last three sessions, LM said ten sentences in conversational speech that expressed either an agent-action or an action-patient relational meaning using the appropriate word order, indicating that he had induced the rule.

Teaching Example 2

The induction teaching approach can be further explained by continuing the narrative of LM's treatment history. At this point, some of LM's utterances expressed a relational meaning but, in these utterances and in one-word utterances, he used a lexicalized NP for all cases of reference, even when the context required the use of a pronoun. For example, he said *mommy go* in a context in which reference to his mother had been established, thus making *she* the more appropriate form. As in the example given previously, LM appeared not to know the pronominalization rule. The one pronoun that LM used was *me* as in *me throw*, but this fact would not argue against the interpretation that LM lacked pronominal rule knowledge. The use of a pronoun to refer to self is not rule governed as are pronouns referring to other people, objects, or events. The contexts in which one refers to oneself by name are quite limited or unusual (e.g., *My name is Jane* and *This is not going to be one of Jane's best days*). There is no alternation between the use of one's name and the use of first-person pronouns (*I, me, my, mine, myself*) that would be controlled by a rule of contextual variation or any other type of rule. Thus, LM's use of *me* was not a sign of rule knowledge but merely an indication that he had learned a term to refer to himself.

The procedure for teaching the pronominalization rule followed the scenario outlined in the hypothetical description of the normal acquisition of the pronominal rule. To highlight the pattern of alternation that exists between lexicalized and pronominalized NPs, LM was presented with a set of sentences constructed to contrast the form and function of the two types of terms (pronouns and lexical items). These utterances were spoken in contexts in which the "sharedness" of a referenced person or animated cartoon character could be manipulated systematically. Three examples of the 30 pairs of sentences and their contextual manipulations used in the teaching process are presented in Table 4–5. LM was encouraged to listen to the sentences and look at the pictures in a manner that simulated the way children are read to by their parents. He was asked to repeat part of the sentences spoken by the teacher to ensure that he attended to the contrast. As indicated before, evidence of the efficacy of using imitation as part of induction teaching is presented in a later section. Table 4–6 is a transcript of one of the exchanges between the

TABLE 4–5 Sentences and Pictures Used to Teach the Pronominalization Rule

	Utterance	*Context*
1a.	Here is a little girl.	Picture of a young girl wearing a hat
1b.	A dog is chasing her.	Picture of the same girl being chased by a dog
2a.	Peter is going to school.	Picture of a young boy going out the door
2b.	The bus driver gives him a ride	Picture of the same boy getting on a school bus
3a.	A dog is chasing Paula.	Picture of a dog chasing a little girl
3b.	A cat is licking her.	Picture of a cat licking the same little girl's face

teacher and LM concerning the three pictures described in Table 4–5.

Notice that the teacher's intention is to focus LM's attention on the contextual contrast between the lexical and the pronominal reference made twice to the same person. This is evident in the part of the exchange in which LM omitted a pronoun in his response *giving a ride* to the request to say *giving him a ride*. The teacher repeated the model with emphasis on the word *him* to ensure that he attended to this form particularly. LM's omission of the article *a* in his response to the new model was of no concern to the teacher because her primary goal was to

TABLE 4–6 Teacher–Student Exchange for Teaching the Pronominalization Rule

Teacher	*LM*
Here, LM, look at what is happening here. Here is a little girl. Can you say "a little girl"?	Little girl
Now look, a dog is chasing her. Can you say "chasing her"?	Chasing her
Yes, now what is this? Peter is going to school. Can you say "Peter"?	Peter
Yes, that is. Now look here, the bus driver is giving him a ride to school. Can you say "giving him a ride"?	Giving a ride
Say "giving *him* a ride."	Giving him ride
Yes, he is. Now look at this picture. Look, a dog is chasing Paula. Can you say "chasing Paula"?	Chasing Paula
Yes, and now here a cat is licking her. Can you say "licking her"?	Licking her

obtain LM's attention to the contrast between *Peter* and *him* and the contexts in which they were used.

There are three aspects of this teaching interaction that deserve particular comment. Notice that the contrast was made between third-person objective-case pronouns and lexical reference and not other pronoun cases. The choice not to use the possessive (e.g., *her, his, their*) was arbitrary and was the next step in teaching the pronoun system. In the course of normal acquisition, the possessive and the objective case appear to be learned first and simultaneously (Brown, 1973). In order to simplify the teaching task, though, only one of the two was taught. The subjective (nominative) case of pronouns is not acquired until much later (approximately Brown's stage II). The teaching of this case proved to be quite difficult and was finally taught with a modified approach that is described in detail in a later section.

Notice also that syntactic roles played by the lexically referenced NPs were different in the three pairs of sentences. In the first pair, *the girl* served as the complement of the copula verb *is*; in the second pair, *Peter* served as the subject of *going*; and in the third pair, *Paula* served as the direct object of *chased*. The reason for this difference was to demonstrate to LM that the pronominal rule was not restricted to lexicalized NPs that have a particular position or play a particular role in a sentence. In other words, the role played by the lexicalized NP was intentionally varied to demonstrate that role was not a possible factor in the application of the pronominalization rule.

Lastly, notice that the two different genders were coded in the pronouns. Although it was not necessary to construct the situation this way, it was decided that an additional contrast could be incorporated into the sentences without making the learning task too difficult for LM. If this prediction had not proven to be correct, the gender distinction could have been removed and the teaching interaction could then have been repeated with only one gender. Because gender was part of the contrast, an additional aspect of the rule was actually being taught at the same time as the main part of the rule: that the gender of the person referenced by the NP can be coded in the pronoun form (of course this only applies to the third person singular, but this is the only part of the pronoun system addressed at this point). Thus, the following rule was taught: *"Replace an NP with a pronoun form corresponding to the gender of the referenced person when reference to that person is shared between the speaker and listener."*

Additional Aspects of Pronoun Teaching

This gender addition to the rule is one of the many additions that would have to be made in process of teaching an adultlike knowledge of the pronoun system of English. Table 4–7 depicts the full system of English pronouns. As can be seen, the gender distinction added to the rule would only account for a relatively small part of the entire system, the part that could be described as the third-

TABLE 4–7 The System of English Pronouns

Person	*Case*					*Number*
	Nominative	*Accusative*	*Genitive*		*Reflexive*	
			Modifier	*Replacive*		
1	I	Me	My	Mine	Myself	Singular
2	You	You	Your	Yours	Yourself	Singular
3 (shows gender)	He/she/it	Him/her/it	His/her/its	His/hers/its	Himself/herself/itself	Singular
1	We	Us	Our	Ours	Ourselves	Plural
2	You	You	Your	Yours	Yourselves	Plural
3	They	Them	Their	Theirs	Themselves	Plural

person-singular portion. Person (first, second, and third), number (singular and plural), case (nominative, accusative, genitive, and reflexive) and genitive function (modifier and replacive) are all distinctions that would eventually have to be incorporated into the rule. The teaching of many of these distinctions could follow the same format as that used to teach the gender distinction and, in fact, was used with LM. For example, the singular–plural distinction was introduced by adding sentences to the teaching interaction that contained reference to multiple people, thereby, incorporating *them* into the system of pronoun forms. Similarly, sentences containing reference to inanimate objects such as a ball were added to the interaction to incorporate the genderless *it* into the system.

The modifier–replacive distinction was introduced by a three-part interaction, as opposed to the two-part interaction that was used for the previous pronoun teaching. Table 4–8 exemplifies this process.

The third part of the interaction provided LM with the information that genitive (possessive) pronouns can be used in sentences to comment on the possession of a NP referenced earlier in a sentence and that, in such cases, it is not followed by the noun.

As mentioned earlier, the first- and second-person pronoun forms are not controlled by the pronominalization rule as are the third-person forms. This is because there is no alternation between a lexicalized NP and a first- or second-person pronoun as there is with third-person pronouns. One could say that first- and second-person pronouns are always used when reference is made to self (*I, me, my, mine, myself*) or to the listener (*you, your, yours, yourself*). These forms are called *deictic forms*, because their meaning is tied to the roles of speaker and listener in a communication event. That is, the forms code the speaker and listener roles in addition to identifying the person being referenced. *I* means "John Smith, who is the speaker" in the sentence *I am here* spoken by John Smith. In contrast, the meaning of *he* in *He is John Smith*, means only reference to the person John Smith.

TABLE 4–8 Modifier–Replacive Dialogue

Teacher	*LM*
Let's look at this picture. This boy's name is John. Can you say "John"?	John
This is his dog. Can you say "his dog"?	His dog
Yes, it is his. Can you say "his"?	His

LM did not require any teaching on first- and second-person pronouns, because he used *me* soon after he was saying sentences and he used *you* soon after he began using third-person pronouns. Thus, he had a three-person distinction in the singular at least. There was no evidence that the contrasts were maintained in the plural, and these distinctions were considered less important at the time and were temporarily placed aside in favor of the case distinctions.

Before addressing the problem of teaching case distinctions, perhaps it would be informative to discuss the kind of teaching that might have been used had LM required person distinction teaching. The first problem that such teaching would raise is that imitation as a teaching procedure would have to be abandoned. The deictic nature of the *me–you* contrast makes it impossible for a child to learn by repeating verbatim the words of a speaker, because the reference the speaker makes in sentences about self (e.g., *I see a dog*), are inappropriately used when the listener repeats the utterance verbatim. The *I* in the modeled sentence takes on a different meaning in the imitated sentence, and this shift in meaning, that is the essence of deixis, would confuse the learner who knew nothing about the pronoun deixis system. It seems that the only way such a system could be taught is by having the learner observe the contrast between *me* and *you* in the speech of others and not participate until the system is partially acquired.

Pronoun Teaching Problems

LM's pronoun system now had all the major contrasts: number, gender, person, and case. The case distinction was only partial, though, because it was between the accusative and the genitive only. There was no evidence in LM's speech samples that he knew the nominative case distinction that marks the subject of sentences.

The fact that pronoun case is not used to distinguish the syntactic role played by NPs could be interpreted as evidence that LM did not know abstract syntactic structure. The pronouns in the subject position of his sentences could be considered to be caseless, because there is no evidence that an alternation existed between the nominative (subject) and accusative (object) case (e.g., she/her, or me/I). It appears then that LM would benefit from being taught a pronoun case addendum to his pronominalization rule. The teaching of this rule was approached in two ways, one unsuccessful and one successful. The first way was to alter the rule that was to be taught (the pronoun case rule) to a rule that might be learned more readily by means of the procedures of induction teaching. The rule was changed to a semantic rule. It could be stated as follows: "A PN serving as agent receives the nominative case, and nonagent, nongenitive PNs receive the accusative case."

The teaching of this rule was approached in much the same manner as before. The strategy in this case was to alternate systematically between agent and patient roles for the same referent, as in the examples of semantic relation rule teaching in (3) of Table 4–4. In this case, word order related to pronoun case; in the previous case, word order related to semantic role. Thus, the essence was actually that semantic role related to pronoun case. Table 4–9 is an example of the teaching interaction.

Notice how the shared new distinction is maintained in the interaction to comply with the general requirements of the pronominalization rule. The pictures previously used to teach the semantic relation rule—the reversible pictures—had to be modified in order to teach this case addendum to the pronominalization rule. In order to have only one pronoun in each appear in a sentence, the agent that kisses the worm in the last part of the interaction could not be the frog whom the worm kissed just before, because the second reference to the frog would have to be pronominal. Adding a second pronoun (*he*) to the sentence that presents the contrasting pronoun *him* (e.g., *He is kissing him*) would divert the learner's attention from the fact that the same object (worm) is being referenced by two different pronoun forms (*he* and *him*), based on the semantic role the referent plays in the two sentences. As before, the sentences were constructed to have no unnecessary clutter that might lead LM astray in his search for an explanation for the case distinction.

TABLE 4–9 Alternation Between Agent and Patient Roles

Teacher	*LM*
The worm is my friend. He is kissing the frog. Can you say, "He is kissing"?	Him kissing
Can you say, "He is kissing"?	Him kissing
Say "he."	He
Say, "He is kissing."	He kissing
Now look at this, the dog is kissing him (the worm). Can you say "kissing him"?	Kissing him

As indicated previously, this teaching approach ultimately failed; LM's spontaneous conversation continued to have no evidence of nominative case pronouns during the weeks this teaching approach was implemented. All preverbal pronouns in his sentences continued to be the accusative case. There was a decrease in the number of preverbal pronouns in LM's speech during this teaching episode. This might have been an indication that he was avoiding the use of pronouns in this position because of a new confusion about preverbal forms, but there was no evidence of case learning.

Two possibilities were considered to explain the failure of this procedure. It may have been related to the fact that the rule that was taught was not in fact the pronoun case rule of English. LM may have hypothesized the semantic case rule described above, found that was inadequate, and consequently discarded it. The teachers were concerned that this might happen before teaching had begun, but they elected to teach the modified rule anyway because the actual rule appeared to be very difficult to teach, especially to a learner who knew nothing about the factors that compose the rule. The actual rule for pronoun case adds something like the following to the pronominalization rule: "PN serving as the subject of sentences receives nominative case, and nonsubject, nonpossessive PNs receive accusative case."

The fact that it was decided that this rule could not be taught simply through induction teaching has important implications for explanations of normal language acquisition as well as language teaching. The problem that would be encountered in teaching such a rule is that there is no obvious way to create a systematic meaning and form alternation when the form to be taught—nominative case—makes no contribution to meaning. In order to use induction teaching as it has been in the examples thus far, to highlight a pattern and an explanation of the pattern, a contrast has to be constructed between alternate forms that have some meaning consequence. The abstract syntactic nature of the nominative case of pronouns can be seen in these pairs of sentences:

1. She is the one.
   Her the one.
2. Me like it.
   I like it.
3. I know he did it.
   I know him.

The only consequence of using *her* as a replacement for *she* in the first pair of sentences is a loss of grammaticalness and not a difference in meaning. The same can be said of the sentences in (2). In (3), the alternation between *he* and *him* illustrates the abstract nature of the grammatical distinction coded by pronoun case. In the second sentence of the pair, the subject of the embedded sentence (*he*) receives the nominative case even though it follows the verb of the main sentence. Thus, the order of words in the surface sentence is not the critical factor in determining the case of a pronoun; rather, it is the syntactic function the NP plays in the abstract structure of the sentence.

Perhaps the following hypothetical teaching interaction can clarify the difficulty that would be encountered in teaching the actual syntactic rule.

Teacher: Let's look at these pictures. She is a big girl. Can you say, "She is"?
LM: She is.
Teacher: Look at this. The dog is chasing her. Can you say "chasing her"?
LM: Chasing her

In this interaction, although the two forms (accusative-case and nominative-case forms) that need to be contrasted can be presented, there are no data given to inform the learner of the reason for the alternation between the cases. It is possible that the learner, when comparing the two contexts, decides that the nominative case is used when the referenced object comes first in an utterance, but this can be easily contradicted by sentences such as (3) in the list above (*I know he did it*), in which the nominative case *he* follows the verb *know*, as well as by sentences such as *Now I see three dogs*, in which the nominative case *I* follows an adverb. There is no solution to the variation except for the abstract rule stated above.

The essence of the claim being made is that the search for this solution would be made no easier by interactions like that described above. In the end, this approach would have a fatal weakness that is different from the failed approach described previously. The fatal weakness of the failed approach appeared to be that the rule that it encouraged LM to learn was inadequate. The fatal weakness of the approach described in the hypothetical interaction would be that it would not encourage LM to learn a rule at all. As has been argued, the strength of induction teaching lies in its capacity to highlight the proper solution by the contrasting pairs of utterances and meanings. The learner is biased towards the proper solution because alternative solutions have been eliminated while the proper solution is highlighted. Without this highlighting capacity, the procedure provides no assistance in the second step of induction learning—explaining the pattern identified. With the elimination of the second component of the approach, the learner is left on his or her own to search for solutions, a situation like that described for normal children in the natural language learning process. Normal children appear to have the capacity to solve such problems on their own, but, given LM's failure to learn certain rules in a natural environment, it is not surprising that he would fail to learn an abstract rule when the teaching procedure provided no assistance in such a critical area.

The issue that language teachers face when confronted with rules to teach that have no contextual solutions is essentially the same issue faced by theoreticians who are attempting to explain natural language acquisition. Neither the teacher of a SLI child nor the environment of a normal child can provide the kind of input that would be useful in learning an abstract syntactic rule. If neither teaching nor natural situations can provide a learner with the kind of information needed to explain a language pattern, the only logical explanation would seem to be that acquisition is guided by an innate knowledge of language. The logic of this argument is that if information critical for the performance of a process cannot be identified in the input data, then the information must already have been available to the process.

Given this nativist perspective, the second explanation that was considered for the failure of the semantic, pronoun-case-rule teaching approach was that the information provided by the teaching interaction was not sufficient to trigger LM's native knowledge about abstract syntactic explanations of linguistic patterns. This explanation leads to a different approach to teaching. Rather than providing information that is necessary and sufficient for the learner to explain a linguistic pattern from external experiences, the teaching approach that this suggests is to provide information that allows the learner to find an explanation of a linguistic pattern from within his own language capacity. (This point will be expanded upon shortly.)

This kind of approach would be closely allied with theories of language acquisition that propose that children have an innate bias towards the proper solutions to complex language problems. There is a rich tradition in theoretical linguistics on this topic. Chomsky's (1981) parameter-setting model of acquisition is perhaps the most well-known nativist theory. Like any nativist theory, its validity rests to a large extent on how well a universal grammar (UG) can be supported, because any sensible claim about preexisting language knowledge cannot be specific to any one language. A UG must contain principles that are sufficiently abstract to guide the acquisition of all languages. In the parameter-setting model of acquisition, the UG makes available a set of linguistic options or parameters that a child rather automatically sets by referring to the input language. The options available to a child correspond to the finite variation that is observed among the world's languages. With the options made available by the principles of the UG, the learner successively approximates the language spoken in the environment by using relatively simple aspects of the language to guide his search (set his parameters). Language learning, thus construed, is a process of progressively narrowing options, in contrast to the unguided trial-and-error process of induction described thus far.

However, even the strongest nativist model (e.g., Chomsky, 1981; Lightfoot, 1982) recognizes the need to invoke induction learning mechanisms to account for aspects of language that are nonuniversal, that is, idiosyncratic to specific languages. For example, if language input merely serves to set options made available by UG, there must be some mechanism to allow a child to recognize where the triggers needed for option-setting are situated in the input. All that a child hears is a sequence of speech sounds, and the UG does not, as it is presently conceived, help the child segment them into useful categories. In other words, before a learning mechanism can begin to match preexisting categories to input data, units in the speech stream have to be induced and correlated to meaning (Pinker, 1984; Gleitman and Wanner, 1982). The results of this preliminary inductive analysis would then provide the triggers for the syntactic options that guide the acquisition of a specific language.

The parameter-setting model has recently been used by Hyams (1986) to explain data on the acquisition of the verb inflection systems of several languages. The explanation rests on the distinction the model makes between core and peripheral grammar. Core grammar is that part of a language that is acquired by setting the parameters of the universal grammar. As a consequence, the core acquisition process is rapid and relatively errorless. Aspects of the peripheral grammar, on the other hand, are acquired only by making exceptions to the established settings of the parameters; as a consequence, they are learned laboriously and with errors.

Hyams claims that the reason children have such difficulty acquiring the verb inflection system of English is because the system has been delegated to the peripheral part of the grammar by a parameter called the *stem parameter*. This parameter is set for English learners by input data that indicate that verbs can occur without inflections (e.g., *Sit down and eat your cereal*). The concept of a parameter for English is illustrated in Figure 4–2. The parameter can be conceived of as a switch that selects one of two options, depending on the output of the preliminary analyzer. The preliminary analyzer searches the language input for data that it can recognize. In this case, it searches for verbs. The verbs are then analyzed to determine whether they can occur without inflections. Because English verbs can do so, the switch is set to the minus (−) inflection setting. Thus, the English learner conceives of his language as one that has no verbal inflections. The fact that English actually has some verbal inflections, specifically the past, progressive, and third-person-singular morphemes, complicates the situation for the English learner. The parameter setting does not allow the UG to assist in the acquisition of these items, and consequently their acquisition is difficult. The basic argument is that this setting complicates the learning of verb inflections, because the learner has to counteract a strong tendency (a parameter setting) to learn a language with entirely inflectionless verbs.

Hyams supports her claim with evidence of the rapidity and errorlessness with which Italian children acquire the complex Italian verb inflection system at approximately age 2;0. These children are claimed to set the stem parameter in the opposite direction from English learners, as illustrated in Figure 4–3, the setting that dictates that verbs cannot occur without inflections. As depicted by the larger circle representing this option, this setting is thought to be the most natural one for the learner to take, and this one will be taken automatically if no data such as the English data are provided. As a result of the + inflection setting, verb inflections are delegated into the core grammar and are acquired rapidly with the assistance of UG.

Teaching Subject Properties

This model of language was employed in the approach taken to teaching LM the case of pronouns after the failure

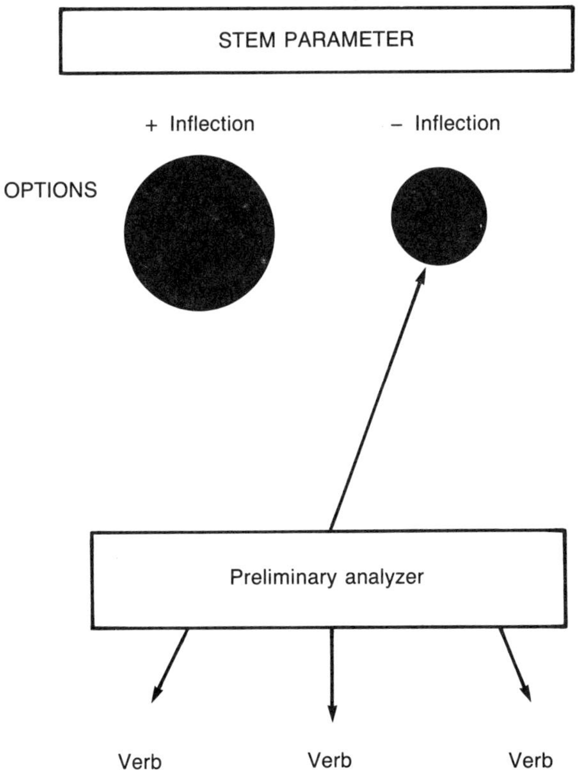

Figure 4–2 An illustration of the setting of the stem parameter for English.

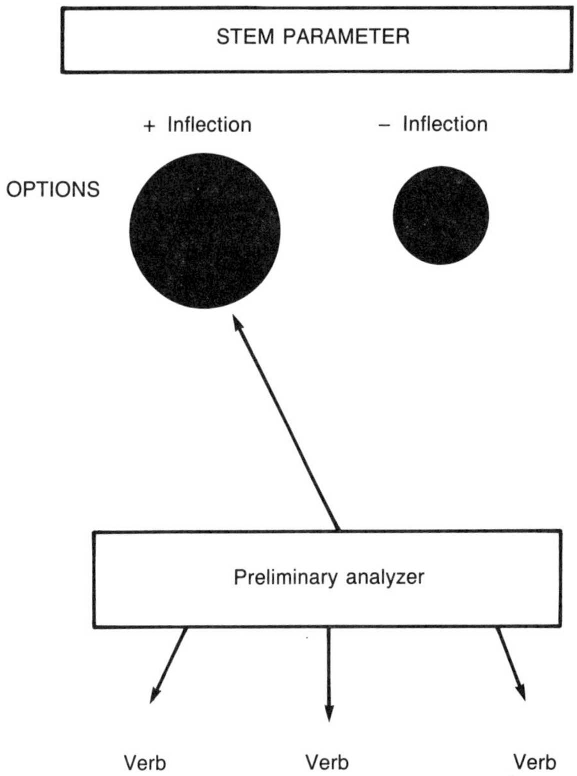

Figure 4–3 An illustration of the setting of the stem parameter for Italian.

of the semantic rule approach. The procedure followed exactly the teaching approach used by Connell (1986b) to teach a group of language impaired children who also had difficulty acquiring the case system of English. Because the procedures used with these children were essentially identical and the results of teaching were very similar, the subjects of the study are used as examples for describing the procedure. The subjects of this study were very similar to LM in their level of language development. They were diagnosed as having SLI, and their problem was described as having failed to learn language elements called subject properties. These properties include nominative case as well as copula, auxiliary *be*, and third-person-singular indicative (e.g., *he hits*), elements that are related only by the fact that their grammatical function is to create a number and person agreement between the subject of a sentence and its predicate. Table 4–10 contains a list of these subject properties and the errors that the children made in each of the areas. The morphosyntactic elements have already been listed above. These are contrasted with the transformational properties in the table because of the fundamental difference between the two types of properties. *Morphosyntactic properties* code agreement relations between the subject and the predicate of a sentence, whereas *transformational properties* are sentence-structure-changing rules that use the subject in their operation. The inversion rule of question uses the subject as a pivot around which the auxiliary element is rotated, as can be seen in the movement of *would* in the question example. The uninverted question spoken by a child with SLI represents a failure to move the modal around the subject. All the errors described in Table 4–10 reflect the abstract syntactic problem previously described for children with SLI.

The approach taken to teaching was slightly different from the examples of induction teaching described thus far. In this case, the approach was to identify a likely trigger for setting the parameter that controls the subject characteristics of languages and then provide this trigger to the children within an induction teaching format. The logic underlying this approach was that, if these children, who could be described as speakers of a subjectless language, were systematically exposed to the appropriate trigger, they could set their subject parameter appropriately, and the acquisition of the subject role and subject properties would become part of the core grammar and thus be easily acquired. This goal of the approach is quite different from the approaches described to this point. The goal of the approach is not only to have the learner identify and explain a pattern in the data and hypothesize a rule, but also to use this entire induction process as a trigger to change the setting of a parameter.

A potential trigger for the parameter was found in Givon's (1976) analysis of certain pidgin and creole languages that are in the process of acquiring subjects. In a developing language, it seems that the functional need to reference a topic strongly by left-dislocating it, as in *Her, she is walking* leads to the development of subject argument (*she*) that plays a unique and novel role in sentence structure. (The form and function of left dislocation is described below.) It seems that after a language gains this new sentence role, morphemes and grammatical operations related to the role evolve.

In an attempt to duplicate this situation, pairs of sentences containing left-dislocated topics were used in teaching interactions. An example of the interactions is presented in Table 4–11.

Notice that there is a left-dislocated topic in the first model given by the teacher: *Her, she is feeding*? The *her* is referred to as being dislocated because it is assumed that it is a form that originated from the NP slot occupied by the subject (*she*). The movement of the form to the beginning of the sentence is a transformational process based on the contextual conditions. The condition that was exploited in the teaching interaction was cases in which the identity of the NP filling the subject slot has the potential of being ambiguous. In the picture that is the theme of the first exchange, there are several children near the fawn. One would have to look quite carefully to notice that one of the children, a girl who is sitting with the other children around the fawn, has a small piece of bread in her hand. On this basis, it can be inferred that she is the one who is feeding the fawn and not the other children. A sentence referencing the girl as the subject of the verb *feeding* would be an appropriate response to the question *Which one is feeding the fawn*, posed by the teacher about the picture in question. A sentence containing a left-dislocated topic (*Her, she is feeding the fawn*) would be appropriate for the situation, because the topic pronoun encodes the potential ambiguity that the situa-

TABLE 4–10 Subject Properties Analyzed

Subject Properties	*Examples*	*Errors*
Morphosyntactic		
Agreement morphemes		
Auxiliary *be*	She *is walking*.	Her walking.
Copula	She *is* big.	Her big.
Third-person-singular present tense	She walks.	Her walk.
Pronoun/nominative case	*He* hits me and *I* hit him.	Him hit me and me hit him.
Transformational		
Question	Would you go?	You would go?

TABLE 4–11 Teaching with Left-Dislocated Topics

Teacher	*Student*
Look at this picture (referring to a picture depicting a girl sitting with a fawn and feeding it in the midst of several children who are playing several games). Look at all the children. Which one is feeding the fawn? That girl, her (pointing to the image of the girl), she is feeding the fawn. Can you say, "Her (pointing to the image of the girl), she is feeding"?	Her (pointing to the image of the girl) feeding
Can you say, "Her (pointing to the image of the girl), she is feeding"?	Her (pointing to the image of the girl), she feeding
That's what she is doing all right. Now look at this picture (referring to a picture of a different girl by herself in a park feeding the fawn). Now what is this girl doing? She also is feeding the fawn. Can you say, "She is feeding"?	Her (pointing to the image of the girl) feeding
Yes, she is the only one in this picture, isn't she. Can you say, "She is feeding"? (pulling the picture out of the reach of the child).	Her feeding
Can you say, "She is feeding"? Yes, she is, she is feeding the fawn. Now let's look at this picture.	She feeding

tion presents in terms of which female child of the several pictured is actually feeding the fawn. Saying the left-dislocated pronoun while pointing to the image of the referenced girl would clarify the reference further. Thus, these two events, the left-dislocated pronoun and the pointing, are devices that counteract ambiguity of reference in certain situations.

This type of sentence was paired in a teaching interaction with a sentence that did not contain a left-dislocated topic: *she is feeding*. This sentence emerged in the interaction in reference to a second picture. This picture contains none of the factors that led to the potential ambiguity of the first picture because the girl is alone. Thus, both the context and the form are different.

The contrast between the two situations and the sentences describing them provided the data necessary for the children to hypothesize a rule. This means that there were sufficient data about the alternation of form to identify a pattern. The pattern was the presence and absence of the left-dislocated pronoun. It also means that this pattern could be explained. The ambiguous situation corresponded to the presence of the left-dislocated pronoun, and the unambiguous situation corresponded to its absence. The rule that could have been hypothesized is this: *"A reference to an NP can be pronominalized and positioned before the sentence to denote ambiguity of reference."*

There is an addendum to this rule that is made necessary by the form of the sentences used in teaching. The pronoun form used to reference the NP in the preposed position is different from the pronoun used to reference the NP in the immediately preverb slot. This change in form is systematic, in that the dislocated pronoun (the added pronoun) has one form and the other pronoun has the other. This pattern could be explained by the fact that the *her* form corresponds to the referencer that clarifies, and the *she* form corresponds to the other one. This addendum could be made to the ambiguity rule.

The addendum is claimed to be the trigger that a learner needs in order to acquire knowledge of the subject role in sentences. The contrast that is created between the two pronoun forms is actually the contrast between the accusative and nominative cases. By creating the contrast between a topic and a nontopic, the motivation for including a subject position in sentences is understood. Thus, what is thought to trigger the parameter setting that there are subjects in the language is information that there are preverbal NPs that play a role other than denoting the topic of a sentence.

There are some additional important points to make about the teaching interaction. The first is that the goal of teaching was to contrast the use of *her* with the use of *she*. This is shown in the teacher's response to the student's failure to imitate the *her* and the *she* together at first. She immediately repeated the model to get at least the *her she* string repeated. The second is the teacher's emphasis on maintaining the communication needs related to describing the two pictures. The student was encouraged to point to the girl in the potentially ambiguous situation. In the unambiguous situation, the teacher removed the picture from the reach of the student after the student pointed to the girl as if clarifying reference to the girl. The teacher was trying to establish a clear difference between her communication needs when ambiguity was present and when it was not.

As a result of this teaching interaction provided four or five times daily concerning a set of ten situations, the children first learned to use nominative-case pronouns to encode the new subject role in their spontaneous sentences and later learned to use all the subject properties being measured. Obvious changes occurred over time in the percentage of correct use of subject properties by each of the four subjects, indicating that the learning of subject properties (copula, auxiliary *be*, case, question inversion, third person singular) was dependent on learning the subject role. Also, learning only occurred in periods during and after the teaching interval, thus providing evidence that the teaching regimen was causally related to the learning. It appears that once the specific parameter that was sensitive to the presence or absence of the subject role in the input language was set properly for these delinquent English learners, they learned the properties associated with the role as rapidly as Italian children learn the complex system of verb inflection.

EMPIRICAL RESEARCH ON INDUCTION TEACHING

Two recent studies have been performed to examine certain aspects of the induction teaching approach (Connell, 1986b, 1987a). These studies have examined alternative methods for providing information about the contrast between forms and meanings of rules in an attempt to determine the best teaching methods. In the study in which LM was a participant, six approximately 3-year-old children with SLI who were in the one-word stage were taught the semantic phrase structure rule described earlier, using procedures that focused either on production of sentences or on comprehension without production. The initial segment of production teaching involved having the subjects repeat paired sentences (LM was one of these) that were spoken by the teacher during a teaching interaction. After the imitation segment of teaching was over, these children were required to say the sentences without models from the teacher during the interactions. Comprehension teaching involved having the child select and look at a picture chosen from a pair of pictures that represented the meaning expressed by a sentence spoken by the teacher. The children were not encouraged (in fact, were not allowed) to repeat these sentences or at any time to say them aloud. They were asked simply to listen while the teacher said the sentences and then to point to relevant pictures.

Experimental control was applied in this study by a multiple baseline design across pairs of subjects. Teaching was given sequentially to the subjects, and it was found that only one kind of teaching—that which used production—was effective. The results of the study were that the children did not induce the semantic phrase structure rule unless they were required to say the sentences aloud during teaching sessions (by imitation at first and subsequently without a model); that is, they appeared to make no use of language input that they merely heard.

In order to determine whether failure to learn through nonimitative procedures was a characteristic of children with SLI that differentiated them from normal children, a follow-up study was performed in which 40 children with SLI were compared to 40 age-matched 3- to 6-year-old normal children in terms of how much induction occurred as a result of saying or not saying the input sentences. In order to compare the two types of children, it was necessary to invent a language rule so that the normal children would not have an advantage because they knew more about English. The rule was a morphological rule that placed the suffix—/a / on nouns to express the meaning "part of."

The children were taught following the same principles as described above. A network of correspondence was established between two form–meaning pairs. The contrast between form and meaning was presented while viewing pictures and hearing a noun or a noun plus a suffix spoken by the teacher. Half the group of subjects merely listened and looked at the pictures and the other half listened, looked, and repeated the words. The results indicated that children with SLI induced the rule as a group better if they were allowed to say the words than if they merely heard them. On the other hand, normal children as a group induced the rule better when they merely heard the data and did not have to repeat it.

Repeating apparently inhibited the induction of normal children, but it enhanced the induction of children with SLI. Thus, children with SLI seem to need more assistance in identifying pertinent data from which to form a pattern or in finding data to explain the pattern, but once the pattern was explained, they appeared to be able to induce a rule as well as normal children.

SUMMARY AND CONCLUSIONS

When one chooses to teach language according to the induction teaching approach, a commitment must be made to the model of language and the model of language acquisition that it assumes (Connell, 1987b). The emphasis of teaching must be on careful structuring of the language input given to a child during meaningful interactions. The input must provide sufficient information for the learner to identify patterns, explain them, and consequently hypothesize a rule. The kind of structuring that needs to be done is based on the teacher's conception of language elements that the child needs to learn, that is, on whether pragmatic, semantic, or syntactic aspects should be given prominence. Regardless of the content to be taught, the input must be tailored to contain the kind of information that a language impaired child can use to induce the kinds of linguistic categories or rules selected. The patterns embodied in the input data would probably have to be especially salient so that a child who apparently has difficulty identifying such patterns can do so easily. Thus, the teacher's main concern is finding ways to highlight and emphasize the language patterns sufficiently so that an inefficient pattern-recognizer and pattern-explainer can process them. In essence, the teacher's emphasis needs to be placed on the *sufficiency* and the *saliency* of the input data. Implicit in this approach is the assumption that the learner is capable of applying the induction learning mechanism as long as the sufficiency and the saliency of the input have been attended to by the teacher. Certainly, there are groups of children for whom this assumption will prove false; that is, there are children who do not have the learning capacity to acquire the rules of language. By definition, though, children who have been identified as having SLI are not members of this group.

As is evident from the previous description of subject property teaching, the deduction-acquisition model suggests an approach to teaching that is, in most respects, in concert with the induction-acquisition model. Both models suggest the need to acquire rules through interaction with the environment. Although the goals might be similar, the expected effects of teaching are quite different. In the induction case, the goal of teaching is for the child to hypothesize a rule and then to use it in the sentence formation process. In the deduction case, the effect of teaching is for the child to hypothesize a rule that consequently changes his conception of the language. In the subject property example, the effect of learning the pronoun case distinction led to the realization of subjecthood and changed the children's conception of English from a subjectless language to a subject language.

The expected effects of such changes are much more far-reaching than the anticipated effects of the other kinds of induction teaching described. The effects of parameter setting extend as far as the UG allows it, in this case across several linguistic elements whose relation is quite distant. As linguistic research uncovers more about the parameters that compose the UG, methods used to teach children with SLI will become more effective.

The comparison between the induction and deduction models raises an important question about specific-language-impaired children. Is their language learning problem one of ineffective deduction or induction, or is it one of not having the innate linguistic knowledge that underlies these learning processes? One possibility is that they know the same about language as normal children when beginning language acquisition but that they are less adept at correlating this knowledge to the input they receive (deduction) or at recognizing patterns (induction) in the input that eventually lead to deductions. The second possibility is that they begin with a linguistic knowledge that is less extensive than that of normal children, making the product of their inductive and deductive processes limited to some degree. Of course, there would be a third possibility: that both knowledge and learning processes are deficient. At present there is no compelling evidence to bring to bear on any of these options, but recognizing them seems essential to arriving eventually at an understanding of SLI.

This issue and the rationale for the approach to teaching being advocated here demonstrate the importance of considering theoretical issues when performing clinical work. Only by understanding the differences in theoretical orientation to the study of language and language acquisition and the impact these orientations have on language teaching is it possible to understand the significance of such questions. Progress in clinical language teaching can only be made if teachers recognize the complex theoretical nature of the language problem facing the children they teach. These children cannot be taught by resorting to simplistic solutions as if they needed to learn a golf swing. The problems are complex, and therefore the solutions cannot be simple. Children must be taught in full recognition of the fact that they are learning a complex system of knowledge, a set of abstract rules that are used to generate sentences. The teacher's efforts should not be focused on simplistic issues such as whether the learner is getting immediate feedback after emitting a certain behavior, but rather on important issues such as whether the learner is receiving and attending to the kind of linguistic input that would lead to deducing or inducing the appropriate rule. The teacher's attention should not be focused on what the learner does as much as on whether he or she constructs solutions to the grammatical problems presented by the language experience. The teacher's goal should be to create a learner who solves grammatical problems efficiently and thereby constructs an appropriate grammar, rather than a learner who increases the frequency of his or her responses. A teacher of this sort is one who truly understands the nature of the task of teaching a first language.

REFERENCES

Aram D, Ekelman B, Nation J. Preschoolers with language disorders: 10 years later. J Speech Hear Res 1984; 27:232–244.

Baer D, Guess D. Teaching productive noun suffixes to severely retarded children. Am J Ment Defic 1973; 77:498–503.

Bates E, MacWhinney B. A functionalist approach to the acquisition of grammar. In: Ochs E, Schiefflin B, eds. Developmental pragmatics. New York: Academic Press, 1979:167.

Bates E, MacWhinney B. Functionalist approaches to grammar. In: Wanner E, Gleitman L, eds. Language acquisition: the state of the art. Cambridge: Cambridge University Press, 1982:173.

Berko Gleason J. Some notes on feedback. In: Snow C, Ferguson C, eds. Talking to children: language input and acquisition. Cambridge: Cambridge University Press, 1977:216.

Bloomfield L. Language. New York: Henry Holt, 1933.

Bohannon J, Warren-Luebecker A. Theoretical approaches to language acquisition. In: Berko Gleason J, ed. The development of language. Columbus, OH: Charles E. Merrill, 1985:175.

Brown R. A first language. Cambridge, MA: Harvard University Press, 1973.

Chomsky N. Syntactic structures. The Hague: Mouton, 1957.

Chomsky N. A review of B.F. Skinner, *Verbal Behavior*. Language 1959; 47:26–57.

Chomsky N. Lectures on government and binding. Dordrecht, Netherlands: Foris Publications, 1981.

Connell P. Teaching subjecthood to language disordered children. J Speech Hear Res 1986a; 29:481–492.

Connell P. Acquisition of semantic role by language-disordered children: differences between production and comprehension. J Speech Hear Res 1986b; 29:366–374.

Connell P. An effect of modeling and imitation teaching procedures on children with and without specific language impairment. J Speech Hear Res 1987a; 30:105–113.

Connell P. Teaching language form, meaning, and function to specific language-impaired children. In: Rosenberg S, ed. Advances in applied psycholinguistics. Vol. I: disorders of first language acquisition. Cambridge: Cambridge University Press, 1987b:40.

Ellis Weismer S. Constructive comprehension abilities exhibited by language-disordered children. J Speech Hear Res 1985; 28:175–184.

Givon T. Topic, pronoun, and grammatical agreement. In: Li C, ed. Subject and topic. New York: Academic Press, 1976:151.

Gleitman L, Wanner E. Language acquisition: the state of the state of the art. In: Wanner E, Gleitman L, eds. Language acquisition: the state of the art. Cambridge: Cambridge University Press, 1982:3.

Hyams N. Language acquisition and the theory of parameters. Dordrecht: D. Reidel Publishing, 1986.

Johnston J, Kamhi A. Syntactic and semantic aspects of the utterances of language impaired children: can same be less? Merrill-Palmer Quarterly 1984; 30:65–85.

Lightfoot D. The language lottery: toward a biology of grammars. Cambridge, MA: MIT Press, 1982.

Maratsos M. The child's construction of grammatical categories. In: Wanner E, Gleitman L, eds. Language acquisition: the state of the art. Cambridge: Cambridge University Press, 1982:240.

Nelson K. Facilitating children's acquisition of syntax. Devel Psychol 1977; 13:101–107.

Pinker S. Language learnability and language development. Cambridge, MA: Harvard University Press, 1984.

Rosenberg S. Disorders of first language development: trends in research and theory. In: Gollin ES, ed. Malformations of development: biological and psychological sources and consequences. New York: Academic Press, 1984:195.

Skinner B. Verbal behavior. Englewood Cliffs, NJ: Prentice-Hall, 1957.

Warren S. Clinical strategies for the measurement of language generalization. In: Warren S, Rogers-Warren A, eds. Teaching functional language. Baltimore: University Park Press, 1985:197.

Chapter Five

GENERALIZATION IN THE TREATMENT OF STUTTERING

JANIS COSTELLO INGHAM, Ph.D.

DESCRIPTION OF STUTTERING

Stuttering is a disorder of speech production characterized by various forms of interruption to the continuous flow of speech. It is usually readily noticeable to listeners and is disagreeable to listeners and speakers alike. Persons who stutter may repeat initial sounds and syllables of words, especially words that occur at the beginning of utterances; they may prolong the duration of speech sounds, sometimes producing unusual pitch changes during those prolongations; they may appear to "get stuck" in the production of a sound by silently holding an articulatory position without producing the sound aloud. Although these forms of behavior can also be observed in the speech of nonstutterers, they occur with much greater frequency and duration in the speech of persons who stutter and are oftentimes accompanied by signs of struggle, marked by facial grimaces and bodily gestures, and by attempts to avoid or escape those situations or particular words that the speaker anticipates will produce those behaviors. Further, persons who stutter often report that they feel a loss of control over their speech mechanism when these behaviors are occurring.

One of the many mysteries of stuttering is its variability. That is, for a given stutterer the occurrence of stuttering may vary considerably over time (e.g., good days and bad days), across situations (e.g., no stuttering when speaking to an infant; lots of stuttering when speaking to a superior), among speaking tasks (e.g., little stuttering during reading or when producing short utterances; more stuttering during extended conversations), across settings (e.g., little stuttering while conversing with the family at the dinner table; severe stuttering when talking on the telephone), and even across words (e.g., a speaker may stutter on a given word the first time it occurs in an utterance, but produce it fluently every other time it occurs). Further, individual stutterers may be quite different from one another in terms of the forms their stuttering takes and the conditions under which it varies.

The cause of stuttering is unknown, and theories abound, including the belief that stuttering is the product of an inadequate neuromuscular speech production mechanism, that stuttering is an extreme aberration of normal disfluencies aggravated by the speaker's belief that these normal disfluencies are abnormal and unacceptable, or that stuttering is a by-product of speech anxiety and the stutterer's communication attitudes. For some stutterers, a genetic predisposition appears likely. Stuttering typically begins in early childhood (between the ages of 3 and 8 years) and occurs more often among boys than girls (approximately 3:1).

IMPORTANCE OF GENERALIZATION TO STUTTERING TREATMENT

Irrespective of the unsolved mysteries of stuttering, clinical experience and empirical research have produced evidence that stuttering is alterable and that significant improvement can be made in the speech produced by children and adults who stutter. In fact, treatment research in stuttering has been so prolific in the last decade or so (cf. Bloodstein, 1987; R. Ingham, 1984a) that clinical research in stuttering has naturally moved toward the study of generalization, perhaps because stutterers have made themselves renowned for their reluctance to display the phenomenon. That is, although previous research on various treatment strategies has demonstrated major reductions in, and even seemingly complete elimination of, stuttering in laboratory and clinical settings, newer studies are beginning to address whether those positive treatment effects spread beyond those settings. When that question of generalization has been asked, answers appear to be ambiguous at best; and clinicians are all too familiar with the stuttering client whose speech is stutter free during treatment in the clinic room but who steps outside the treatment room door at the end of the session and says, "SSSSSSSSee you n-n-n-next wa-wa-wwwweek."

Procedures that produce significant improvement in the speech of persons who stutter are, of course, interesting and important both because of the contributions they make to theories of stuttering and to the elimination of stuttering through effective clinical treatments. However, treatments that produce only clinic-bound effects have limited value in the latter arena, wherein producing durable behavior change that takes place in a client's "real life" is the ultimate goal. This realization has turned much current research toward the objective of producing and understanding generalization of treatment effects.

The investigation of generalization is not simple and straightforward: generalization is difficult to define in all of its variations; it is difficult to produce; it is difficult to understand and explain when it does occur, let alone to predict; and the research designs required to investigate it experimentally are difficult to conceive and arrange. Undaunted by these caveats, the pages that follow attempt to develop criteria by which the occurrence of generalization can be judged, to review what is currently known about generalization phenomena in relation to stuttering treatments, to suggest some underlying explanatory principles, and to offer directions for clinical activities that appear to promote generalization.

The generic term *generalization* can be defined in several different ways, three of which are tackled in this chapter: *response generalization, generalization across settings*, and *transfer*.

RESPONSE GENERALIZATION IN STUTTERING

Stuttering as a Response Class

Response generalization occurs "when the effects of learning a particular behavior during treatment spread to other behaviors of the learner" (Costello, 1983a, p. 276). The concept of response generalization in stuttering has parallels to similar phenomena in child and adult language and articulation, and it appears to have been studied more thoroughly in those domains. For example, when a child has been taught correct articulation of /s/ in certain words and, because of that treatment, also becomes able to produce correctly /z/, /ʃ/, and even /θ/ when no treatment has been offered for those phonemes, response generalization can be said to have occurred. As another example, if an aphasic patient was taught to produce correctly 25 words that were names of furniture and then, as a by-product of that treatment, the patient was able to name other furniture pieces and perhaps also previously difficult food names or elusive names of persons, response generalization could be said to have occurred.

Response generalization has been shown to occur when stuttering has been the treatment target. One example appears in the work of Costello and Hurst (1981). In this study we* were interested in determining whether different types of stutters, such as sound prolongations, syllable repetitions, and inhalation interjections, were independent behaviors in stutterers' individual repertoires or were part of the same response class. We attempted to answer this question by applying treatment only to one particular form of stuttering for a given subject, thus providing the opportunity to observe whether the treatment effects would spread to other types of stutters in the subject's stuttering pattern. Figure 5–1 provides a sample of the results. Condition A displays the baseline rates of two forms of stuttering that occurred for one subject: stutters that contained lip tremors and part-word repetitions. When a 10-second period of time-out from talking was introduced contingent *only* on occasions of tremors (condition B), tremor-type stutters decreased, as expected, *and so did untreated part-word repetitions*. This covariation between treated and untreated forms of stuttering was replicated when the contingency for tremors was withdrawn and both behaviors increased (the next condition A). It was reinstated in the next condition B, both behaviors once again decreasing when only tremors were directly manipulated. The phenomenon was replicated with two other sub-

* For the confused reader: J. Costello = J. Ingham.

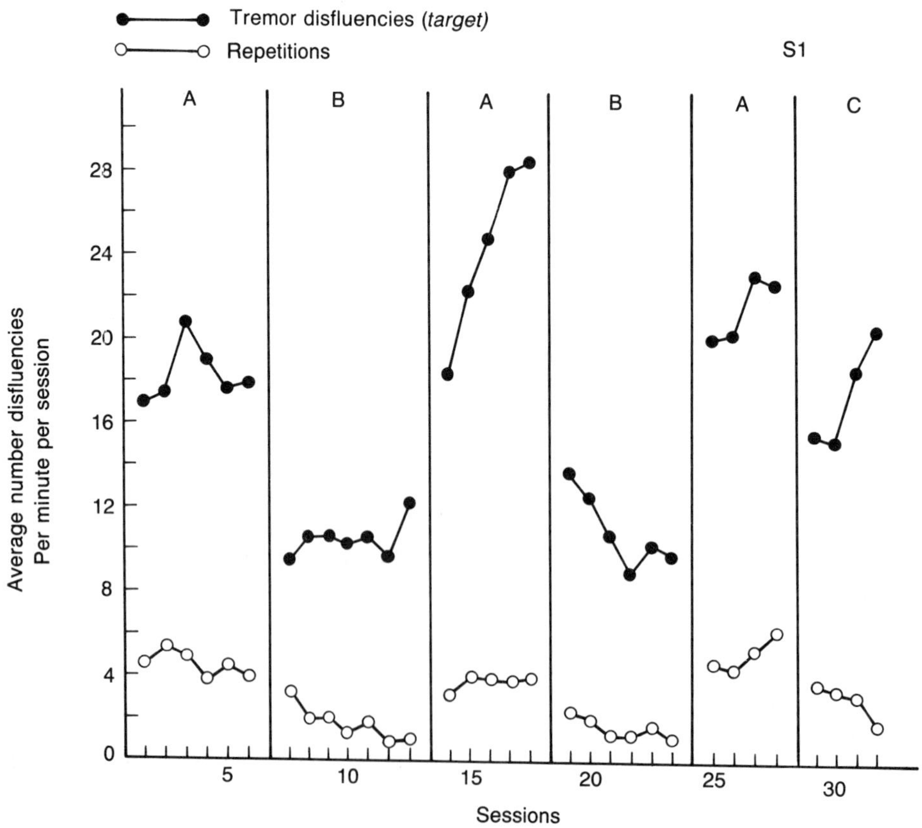

Figure 5–1 Average number of stutters per minute in baseline (*A*), time-out contingent on tremor-type stutters (*B*), and time-out contingent on part-word repetitions (*C*). Closed circles = tremor-type stutters; open circles = repetitions. (Costello JM, Hurst MR. An analysis of the relationship among stuttering behaviors. J Speech Hear Res 1981; 24:247–256. Reprinted by permission.)

jects on different forms of stuttering behaviors (three for each).

This demonstration of response generalization suggests that, whatever the surface form of behaviors perceived as stutters, all appear to be part of the same response class, because modification of one produces concurrent changes in the others. In regard to stuttering theory, these data could suggest that the many forms stuttering takes within a given speaker are all related to the same source and are susceptible to the same treatment. This finding is in opposition to Brutten and Shoemaker's (1967) two-factor theory of stuttering, which hypothesizes that certain forms of stuttering (the so called "kernel characteristics" described by Wingate [1964a]) are produced by anxiety conditioning, and that other forms (Wingate's "accessory features," Van Riper's "secondary mannerisms") are produced by instrumental conditioning. Brutten and Shoemaker suggest the use of different treatment strategies for each of these assumed independent classes of behavior, whereas the findings of Costello and Hurst suggest that all forms of stuttering may be modifiable by direct contingency manipulations.

Intratherapy Generalization

Intratherapy generalization (Costello and Bosler, 1976) or *intratherapy contextual generalization* (Rockman and Elbert, 1984) is a variant of response generalization that has been shown to apply to the treatment of stuttering as well as other disorders. It occurs, for example, when a misarticulating child is taught a target phoneme in the initial position of selected nonsense syllables, and thereby becomes able to produce that sound at "more complex" levels, such as in words and phrases. This variety of generalization can also be seen in stuttering when the client who has learned stutter-free productions of short utterances is then able to produce longer utterances without stuttering (Costello, 1983b), or when the client who has acquired stutter-free speech through monologue tasks in the clinic is subsequently able to use fluent speech in reading and conversation tasks. Such *across-modality generalization* was noted as a consequence of a time-out treatment applied to the stuttering behavior of three young adult stutterers in our laboratory (Costello, 1975). Their pretreatment and posttreatment stuttering frequencies are shown in Figure 5–2. The modality in which treatment was given is asterisked. Pretreatment stuttering frequencies are shown in solid blocks, and posttreatment data are shown in open blocks. Brett received treatment in reading and monologue and generalized his reduced stuttering to conversation. David and Tom were treated through monologue tasks and showed generalization of comparable levels of stuttering reduction to reading and conversation modalities.

Clinical Implications

Generalization of this nature is important to note because it illustrates that, contrary to some still popular notions, stuttering is a set of behaviors that responds much like other behaviors under treatment conditions. And, just like other behaviors, the need exists to continue the search for explanations about why such intratherapy generalization occurs to different degrees for different subjects, or not at all for some subjects and quite completely for others.

The lesson for clinicians in the meantime is that generalization of treatment effects across stuttering behaviors and across levels of treatment tasks is to be expected, but that the extent of such generalization remains unpredictable. Therefore, clinicians cannot *assume*, but must *assess* the nature and extent of response generalization that occurs for each client at different stages of treatment. Such assessments are most readily achieved by periodically probing the client's speech performance under a variety of untreated conditions. If it is found, for example, that improvement stemming from treatment applied during reading tasks has not generalized to a client's self-formulated speech, then direct treatment during monologue or conversation would appear appropriate. On the other hand, clinical experimentation may indicate (as it has in our clinic) that improvement gained from treatment carried out during connected speech activities readily generalizes to reading tasks for some clients. Such information would probably lead a clinician to determine that treatment ought to be given first in connected speech and only later in reading, if the generalization assessment data indicated that stuttering continued in reading.

In summary, clinicians should be able to take advantage of response generalization, when it occurs, and begin to recognize treatment strategies that facilitate its occurrence, thus increasing the efficiency of their stuttering treatments.

ACROSS-SETTINGS GENERALIZATION IN STUTTERING

A more often studied area of generalization is *across-settings generalization*, also known as *carry-over, extratreatment generalization, extratherapy generalization, beyond-clinic generalization*, and so on. Perhaps the number of terms that have evolved to label this process is indicative of the extent of its significance to a discipline that espouses a special attraction to applied or clinical research.

Rather than proposing yet another definition of this term, the oft-quoted one of Stokes and Baer (1977), described in other chapters in this book, is reiterated here. Stokes and Baer say,

> [Generalization is]...the occurrence of relevant behavior under different, nontraining conditions (i.e., across subjects, settings, people, behaviors, and/or time) without the scheduling of the same events in those conditions as had been scheduled in the training conditions. Thus generalization may be claimed when no extratraining manipulations are needed for extratraining changes; or may be claimed when some extra manipulations are necessary, but their cost or extent is clearly less than that of the direct intervention. Generalization will not be claimed when similar events are necessary for similar effects across conditions (p. 350).

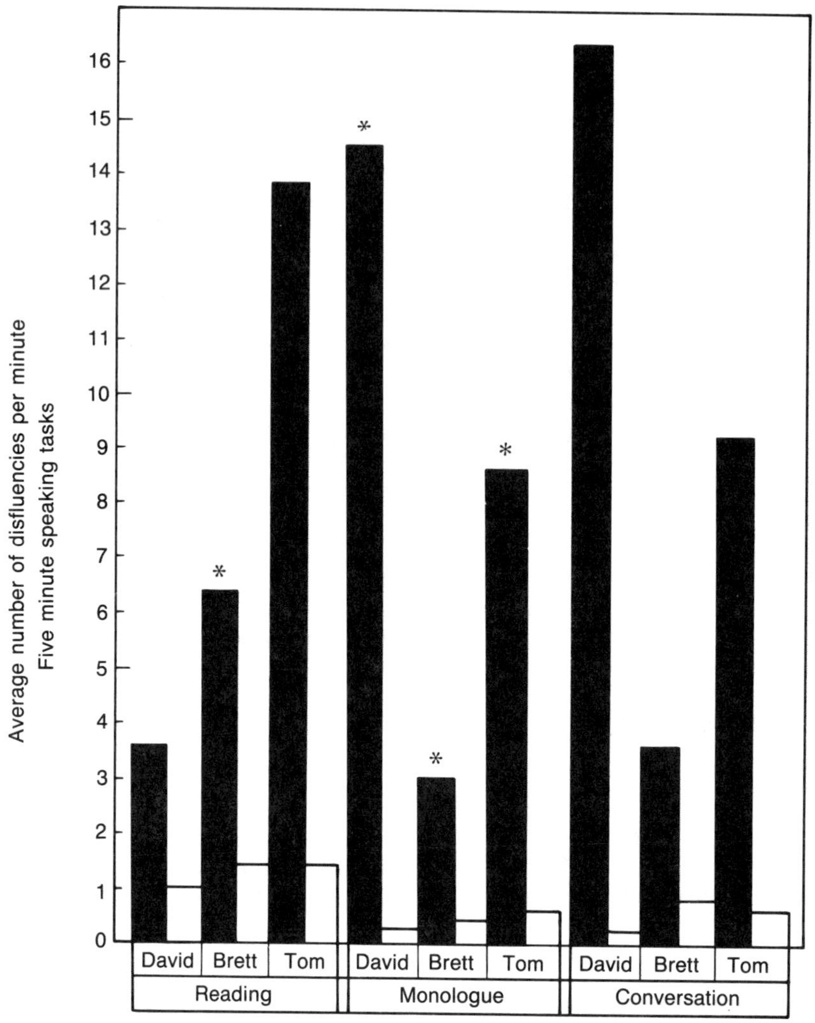

Figure 5–2 Average number of stutters per minute in pretreatment (*solid blocks*) and posttreatment (*open blocks*) reading, monologue, and conversation samples for David, Brett, and Tom. Treatment modalities are asterisked. (Costello JM. The establishment of fluency with time-out procedures: three case studies. J Speech Hear Disord 1975; 40:216–231. Reprinted by permission.)

In other words, across-settings generalization can be said to have occurred when a target behavior that was taught in one environment (e.g., a clinic room) is observed to occur in a different environment (e.g., the classroom or home), in the absence of the teaching procedures that were used to establish the behavior in the first setting (i.e., without imitative models, prompts, instructions about how to produce the correct response, carefully planned evoking stimuli such as picture cards and word lists, the presence of the clinician, and, most especially, arranged reinforcement and punishment contingencies). This variety of generalization is an aspect of *stimulus generalization* (in contrast to *response generalization* discussed above), wherein generalization is said to happen when the occurrence of the behavior of interest spreads to new stimuli (rather than when behavior change spreads to new responses).

While Stokes and Baer's definition of generalization has become a standard, some refinements appear necessary. The definition encompasses at least two phenomena that deserve separate recognition because they appear to be different processes. The first refers to the part of the definition that reads, " .. when no extratraining manipulations are needed ... or ... when some extra manipulations are necessary, but their cost or extent is clearly less than that of the direct intervention" (Stokes and Baer, 1977).

It is certainly not news that hoped-for generalization across settings is oftentimes not the result of a given treatment. It then becomes the responsibility of the clinician or experimenter to devise extended and continued treatment procedures to produce that generalization. Sometimes these "extra manipulations" are relatively small and easy to arrange, such as asking a child's classroom teacher to provide a certain number of opportunities each day for the child to ask questions. However, at other times these "extra manipulations" may be much more extravagant and time consuming, such as establishing a token reinforcement system in the home and teaching a child's parents to recognize and reinforce occurrences of the target behavior whenever and wherever they occur.

It is not clear where one draws the line regarding the "cost or extent" of such "extra manipulations," but it is clear that they are above and beyond the procedures used to establish the behavior in the original treatment setting and should be recognized as such. For that reason, some have labeled such procedures, irrespective of their cost or extent, *planned* or *programmed generalization*, or *transfer procedures* (Costello, 1983a), emphasizing the active nature of the process. It seems that if there are, indeed, two factors to contend with—first, within-clinic procedures used to establish new behaviors, and second, "add-on" procedures to facilitate the occurrence of those behaviors in the natural environment—and if the procedures used for each process are not necessarily the same, the differences are made clearer and the concepts are kept distinct by giving them different names. Thus, this chapter uses the term *transfer* to indicate across-settings behavior change promoted by procedures beyond those used to establish the target behavior in the original clinic setting.

The second needed refinement to Stokes and Baer's definition of across-settings generalization refers to the part of the definition that reads, " ... the occurrence of relevant behavior under different, nontraining conditions (i.e., across subjects, settings, people, behaviors, *and/or time*) ... " (italics added). It has been suggested, particularly by R. Ingham (1981), that the spread of newly acquired behavior across settings (generalization) and the durability or longevity of newly acquired behavior across time (maintenance) are probably separate phenomena and may require different procedures to produce them (as well as different names to distinguish them). For example, studies that measure "generalization" by having subjects return to the clinical environment at some later time for follow-up evaluations are more likely assessing *maintenance* and do not shed light on across-settings generalization because they do not measure behavior in nontreatment settings. Conversely, it is possible for behavior learned in a clinic setting to *generalize* to extraclinic environments but not be *maintained* in those environments long enough for that generalization to be noted (Koegel and Rincover, 1977). For example, a client may leave a successful clinic session speaking quite fluently in all environments and with all persons, only to find that fluency to be transient, evaporating completely 2 hours later. This would be a case of generalization without maintenance.

A growing body of research on maintenance of stutter-free speech is beginning to appear (Boberg, 1981; Boberg, Howie, and Woods, 1979; Howie, Tanner, and Andrews, 1981; R. Ingham, 1980, 1981, 1982). It is research that asks whether newly acquired speech patterns are maintained for substantial periods of time following completion of treatment (a passive, measurement-oriented view of maintenance), and research that attempts to operationalize and evaluate procedures designed to *produce* durable, maintained behavior change (an active perspective regarding maintenance).

CRITERIA FOR JUDGING THE ADEQUACY OF THE EXPERIMENTAL TREATMENT OF STUTTERING

Perhaps a logical place to begin an overview of research on across-settings generalization is to suggest a set of criteria for studies attempting to evaluate treatment outcome, including the occurrence of generalization (Costello and R. Ingham, 1984; R. Ingham and Costello, 1984). These criteria apply equally to research and clinical activities aimed at producing across-settings generalization.

Selection of Valid Dependent Variables

Obviously, if the dependent variables measured are not deemed to be sensitive reflections of the target behavior of interest, whether or not they generalize is of little consequence. In the stuttering literature, the consensus appears to be that at least two aspects of behavior must be measured to meet minimum validity requirements: frequency of stuttering, usually reported as percentage of syllables stuttered (%SS), and speech rate, usually reported as syllables per minute (SPM).

Stuttering Frequency

Because essentially all therapies have as a goal the reduction, if not the complete elimination, of moments of stuttering, frequency of stuttering is obviously a relevant measure; however, various researchers, clinicians, and individual stuttering clients themselves have differing views about acceptable %SS levels (in our clinic, the goal is less than 1%SS). Although any reliable reduction in stuttering that occurs in beyond-clinic settings might be considered an occasion of across-settings generalization for research and theoretical purposes, clinically significant across-settings generalization would not be considered to be achieved unless stuttering frequency in nontreatment settings reached those "acceptable" %SS levels.

Speech Rate

It is well known that prolonged speech and even considerably less drastic reductions in speaking rate can produce reduced stuttering, so the inclusion of speed of speech information is important to get a full picture of a talker's speaking performance. For example, 0%SS associated with a "normal" speaking rate of 200 SPM tells a very different story than 0%SS and 90 SPM.

Speech Naturalness

Another aspect of the treated speech of stutterers that is fast becoming a critical dimension to measure is the notion of speech naturalness. Stuttering outcome research has made it abundantly clear that for some stutterers and some treatments, the posttreatment stutter-free speech of stutterers, even while being produced at normal speech rates, remains distinguishable from the speech of nonstutterers. The elusive quality of the "naturalness" of that speech seems to be the essence of the difference. Fortunately, recent research appears to have been successful in making available a reliable and highly discriminating measure of speech naturalness (R. Ingham, Gow, and Costello, 1985; R. Ingham, Martin, Haroldson, Onslow, and Leney, 1985; R. Ingham and Onslow, 1985; Martin, Haroldson, and Triden, 1984). This method requires the stutterer to speak continuously while a listener (e.g., clinician or client) makes periodic ratings of the client's speech naturalness (usually at 15-second or 30-second intervals) on a 9-point scale, wherein 1 = highly natural and 9 = highly unnatural. Speech naturalness ratings between 1 and 3 typify the speech of normally speaking adults (mean = 2.12, standard deviation = 1.17) (Martin, Haroldson, and Triden, 1984) and would thus be an appropriate goal for the treated stutterer as well. Further, it would seem that speech naturalness measurements made by a stutterer's peers, family, or untrained laypersons might well serve to assess the "social validity" of the treatment outcome, a concept first described by Wolf (1978).

This tripartite set of measures—stuttering frequency, speech rate, and speech naturalness—offers the opportunity to obtain a sensitive and valid composite picture of a speaker's speech pattern and its degree of normalcy, the kind of assessment that is clinically desirable for the measurement of across-settings generalization. An added advantage of these measures is that they can be obtained "on-line," i.e., while the client is speaking. (See Fowler and R. Ingham [1986] for a description of a computer software package that makes this readily possible.) Therefore, these measures not only are valid measures of relevant speech behaviors, but also are conveniently obtained.

Other Measures

Another variable of interest, although not so reliably quantified, is an assessment of clients' *satisfaction* with their posttreatment speech in terms of how it sounds and feels to them, and how much effort is required to maintain or monitor it. Some authors (e.g., Perkins, Rudas, Johnson, Michael, and Curlee, 1974; Webster, 1979) have included questionnaires to tap these aspects of subjects' posttreatment behavior, but the validity of such measures has yet to be studied. Further, any other behaviors (such as "gentle onset" or "regulated breathing") or constructs (such as "communication attitude" or "anxiety") that are central to a particular treatment under study would be logical candidates for measurement in the course of evaluating across-settings generalization.

Reliable Measurement of Dependent Variables

That reliable measurement of the dependent variables of interest is a crucial aspect of any behavioral research should not have to be stated. However, all too often this aspect of research methodology is overlooked by clinical researchers. Add to this the fact that even the simple recognition of a given moment of stuttering is not a particularly straightforward task (Curlee, 1981; MacDonald and Martin, 1973; Martin and Haroldson, 1981; Young, 1969), and one would probably conclude that not much stock can be attributed to generalization findings from studies that do not report reliability of measurement or that do not do so in a satisfactory manner.

This aspect of measurement is even more often overlooked in everyday clinical activities, and it is just as important there as in research endeavors. Clinicians can periodically check the reliability of their measurement of stuttering frequency, speech rate, and speech naturalness to assure themselves (and their employers and clients) that the data on which treatment effectiveness is being judged and treatment decisions are being made are not influenced by familiarity, bias, or carelessness. Such reliability checks can be rather easily obtained by asking other clinicians to measure the same behaviors from tape recordings of a client's speech that have been assessed by the clinician. Percentage agreement comparisons of the data collected by the clinician and the observer can shed light on the matter of reliability and are particularly important to obtain from samples that evaluate across-settings generalization, a treatment's ultimate goal.

Periodic Measurement of Dependent Variables

When one is hoping to discern the influence of a given treatment procedure on generalization, the more frequent the assessment of generalization, the more likely one is to learn about the relationship between the treatment and the spread of its effects, as exemplified in time-series experimental designs. For example, if no generalization is noted consistently until particular transfer activities have been introduced (e.g., Resick, Wendiggensen, Ames, and Meyers, 1978; Ryan, 1974), one would no doubt begin to recognize the importance of such activities to the generalization process. However, when generalization measures are made only at the end of treatment, or more loosely, after a maintenance period of some weeks or months, it becomes impossible to attribute generalization effects to a particular treatment or components of a treatment. Periodic generalization probes conducted prior to treatment, during treatment, immediately following the termination of treatment, and at extended follow-up periods provide timely information about the spread of treatment effects beyond the clinic setting and offer data upon which to base treatment decisions.

Measures of Dependent Variables in Multiple, Ecologically Valid, Beyond-Clinic Nontreatment Environments

Stutterers are notorious for the variability of their behavior over time and across conditions. The data displayed in

Figure 5–3, collected from a 4-year-old stuttering boy, are illustrative. This figure shows %SS calculated from weekly standard talking samples, recorded in six different conversation settings. Blatantly noticeable is the variability of stuttering frequency both across talking settings in any given week and within each condition across time. Further, variability is present not only during baseline but for a considerable period of time after the initiation of treatment (right of the solid vertical line), even when the child and clinician conversed in the clinic (open circles), a task quite similar to the task going on during treatment. Further, if data from that treatment were to be displayed on this graph as well, one would observe a gradual decline in %SS that reached and stayed below 1%SS at week 12. However, the data from the generalization probes displayed in Figure 5–3 make apparent the fact that that level of stutter-free speech was not even beginning to be mirrored in the child's beyond-clinic performance until several weeks later. In this case, if treatment outcome were to be judged on the basis of within-clinic treatment data, the data would be highly misleading.

It can also be noted from these data that, for this child at least, when across-settings generalization began to occur in a convincing fashion, it occurred similarly and simultaneously in all of the measured (nontreatment) environments, rather than progressively from one to another. Further, the variability observed across the earlier data points was substantially reduced once generalization began to occur.

These data illustrate the importance of obtaining measures of a subject's or client's speech in multiple naturalistic, nontreatment environments—seemingly the only way to obtain valid evidence regarding across-settings generalization. Further, the necessity of obtaining periodic measures from a *standard set* of speaking conditions seems apparent, because one data point obtained from one condition on one occasion does not provide a very complete or accurate picture of the stutterer's overall speech performance. For example, assume that only one pretreatment data point had been obtained and that it happened to be from the child's conversation with his mother in the clinic during week four (closed circle, 3.7%SS). Then suppose that the next beyond-clinic assessment occurred during week 15. If the data had been taken from another conversation with the child's mother, it would appear that he had reduced his stuttering frequency by more than 50 percent (to 1.4%SS); but if the assessment had been made instead by having the child talk with the clinician outside the clinic room (open triangle, 0.5%SS), the data would indicate that his stuttering had been reduced more considerably, even to a clinically acceptable level (less than 1%SS), and perhaps dismissal would be contemplated. On the other hand, if the week-15 sample had been conducted by recording a conversation between the child and his father in the home (closed triangle, 5.6%SS), one might conclude that the treatment had worsened the child's stuttering, and major changes in the treatment regimen might have been considered. The moral of the story is that single samples can provide misleading indicators of the stutterer's speech performance when assessing treatment outcome in regard to across-settings generalization.

Once one becomes convinced of the value, even the absolute necessity, of gathering data from multiple settings, one must decide which settings are appropriate. Little or no research has been conducted in this area. We have suggested (Costello and R. Ingham, 1984; R. Ingham and Costello, 1984) that the settings be representative of genuine talking conditions and talking partners, but interesting questions arise about how to determine the representativeness of a given talking setting. Perhaps it would be useful to gather pretreatment data through talking logs, noting the talking occasions encountered by a client and how talkative the client is in each, and then selecting standard talking sample conditions accordingly.

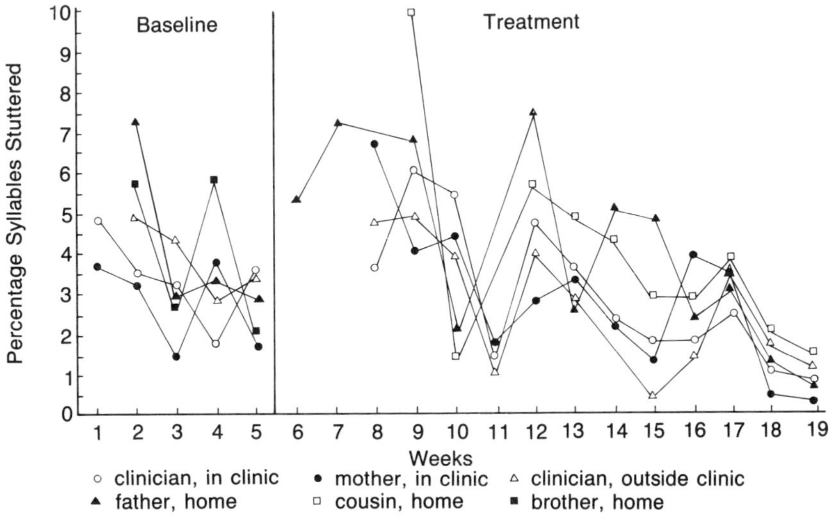

Figure 5–3 Percentage syllables stuttered by a 4-year-old boy in 10-minute samples of conversation pretreatment (baseline) and during treatment.

It would be interesting to see whether generalization, should it occur, would spread equally across talking conditions that are encountered more and less often. Further, if transfer treatment were extended to the natural environment(s), as is often the case—an example of Stokes and Baer's (1977) techniques of *training sufficient exemplars* and *sequential modification*—it would be interesting to evaluate whether greater generalization is produced by introducing treatment first into frequently occurring natural talking environments or into environments in which the client was particularly talkative.

The stuttering study that appears to have collected the greatest amount of beyond-clinic data to date was conducted with a single subject by R. Ingham and Packman (1977). This adult woman tape-recorded all of her speech every other day for more than 9 months. In their attempt to present these generalization data in a coherent fashion, Ingham and Packman pointed out that the subject's talking could be divided into various descriptive categories (such as talking on the telephone, talking with her husband at home, talking with people at work) or by divisions of time (such as morning, afternoon, and evening), but they recognized that all of these categories were arbitrary and not necessarily functional classes of talking behavior for the subject. Research has yet to address the question of whether stutterers might have groups of talking situations that are functionally related. However, as generalization research that relies on multiple talking samples from beyond the original treatment setting continues, these issues are bound to become topics for investigation.

Nonreactive Measurement of Dependent Variables

Admittedly, it can be logistically difficult to obtain frequent samples of a subject's speech in multiple natural settings. The task is made easier by enlisting the aid of the subject or the subject's parents to arrange for these periodic standard samples to be recorded and then to hand the tape recordings over to the clinician or experimenter for analysis. However, the nature of these tasks, i.e., that they be conducted periodically, for some substantial period of time, among the same persons, and that they provide talking samples of adequate length, demands that they be conducted overtly. But what about the reactivity of such overt measures? That is, when subjects are aware that speech samples are being made for the purpose of assessing their current speech production, might that awareness, coupled with the presence of a tape recorder, influence their speech so that it is not a sample representative of their truly spontaneous, natural speech?

This question has been studied, but the answer remains ambiguous. When data from covertly obtained speech samples have been compared to comparable data collected from overtly obtained speech samples in the same time period, some studies (e.g., R. Ingham, 1975) have found that speech was better in the overtly obtained samples, whereas other studies have found no difference between the two methods of sampling (e.g., Howie, Woods, and Andrews, 1982). It may be that early in the treatment and posttreatment periods the comparison of data collected from both procedures would give a different picture than the same comparison collected during follow-up several months or even years later. At this time the most conservative procedure would be to ensure that some occasions of covertly sampled speech are obtained, in order to provide an accurate picture of the presence or absence of across-settings generalization.†

Judgment of the Potency of Treatment

It might logically be expected that certain treatments would be unlikely to produce generalized effects, because their direct effects appear frail. That is, a treatment that was based on unsound or untested principles, that was employed only for a short period, that produced only a 50 percent reduction in stuttering, or that left clients with slowed, labored, or unnatural-sounding speech might not be expected to produce generalization. Thus, a lack of generalization associated with such treatments might not be considered particularly telling in regard to our understanding of the generalization process.

On the other hand, a lack of generalization associated with a treatment based on well-established principles, shown to produce substantial treatment effects in the clinical setting, and applied over an ample period of time might arouse a greater puzzlement, because such a treatment would no doubt be assumed to be more likely to produce generalized effects.

The role in generalization played by the power of a given treatment to establish stutter-free (or improved) speech in the clinical setting has received little study. Of course, the question of how to operationalize the relative power of different treatments is daunting. One attempt has been to use meta-analysis (Andrews, Guitar, and Howie, 1980), a method of estimating the magnitude of a treatment effect (*Effect Size*) from a statistical comparison of treated and control group mean scores or group mean pretreatment and posttreatment scores. Effect Sizes across treatment strategies are then compared, typically across published studies. This procedure seems inadequate in its underlying rationale, which takes all data at face value and thus obviates any kind of evaluation of the quality of the data obtained by the methods of a given study. Further, meta-analysis procedures necessarily ignore a substantial number of important treatment studies (i.e., the single-subject, response-contingent studies). The method has been roundly criticized by Eysenck (1978), who entitled his comments, "An Exercise in Mega-Silliness."

Although the influence on generalization of the effectiveness of the particular treatment procedure used to es-

† We have dealt with the thorny problem of clients' rights to know when their speech is being recorded and/or evaluated by explaining at the beginning of treatment the rationale for covert evaluation during and following the period of treatment and obtaining written consent from each client. Clients are also told that they may examine their records at any time during and following treatment. Common courtesy regarding clients' privacy and the nature of covert assessments (e.g., telephone surveys, surreptitious tape recording by parent or spouse) is, of course, observed.

tablish improved speech continues to appear to be an important variable for consideration, a broad overview of the many stuttering treatment strategies that have been reported in the literature makes obvious the complication that this variable presents and attempts to determine the nature and extent of generalization effects in stuttering treatment. Table 5–1 lists general categories of treatment strategies that are described in the stuttering treatment literature. The length of this list is further complicated by the fact that many reported treatment studies employ combinations of these general techniques. Further, within each treatment category there exist published studies that do and do not illustrate convincing treatment effects. Consequently, the connection to be drawn between the nature of the treatment used and its ability to produce across-settings generalization remains unknown. However, it seems logical to assume that a minimum requisite would be the use of a treatment that produces a clinically acceptable level of stuttering reduction within the boundaries of the clinical setting.

TABLE 5–1 Stuttering Treatments Reported in the Empirical Literature

Attitude adjustment
Delayed auditory feedback
Extended length and complexity of utterance
Electromyographic biofeedback
Gentle onset of phonation
Masking
Metronome conditioning
Prolonged speech
Regulated breathing
Response-contingent feedback for stuttering and/or stutter-free utterances
Self-monitoring and/or self-presented response-contingent consequences
Shadowing
Slowed speech
Stuttering modification
Systemic desensitization

Inclusion of Transfer Activities

Another issue to consider is whether a given treatment includes activities directly aimed at producing generalization, i.e., a transfer phase. It appears that the inclusion of such direct transfer treatment, at least for adult and older child stutterers, is mandatory if any degree of across-settings generalization is to occur (e.g., Resick et al, 1978; Ryan, 1979). In other words, you can train and you can hope, but the "train and hope" strategy, so aptly named by Stokes and Baer (1977), does not appear to do the job. (More about transfer below.)

Assessment of Maintenance

The current status of knowledge regarding the maintenance of stuttering treatment effects is well stated (and sadly, too) by R. Ingham (1986):

> A strong case could be made for the claim that generalization is negatively correlated with the extensiveness of therapy evaluation: the more substantial the evaluation, the less likely we will find evidence of successful generalization, especially over time ... There is overwhelming evidence that the longer the follow-up, the poorer the outcome (Ingham, 1984a).

Although studies that *assess* long-term maintenance are few and far between, experiments that attempt to *produce* maintenance are even less frequent (R. Ingham, 1980; 1982). The logistic problems associated with the conduct of studies of this nature—the need for long-term follow-up, obtaining many recordings of each subject's speech under natural conditions, keeping track of the subject's whereabouts for extended periods, enlisting confederates to assist in data collection and evaluation, and managing reams of data—make it understandable that researchers and clinicians alike have been daunted by the task; but the evaluation of stuttering treatment outcomes and the discovery of the variables that contribute to generalization and maintenance cannot be complete without these kinds of data.

APPLICATION OF THE CRITERIA

The growing literature on the generalization effects of stuttering treatments has been recently and thoroughly reviewed by R. Ingham (1984b; 1986; R. Ingham and Onslow, 1987), so it seems redundant for J. Ingham to repeat all of that here. Furthermore, it appears that it may be too early to draw meaningful inductions from the currently available literature. Table 5–2 lists the vast majority of treatment studies reported in the literature on stuttering that attempt to comment on the across-settings generalization of their effects. Listed across the top of the table, by number, are the criteria described in the previous pages. A circle indicates that, according to this writer's judgment, the particular criterion was at least minimally met in the study listed. Note that in the table as a whole, there is not a great density of circles! The summary at the end of the table indicates that, although most of the treatments studied have appeared relatively powerful in regard to establishing improved speech in the original clinical setting (item six, 72 percent of the 54 studies listed), and have measured speech status periodically (item three, 67 percent of the studies)—although not necessarily with valid, reliable, or covert measures (items one, two, and five—56 percent, 46 percent, and 20 percent, respectively)—fewer treatments have included those all-important aspects of transfer and maintenance activities (items seven and eight—54 percent and 37 percent, respectively), and fewer still have bothered to assess across-settings generalization by sampling speech in nontreatment environments (item four, 20 percent). Therefore, using these studies to draw conclusions about across-settings generalization effects of stuttering treatment or to pinpoint effective generalization techniques would have questionable validity. There is not yet ample litera-

TABLE 5-2 Evaluation of Stuttering Treatment Research in Regard to Credibility of Reports of Generalization

Report in the Literature	*Criteria**							
	1	*2*	*3*	*4*	*5*	*6*	*7*	*8*
Andrews and Feyer (1985)	o	o				o	o	
Andrews and Ingham (1972a)	o		o		o	o	o	
Andrews and Ingham (1972b)	o		o					
Andrews and Tanner (1982a)	o	o	o					
Andrews and Tanner (1982b)	o	o	o				o	
Azrin and Nunn (1974)			o					
Azrin, Nunn, and Frantz (1979)	o							o
Beattie (1973)						o	o	
Boberg (1980)	o		o			o	o	o
Boberg and Sawyer (1977)	o	o	o	o	o	o		o
Budd et al. (1986)		o	o			o	o	o
Condit (1987)	o	o	o	o	o	o	o	o
Coppola and Yairi (1982)			o					
Cote and Ladouceur (1982)	o	o	o		o			
Craig and Andrews (1985)	o		o			o	o	
Craig and Cleary (1982)	o	o	o				o	o
Craven and Ryan (1984)	o		o			o	o	
Crowder and Harbin (1971)		o						
Curlee and Perkins (1969)						o	o	
Florance and Shames (1980)						o	o	o
Gregory (1972)			o	o				
Guitar (1976)						o		o
Hee and Holmes (1976)								
Herscovitch and LeBow (1973)		o	o			o		
Howie, Tanner, and Andrews (1981)	o	o	o		o	o	o	o
R. Ingham (1980)	o	o	o	o	o	o	o	o
R. Ingham (1981) - Exp. I	o	o	o	o	o	o	o	o
R. Ingham (1981) - Exp. II	o	o	o	o	o	o	o	o
R. Ingham (1982)	o	o	o	o	o	o	o	o
R. Ingham and Packman (1977)	o	o	o	o	o	o		o
James (1981)	o	o	o			o	o	
Marshall and Starch (1984)	o		o			o		
Martin, Kuhl, and Haroldson (1972)	o	o	o	o	o	o		
Perkins et al. (1974)	o	o	o	o		o	o	
Peters (1977)		o				o		
Prins (1970)								
Ramig and Wallace (1987)	o					o	o	
Reed and Godden (1977)	o	o	o			o		
Resick et al. (1978)	o	o	o			o		
Rickard and Mundy (1965)								
Riley and Riley (1979)						o		
Riley and Riley (1983)			o			o		
Riley and Riley (1984)			o			o		
Rustin and Kuhr (1983)							o	
Ryan (1971)			o			o	o	o
Ryan (1974)			o			o	o	o
Ryan and Van Kirk (1974)	o	o				o	o	o
Ryan and Van Kirk (1983)	o		o	o		o	o	o
Shaw and Shrum (1972)		o				o		
Shine (1980)			o			o	o	o
Small (1975)						o	o	
Turnbaugh and Guitar (1981)	o	o	o			o	o	o
Wakaba (1983)								
Webster (1980)	o		o			o	o	
Percentage of studies (of 54)	56	46	67	20	20	72	54	37
Number of studies	30	25	36	11	11	39	29	20

* 1 = Selection of valid dependent variables (minimum: stuttering frequency and speech rate)
2 = Reliable measurement of dependent variables
3 = Periodic measurement (minimum: pretreatment, posttreatment, follow-up)
4 = Multiple measures in ecologically valid beyond-clinic environments
5 = Nonreactive (covert) measurement
6 = Use of a reasonably potent acquisition treatment
7 = Inclusion of transfer activities
8 = Inclusion of maintenance activities

ture addressing these questions from a methodologically sound perspective.

PROMISING GENERALIZATION TECHNIQUES

It is possible to draw from this literature some tentative inferences about variables that appear to contribute to the occurrence of across-settings generalization, as long as the reader is willing to hold these conclusions as conditional until they have been properly tested.

In general, it appears that treatment effects, irrespective of the particular procedure used, do not usually generalize to beyond-clinic settings without the inclusion of specific transfer activities. Although the full range of transfer technologies described by Stokes and Baer (1977) has not been investigated in the stuttering literature, the most frequently used and so far most promising procedures take three forms. Often two or even all three are used concurrently.

Response-Contingent Procedures

To varying degrees, essentially all of the seemingly effective treatments currently described in the literature utilize response-contingent procedures. Typically, treatment is programmed in small progressive steps, for example from monosyllabic, simple, readily stutter-free utterances through utterances of gradually increasing length ultimately to extended durations of connected speech; or from slowed, prolonged utterances to slightly faster speech to approximations of normal speech rate. Advancement from one step to the next is dependent upon behavioral criteria that assume mastery (Costello, 1977; 1980; 1982). Also, moments of stuttering typically produce contingent negative feedback (verbal comment, time-out from talking, presentation of a negative stimulus such as a buzzer or light, the requirement to repeat the utterance, and so on), and oftentimes (although not quite as often) stutter-free utterances produce positive reinforcement as well (commonly verbal praise and token reinforcement). These performance-contingent activities are typically quite dense during establishment of fluent speech in the clinical setting, but they are usually included, perhaps in "looser" form, in transfer and maintenance activities as well.

Specific Use of Transfer Tasks

"Successful" treatments have typically included transfer activities that could be described in the language of Stokes and Baer (1977) as applications of "programming common stimuli," "training sufficient exemplars," and "sequential modification." (See Kearns's chapter in this volume for an in-depth description of those and other generalization technologies.) Attempts at actively promoting generalization through specific treatment activities have typically included procedures that appear to be aimed at incorporating "real world" stimuli into the treatment, so that those stimuli might gain stimulus control over the stutterer's newly learned behavior. In some cases, stimuli from the natural environment are brought into the clinic (e.g., parents, peers, classroom materials). In other cases (or in conjunction), clinical activities are extended beyond the clinic by having the clinician accompany the client into the natural environment for direct talking practice in "real life," or simulated real life, conditions. (Isn't it ironic that speech-language pathologists have fought so long for decent offices away from the noise of playground screams, only to discover now that perhaps the most important part of the treatment process must take place outside of that precious office domain!) Often this kind of procedure takes the form of individualized hierarchies of activities that are ordered according to the frequency of stuttering or the perceived "difficulty" of various speaking activities. Procedures that utilize trained parents, peers, spouses, or teachers as treatment agents in the client's natural environment are also examples of this principle, although they have not been reported very extensively in the literature.

Self-Management Procedures

Self-management techniques, categorized by Stokes and Baer (1977) as "mediating generalization," appear to have potential for facilitating across-settings generalization of stuttering treatment effects. For example, stuttering has been shown to decrease for some stutterers when moments of stuttering are self-recorded (Costello, 1975; R. Ingham, Adams, and Reynolds, 1978; La Croix, 1973). Further, James (1981) showed that an adult stutterer could learn to self-administer a brief time-out from talking in the clinic environment and to apply that same contingency to his stuttering in the natural environment, thus reducing stuttering under those conditions as well. Also, in a brief laboratory study, Martin and Haroldson (1982) demonstrated that self-administered time-out was associated with the maintenance of improved fluency, whereas the effects of externally administered time-out, which was equally powerful in reducing stuttering, were not maintained when the contingencies were removed. The encouraging results of self-management techniques are certainly not peculiar to stuttering treatments. Much of the behavioral literature is looking to these kinds of procedures to facilitate generalization and maintenance (cf. Koegel, Koegel, and Ingham, 1986).

Obviously, giving the capability, the choice, and the responsibility to the client, as is the case when self-management techniques are utilized, should facilitate carry-over into the natural environment, because the treatment then resides with the client. However, this raises an interesting question regarding what it is that is being generalized. That is, when an improved speech pattern is produced in the natural environment, is it that improved

‡ The reader who nonetheless yearns for examples of generalization-oriented procedures is encouraged to consult directly the 29 studies listed as including transfer phases in their treatments. A warning: be prepared for oftentimes sparse descriptions and the appearance of arbitrariness in task selection across studies.

speech pattern that is being generalized, or is it the use of the self-management technique that is being generalized? Further, if the client is, in fact, overtly or subliminally self-recording stuttering moments, or purposefully using a slightly slowed speech rate, or using self-applied stuttering-contingent time-out, or even simply concentrating on and monitoring speech production some significant portion of the time, can this rightly be said to be *generalization*? From the outside looking in, the result may appear to be clinically satisfactory, but is it what we mean by generalization? Is this an example of *no extratraining manipulations* being needed for extratraining changes, or perhaps *some extratraining manipulations of less cost and extent* being required (Stokes and Baer, 1977)? Or is it, in actuality, a way of maintaining a rather full-blown treatment regimen in the natural environment? In an analogous sense, the term *generalization* would not be used to describe what happens when a dysarthric patient with velopharyngeal insufficiency begins producing normal-sounding speech in the natural environment because of the use of a palatal lift. Could the ongoing use of self-management techniques be viewed as a stutterer's prosthesis? And if it turns out that some degree of these kinds of activities is essentially *always* required for the maintenance of stutter-free speech, might we ask if such a thing as generalization (in its clinically relevant, across-settings form) *ever* really occurs?

And, what about the case in which a client is taught self-management techniques in the clinical setting, yet improved fluency does not generalize to the natural environment? Which set of behaviors should be the target for continued treatment: fluency skills or the use of self-management techniques?

One possible solution to this issue that has not yet been explored in the literature (with the exception of the James [1981] study mentioned earlier) is that self-management skills, in the form of self-recording and/or self-consequation, could be introduced early in treatment. Most of the stuttering treatment literature addresses transfer activities as treatment steps that are tacked on to what was intended to be the end of treatment. Perhaps teaching clients from the beginning to recognize moments of stuttering and to present their own consequences for stuttered (and stutter-free) speech would be more likely to make self-monitoring an ingrained and automatic aspect of stutterers' behavior that would be readily and effortlessly available for use in the natural environment. (Perkins [1983a; 1983b; 1984] would suggest that it is *only* the stutterer who knows when a "real" moment of stuttering has occurred anyway.)

From a less behaviorally bound perspective, one might also speculate that an advantage of early opportunities to self-monitor might be that clients would be required to take responsibility for their own stuttering behavior and for its modification from the early stages of treatment. Perhaps the clinic-bound nature of the effects of stuttering treatment stems from the fact that clinicians take rather full command and responsibility for producing behavior change at the beginning of treatment. Then, when it becomes the client's turn, the ability to "do it on your own" has not been acquired. Under these conditions, the missing link between acquisition and generalization might not be an issue of stimulus control but one of cognition.

The potential role of cognitive factors is exemplified by recent interest in the concept of *locus of control* described earlier by Rotter (1966). Some very preliminary studies have indicated that the prediction of relapse following apparently successful stuttering treatment may be associated with whether clients, at the end of treatment, perceive their success as being the result of their own efforts and ability and thus under their personal control (internal locus of control), or whether they attribute their success to luck or to others, such as the clinician (external locus of control) (Craig and Andrews, 1985; Craig, Franklin, and Andrews, 1984; Craig and Howie, 1982). Of course, the problem that faces would-be researchers who wish to study this issue is how to operationalize the concept so that the phenomenon of the client's "taking control" can be measured in some valid and reliable fashion. We are certainly a long way from being able to do that at present, but there is interest in that direction, and it may prove fruitful.

ROLE OF THE METHOD USED TO ESTABLISH IMPROVED FLUENCY

Perhaps this is the time to raise the issue of the influence on generalization of the method used to establish stutter-free speech in the clinic. For adult stutterers, the most popular treatment procedure in use today is prolonged speech or one of its variants (e.g., Andrews, Howie, Dozsa, and Guitar, 1982; Boberg, 1976; Curlee and Perkins, 1969; Goldiamond, 1965; Ingham and Andrews, 1973, Perkins, 1973; Perkins et al, 1974; Resick et al, 1978; Ryan and Van Kirk, 1974; Webster, 1974), probably because these treatment procedures are best able to produce pervasive changes in the speech patterns of stutterers. On the other hand, because these techniques require a major change in the method of speech production, including extended phonation, slowed rate, gentle onset of phonation at voiceless-to-voiced transitions, breathstream management, and the like, it may be that such complicated behavior change is motorically difficult to produce and unlikely to become habitual very readily. That is, something in the nature of the required fluent behaviors may make them particularly resistant to generalization. However, when simpler methods of behavior change have been studied, none has been as effective for the adult stutterer. It may be the case, then, that whatever our future research may develop in the way of new transfer procedures, the generalization problem will remain as long as the crux of treatment requires new behavior patterns of this nature.

AGE OF THE STUTTERER AS A GENERALIZATION VARIABLE

Interestingly, a reliance on prolonged speech treatments has not seemed to be necessary for young stutterers. Although the literature is sparse, some of it is rather convincing in demonstrating that simple contingency management procedures not only are effective in establishing stutter-free speech for children in the clinic (Costello, 1983b) but also that their fluent speech generalizes spontaneously to the natural environment (Martin, Kuhl, and Haroldson, 1972; Reed and Godden, 1977; Ryan, 1971, 1974; Ryan and Van Kirk, 1983; Shaw and Shrum, 1972). Most young children do not appear to find the behavior change process as grueling as do older children and adults. If this finding is upheld in future research, our ultimate understanding of generalization will no doubt be affected. Why should it be that young children (most often, those under the age of 6 years or so) display powerful behavior change under simpler treatment regimens, and why is it that those treatment effects should rather easily generalize?

One model suggests that generalization is the reciprocal, or opposite, of discrimination, and that the way treatment is typically administered necessarily produces discrimination. That is, behavior is taught under one set of conditions (clinic room, clinician, arranged evoking stimuli, unnatural speaking tasks, and response-contingent reinforcers and punishers), and behavior thus becomes *discriminated* in that its occurrence is "hooked" to those conditions, i.e., it is under stimulus control. Because it is under stimulus control, or discriminated, by definition it cannot be generalized. This, of course, leads to the kinds of transfer activities described above, in which attempts are made to expand stimulus control by making stimuli from the natural environment discriminative for stutter-free utterances.

However, the question remains that if discrimination accounts for the absence of generalization in adult treatments, why does the same phenomenon not occur for children? Are we prepared to suggest that stimulus control is a weaker phenomenon for young children? That clinical stimuli are not particularly salient to them? That discriminated behaviors are more difficult for young children to acquire? These premises are doubtful, and studies of early childhood development would certainly seem not to support those contentions.

What, then, could account for generalized learning in children as opposed to adults? And how is this related to the oft-reported phenomenon of spontaneous recovery among children who stutter (Andrews and Harris, 1964; Cooper, 1972; Dickson, 1971; Martyn and Sheehan, 1968; Shearer and Williams, 1965; Sheehan, 1979; Wingate, 1964a; Young, 1975)? It appears that at least some proportion of children reported to "recover spontaneously" from stuttering come into contact with contingencies similar to those they would encounter in treatment, those contingencies being delivered by parents and other "significant others" in the children's environment (e.g., "slow down," "pay attention to what you're saying," "say that word again," etc.). It has been suggested (R. Ingham, 1976, 1983; Martin and Lindamood, 1986) that many reports of so-called spontaneous recovery could be attributed to such informal treatment. Were this to be so, such cases would add to the perception that stuttering behavior is easier to modify in young children than in adults. Perhaps where generalization is concerned, this suggests a model different from the discrimination–generalization reciprocity model elucidated above.

Such a model might reside in a motor learning perspective. Certainly the fashion in stuttering research these days is the conduct of studies aimed at demonstrating or discovering the role of motor or neuromotor (including genetic) variables (Cooper and Allen, 1977; Cross and Luper, 1979; Garber and Siegel, 1982; Kent, 1983, 1984; Kidd, 1984, MacKay and MacDonald, 1984; Moore and Haynes, 1980, Perkins, Bell, Johnson, and Stocks, 1979; Perkins, Rudas, Johnson, and Bell, 1976; Zimmermann, 1980). If stuttering were produced by a frail or slowly developing neuromuscular speech production system, might not this explain why some children spontaneously outgrow their stuttering as their developing systems become increasingly able to render the skills needed to speak fluently? And perhaps other children respond readily and broadly to varying degrees of treatment because stuttering has not become firmly entrenched in their speaking patterns, and their developing motor skills are still reasonably malleable.

On the other hand, for those who receive no treatment as children or for whom stuttering resists early treatment for some reason (probably as much for the quality of the treatment as for the intractability of the stuttering), perhaps stuttering becomes a deeply ingrained habitual motor pattern and therefore eventually requires a different and more powerful treatment. It would also make sense that a motor-based treatment (such as prolonged speech) would be appropriate for a motor-based behavior disorder.

AUTOMATIZATION AS A REPLACEMENT FOR GENERALIZATION

So, one might ask, what is the motor learning equivalent of generalization? It would appear to be what some (e.g., Manning and Shirkey, 1982; Ruscello, 1984; Wright, Shelton and Arndt, 1969) have called *automatization*. Broadly, this term refers to *the production of newly acquired behavior without effort or conscious control under a variety of conditions*.

If one is interested in attempting to assess the "automaticity" of speech perceived as fluent, the measurement of speech across a variety of conditions would seem to be required, just as has been described above for the assessment of generalization. In addition, it would be necessary to assess the amount of "effort and conscious control" used by a subject during speaking tasks. Problems inherent in developing valid operational definitions of these constructs do not seem to be discussed in the relevant (mostly theoretical) literature, but perhaps indirect measures such as the speed and naturalness of speech and subjects' reports of the degree of attention they pay to their speech production under various conditions would shed light on this feature of the definition.

The question then becomes, if one were to observe a treated stutterer speaking natural-sounding, stutter-free speech at normal speaking rates across a variety of "real life" speaking conditions, how could it be determined whether that goal was reached by generalization or automatization? The end product of the two processes appears identical. The answer might be found through periodic observations of behavior change over the course of treatment. Perhaps if behavior had been observed to change gradually across environments, and to change first under conditions that contained particular elements common to the treatment environment (i.e., to give the appearance of spreading stimulus control), one would be led to conclude that generalization had taken place. On the other hand, if behavior were observed to change with similar speed and degree across environments, as though some prerequisite degree of mastery had occurred, then the change might be attributed to automatization. Implicit in this distinction is the assumption that treatment aimed at producing generalization would be different from treatment aimed at producing automatization.

In a recent review of motor learning perspectives regarding speech production, Ruscello (1984, p.135) pointed out the salient features that characterize essentially all theories of skilled motor learning: "practice, stages of motor skill development, cognitive analysis, and feedback processes." Variations on these themes are central to most current stuttering therapies, even though generalization, rather than automatization, appears to be the underlying focus of those therapies. Of those four variables, the motor learning research universally regards *practice* as the dominant, critical feature, especially practice under varied conditions. Again, this describes much of present day stuttering treatment, which is designed to provide extensive stutter-free talking experience, in graded tasks, including transfer activities. From this perspective it could be suggested that the spread of newly acquired stutter-free speech from clinics to natural environments could be accounted for at least as well by automatization concepts as by generalization concepts. Especially when one considers that most transfer tasks are added onto the acquisition stage of treatment, one could hypothesize that the value of such treatment steps is the added amount of motor *practice* they afford, rather than the expanded stimulus control they provide. If it were to be the case that automatization principles, rather than generalization principles, were at the heart of behavior change in beyond-clinic conditions, then it would seem logical to suppose that treatment procedures that were purposely aimed at producing automatization might produce more widespread and enduring behavior change.

Treatment Based on Automatization Concepts

As has been alluded to above, many treatment activities found in current stuttering treatments could be considered automatization activities, especially transfer tasks that provide practice under varied conditions. However, one difference between treatment tasks motivated by automatization versus generalization concepts would appear to be the importance of beyond-clinic variables. That is, procedures that incorporate into treatment stimuli from the natural environment or arrange for elements of treatment to occur in the natural environment—the kinds of strategies typically employed during a transfer phase—seem to be unnecessary from an automatization perspective. Although practice of the kinds of behavior ultimately required of the learner is important in the mastery of a new motor skill, treatment with a motor skill focus would appear to concentrate on practice of speaking under varying motor conditions, rather than on practice of speaking under varying environmental or stimulus conditions, e.g., reading, conversation, fast speech, emotional or excited speech, speech on the telephone, speech that is interrupted, speech that is centered on familiar topics and unfamiliar topics, speech that commands, speech that requests, speech that questions, and so on. In short, automatization-oriented treatment would concentrate on practice aimed at *response generalization* rather than the *stimulus generalization* focus of most current therapies.

One place to look for guidance regarding the selection of therapy tasks that would facilitate automatization is in the theories of motor skill acquisition. However, for the most part, such theories of the development of "motor traces" (Adams, 1971) and "schema" (Marteniuk, 1976a, 1976b; Schmidt, 1975a, 1975b, 1976) and so forth are currently too abstract and untested to lead directly to treatment applications. Yet, most theories do have common threads, stated above by Ruscello (1984), from which therapeutic inferences can be drawn.

Practice of Correct Speech Production

The important role of motor practice has already been rather thoroughly discussed, and varieties of connected speech tasks in which stuttering clients could be engaged for practice were mentioned. Also, treatment geared toward rigorous motor learning could be introduced in earlier stages of therapy. One such tactic might be to increase mastery level performance requirements (pass criteria) early in the treatment program. For example, in early phases of a prolonged speech program, clients might be required to speak using stutter-free speech for 20 consecutive minutes rather than 5, or with no stuttering instead of some small amount of stuttering, or across three treatment sessions rather than just one. The rationale, obviously, is to build strong and resilient fluency skills early on.

Another tactic designed to establish robust motor skills, and suggested for this purpose in some of the articulation treatment literature (Bankson and Byrne, 1972; Kent and Lybolt, 1982), is development of a client's ability to retain stutter-free speech under increased speaking speeds. This is an especially interesting concept where stuttering treatment is concerned, because of the emphasis on slowed speech that pervades much of that treatment. Although reductions in speed of speech may be necessary to establish changed speaking patterns in many persons who stutter, permanently slowed speaking rates may not be the appropriate ultimate target. Treatment that provides practice in maintaining new speech patterns under unusually fast speaking rates may be what is needed to push the client beyond the use of labored speech that requires constant vigilance. (On the other hand, there is the risk that requiring stuttering clients to speak at fast speech rates beyond the motor capabilities of their hypothetically subnormal speech mechanisms could undo the progress obtained by the therapy to that point!)

Use of Stages of Motor Skill Development

As mentioned earlier, most popular stuttering treatments in use today are well abreast of this principle of behavior change, initiating treatment by requesting responses that are motorically and linguistically simple for the client and progressing gradually to more complex and authentic speaking tasks. Little more need be said about this, except to point out that the popular use of this principle indicates that much of current stuttering treatment has motor skill learning at its base, whether or not it is made explicit by those who designed the treatment programs.

Cognitive Analysis

Several motor skill theories stress the important role of the learner's cognitive participation in early, acquisition stages of treatment (Ruscello, 1984). Usually this means that it is important for the learner to have a clear understanding and perception (in the sensory meaning of the word) of the behavior required, such understanding and perception facilitating the client's mental planning, which precedes execution of the response. Although a good deal of such cognitive activity no doubt takes place (subvocally and therefore unobserved and unrecognized) in stuttering treatments, and different authors vary in the attention they pay to the importance of explaining and modeling target behaviors to child and adult clients, the systematic use of mental planning has not been a topic that has received much attention in the stuttering literature.

On the other hand, as reviewed above, the use of self-management activities has been studied in the stuttering literature and shown to have a positive influence on learning. These kinds of activities could be considered cognitive, although they have most often been directed toward the speaker's evaluation of his or her own speech performance after the fact (self-monitoring) rather than beforehand (mental planning). The connection between these two kinds of cognitive activities has not been established, but it seems logical to assume that they are closely linked. That is, the person whose emphasis has been on mental planning before the production of a response probably evaluates afterwards how well that response matched the plan, and the person who has concentrated on evaluation of the quality of a response following its production probably uses that information in planning how best to produce the next response.

It is interesting to note, however, that suggestions for moving newly acquired behavior performance levels from acquisition to automatization often include having the client produce the new behavior under conditions of "distraction." Recall that the definition of automatization requires behavior that is not under conscious control. The kind of mental planning and self-management activities described above would seem to be diametrically opposed to this aspect of automatization. Although such cognitive activities may be required during the acquisition of a new behavior, they must eventually be eliminated before those behaviors can be considered "automatic." It is not unusual to observe a decrease in stutter-free speech when clients first begin using their new speech pattern in conversational speech, presumably because they have difficulty determining *what* they want to say as well as *how* they want to say it. Perhaps this is an example of a talking task conducted under conditions of distraction.

If considerable parts of stuttering treatments are designed, purposefully or inadvertently, to require the speaker's utmost attention to speech production, perhaps later stages of treatment need to be designed to reduce that reliance on cognition. Therefore, the addition of tasks that require the maintenance of stutter-free speech under conditions of distraction would seem to be mandatory (e.g., talking with a radio news broadcast in the background, talking while engaged in a complex motor task such as assembling a model car, answering questions while concentrating on reading a newspaper article).[§]

Use of Feedback Processes

Feedback is a significant component of essentially all theories of motor skill learning. As well, it is a significant component of essentially all effective stuttering treatments and a basic principle of behavior change (i.e., the application of reinforcement and punishment contingencies). However, stuttering treatments tend to rely on externally presented feedback (usually from a clinician), whereas theories of motor skill learning refer primarily to a speaker's internal, sensory feedback system. Kent and Lybolt (1982), proponents of Schmidt's (1975a; 1975b; 1976) schema theory, say it this way:

> The schema ... generates the expected sensory consequences (feedback) for the motor act to be performed, that is, *what the feedback should be*. The *expected* sensory consequences are compared against the *actual* sensory consequences to derive an error signal. The error signal is used to adjust and refine the schema. In this way, the schema is gradually refined until it can cope with many variations in goals and instantaneous conditions (pp. 13–14).

Although clinician-delivered feedback may be appropriate and even mandatory in the acquisition stages of treatment, and passing that feedback responsibility from the clinician to the client through the use of self-management techniques would seem to advance the process further, automatization appears to occur only when neither kind of feedback—clinician-presented or self-presented—is relied upon any longer by the speaker. Several of the tasks described above, such as fast speech, emotional speech, and talking under conditions of distrac-

[§] It is interesting to note that distraction has been suggested as an explanation for why certain conditions reduce the occurrence of stuttering (Bloodstein, 1987, pp. 269–278), quite a different perspective than that presented here.

tion, are tasks that might prevent the occurrence of self-evaluation. If clinician feedback were also withheld (e.g., by requiring clients to engage in tasks in the absence of the clinician), perhaps these kinds of activities could serve as treatment tasks that would contribute to automatization. Additionally, covert assessments of client's speaking performance under varying naturalistic conditions would prevent the influence of clinician-presented feedback and the reactivity of speaking tasks that the client knows are being conducted for clinical purposes.

The assessment of automatization is, of course, a matter of concern. All of the criteria described earlier for judging whether new speech patterns have generalized are equally necessary for judging whether automatization has occurred. However, although speaker's reports are relevant, and judgments of naturalness might be too, there is really no infallible way of knowing when speakers are self-monitoring or using other forms of effort or conscious control. Ultimately, measures of automatization will fall short in this domain. Nonetheless, the kinds of treatment tasks stimulated by viewing the business of treatment from a motor learning automatization perspective may lead to behavior change that will meet the standards set by these criteria.

CONCLUSIONS

This chapter has sought to review, within the confines of stuttering treatment, the concepts of across-settings generalization and automatization, comparing and contrasting the principles that underlie each construct, the nature of the treatment activities each would dictate, and the characteristics required for their assessment. The overlapping nature of these two concepts may effectively prevent their independent analysis. Nonetheless, on the face of it they seem sufficiently different that the systematic study of each would be appropriate. Clinically, at this stage all that can be hoped is that clinicians, understanding the somewhat different theories underlying these two phenomena, will utilize that knowledge to develop creditable treatment regimens for their clients and bolster those treatments with rigorous measurements to assess their adequacy. In the meantime, researchers will, no doubt, continue their study of the phenomena that produce widespread and durable behavior change and will eventually provide the facts needed to harness those phenomena for clinical application.

REFERENCES

Adams JA. A closed-loop theory of motor learning. J Motor Behav 1971; 3:111–145.

Andrews G, Feyer AM. Does behavior therapy still work when the experimenters depart? An analysis of a behavioral treatment program for stuttering. Behav Modif 1985; 9:443–457.

Andrews G, Guitar B, Howie P. Meta-analysis of the effects of stuttering treatment. J Speech Hear Disord 1980; 45: 287–307.

Andrews G, Harris M. The syndrome of stuttering. Clinical Developmental Medicine, London: Heinemann, 1964: 17.

Andrews G, Howie PM, Dozsa M, Guitar BE. Stuttering: speech pattern characteristics under fluency-inducing conditions. J Speech Hear Res 1982; 25:208–216.

Andrews G, Ingham RJ. An approach to the evaluation of stuttering therapy. J Speech Hear Res 1972a; 15:296–302.

Andrews G, Ingham RJ. Stuttering: an evaluation of follow-up procedures for syllable-timed speech/token system therapy. J Commun Disord 1972b; 5:307–319.

Andrews G, Tanner S. Stuttering treatment: an attempt to replicate the regulated-breathing method. J Speech Hear Disord 1982a; 47:138–140.

Andrews G, Tanner S. Stuttering: the result of 5 days of treatment with an airflow technique. J Speech Hear Disord 1982b; 47:427–429.

Azrin NH, Nunn RG. A rapid method of eliminating stuttering by a regulated breathing approach. Behav Res Ther 1974; 12:279–286.

Azrin NH, Nunn RG, Frantz SE. Comparison of regulated breathing versus abbreviated desensitization on reported stuttering episodes. J Speech Hear Disord 1979; 44:331–339.

Bankson NW, Byrne MC. The effect of a timed-correct sound production task on carryover. J Speech Hear Res 1972; 15:160–168.

Beattie MS. A behaviour therapy programme for stuttering. Br J Disord Commun 1973; 8:120–130.

Bloodstein O. A handbook of stuttering. 4th ed. Chicago: Easter Seal Society, 1987.

Boberg E. Intensive group therapy program for stutterers. Hum Commun 1976; 1:29–42.

Boberg E. Intensive adult therapy program. Semin Speech Lang Hear 1980; 1:365–373.

Boberg E, ed. The maintenance of fluency. New York: Elsevier, 1981.

Boberg E, Howie P, Woods L. Maintenance of fluency: a review. J Fluency Disord 1979; 4:93–116.

Boberg I, Sawyer L. The maintenance of fluency following intensive therapy. Hum Commun 1977; 2:21–28.

Brutten EJ, Shoemaker DJ. The modification of stuttering. Englewood Cliffs, NJ: Prentice Hall, 1967.

Budd KS, Madison LS, Itzkowitz JS, Price HA. Parents and therapists as allies in behavioral treatment of children's stuttering. Behav Ther 1986; 17:538–553.

Condit L. The measurement and facilitation of generalization in a young stutterer. Master's thesis. University of California, Santa Barbara, 1987.

Cooper E. Recovery from stuttering in a junior and senior high school population. J Speech Hear Res 1972; 15:632–638.

Cooper MH, Allen GD. Timing control accuracy in normal speakers and stutterers. J Speech Hear Res 1977; 20:55–71.

Coppola VA, Yairi E. Rhythmic speech training with preschool stuttering children: an experimental study. J Fluency Disord 1982; 7:447–457.

Costello JM. The establishment of fluency with time-out procedures: three case studies. J Speech Hear Disord 1975; 40:216–231.

Costello JM. Programmed instruction. J Speech Hear Disord 1977; 42:3–28.

Costello JM. Operant conditioning and the treatment of stuttering. Semin Speech Lang Hear 1980; 1:311–325.

Costello JM. Techniques of therapy based on operant theory. In: Perkins WH, ed. Current therapy of communication disorders. General principles of therapy. New York: Brian C. Decker Division of Thieme-Stratton, 1982:3.

Costello JM. Generalization across-settings: language intervention with children. In: Yoder D, Miller J, Schiefelbusch RL, eds. Language intervention. ASHA Reports No. 12. Rockville:The American Speech-Language-Hearing Association, 1983a:275.

Costello JM. Current behavioral treatments for children. In: Prins D, Ingham RJ, eds. Treatment of stuttering in early childhood: methods and issues. San Diego: College-Hill Press, 1983b:69.

Costello J, Bosler S. Generalization and articulation instruction. J Speech Hear Disord 1976; 41:359–373.

Costello JM, Hurst MR. An analysis of the relationship among stuttering behaviors. J Speech Hear Res 1981; 24:247–256.

Costello JM, Ingham RJ. Assessment strategies for stuttering. In: Curlee RF, Perkins WH, eds. Nature and treatment of stuttering: new directions. San Diego: College-Hill Press, 1984:303.

Cote C, Ladouceur R. Effects of social aids and the regulated breathing method in the treatment of stutterers. J Consult Clin Psychol 1982; 50:450.

Craig A, Andrews G. The prediction and prevention of relapse in stuttering: the value of self-control techniques and locus of control measures. Behav Modif 1985; 9:427–442.

Craig A, Cleary PJ. Reduction of stuttering by young male stutterers using EMG feedback. Biofeedback Self Regul 1982; 7:241–255.

Craig A, Franklin JA, Andrews G. A scale to measure locus of control of behavior. Br J Med Psychol 1984; 57:173–180.

Craig A, Howie PM. Locus of control and maintenance of behavioural therapy skills. Br J Clin Psychol 1982; 21:65–66.

Craven DC, Ryan BP. The use of a portable delayed auditory feedback unit in stuttering therapy. J Fluency Disord 1984; 9:237–243.

Cross DE, Luper HL. Voice reaction time of stuttering and nonstuttering children. J Fluency Disord 1979; 4:661–668.

Crowder JE, Harbin R. The effect of punishment on stuttering: a case study. Psychother Theor Res Pract 1971; 8:179–180.

Curlee R. Observer agreement on disfluency and stuttering. J Speech Hear Res 1981; 24:595–600.

Curlee RF, Perkins WH. Conversational rate control therapy for stuttering. J Speech Hear Disord 1969; 4:245–250.

Dickson S. Incipient stuttering and spontaneous remission of stuttered speech. J Commun Disord 1971; 4:99–110.

Eysenck HJ. An exercise in mega-silliness. Am Psychol 1978; 33:517.

Florance CL, Shames GH. Stuttering treatment: issues in transfer and maintenance. Semin Speech Lang Hear 1980; 1:375–388.

Fowler SC, Ingham RJ. Stuttering treatment rating recorder (software). Santa Barbara: University of California, 1986.

Garber SR, Siegel GM. Feedback and motor control in stuttering. In: Routh DK, ed. Learning speech, and the complex effects of punishment. New York: Plenum Press, 1982:93.

Goldiamond I. Stuttering and fluency as manipulable operant response classes. In: Krasner L, Ullman LP, eds. Research in behavior modification. New York: Holt, Rinehart, & Winston, 1965:106.

Gregory HH. An assessment of the results of stuttering therapy. J Commun Disord 1972; 5:320–334.

Guitar BE. Reduction of stuttering frequency using analog electromyographic feedback. J Speech Hear Res 1976; 18:672–685.

Hee JC, Holmes PA. Elimination of stuttering by a regulated breathing approach. J Commun Pathol 1976; 8:40–44.

Herscovitch A, LeBow MD. Imaginal pacing in the treatment of stuttering. Behav Ther Exp Psychiatr 1973; 4:357–360.

Howie PM, Tanner S, Andrews G. Short and long-term outcome in an intensive treatment program for adult stutterers. J Speech Hear Disord 1981; 46:104–109.

Howie PM, Woods CL, Andrews G. Relationship between covert and overt speech measures immediately before and immediately after stuttering treatment. J Speech Hear Disord 1982; 47:419–422.

Ingham RJ. A comparison of covert and overt assessment procedures in stuttering therapy outcome evaluation. J Speech Hear Res 1975; 18:346–354.

Ingham RJ. "Onset, prevalence, and recovery from stuttering": a reassessment of findings from the Andrews and Harris study. J Speech Hear Disord 1976; 41:280–281.

Ingham RJ. Modification of maintenance and generalization in stuttering treatment. J Speech Hear Res 1980; 23:732–745.

Ingham RJ. Evaluation and maintenance in stuttering treatment: a search for ecstasy with nothing but agony. In: Boberg E, ed. Maintenance of fluency. New York: Elsevier, 1981:179.

Ingham RJ. The effects of self-evaluation training on maintenance and generalization during stuttering treatment. J Speech Hear Disord 1982; 47:271–230.

Ingham RJ. Spontaneous remission of stuttering: when will the Emperor realize he has no clothes on? In: Prins D, Ingham RJ, eds. Treatment of stuttering in early childhood: methods and issues. San Diego: College-Hill Press, 1983:113.

Ingham RJ. Stuttering and behavior therapy: current status and experimental foundations. San Diego: College-Hill Press, 1984a.

Ingham RJ. Generalization and maintenance of treatment. In: Curlee RF, Perkins WH, eds. Nature and treatment of stuttering: new directions. San Diego: College-Hill Press, 1984b:447.

Ingham RJ. Stuttering treatment generalization. Paper presented at the Annual Convention of the American Speech-Language-Hearing Association, Detroit, November, 1986.

Ingham RJ, Adams S, Reynolds G. The effects on stuttering of self-recording the frequency of stuttering or the word "the." J Speech Hear Res 1978; 21:459–469.

Ingham RJ, Andrews G. Details of a token economy stuttering therapy programme for adults. Aust J Hum Commun Disord 1973; 1:13–20.

Ingham RJ, Costello JM. Stuttering treatment outcome evaluation. In: Costello JM, ed. Speech disorders in children: recent advances. San Diego: College-Hill Press, 1984:313.

Ingham RJ, Gow M, Costello JM. Stuttering and speech naturalness: some additional data. J Speech Hear Disord 1985; 50:217–219.

Ingham RJ, Martin RR, Haroldson SK, et al. Modification of listener-judged naturalness in the speech of stutterers. J Speech Hear Res 1985; 28:495–504.

Ingham RJ, Onslow M. Measurement and modification of speech-naturalness during stuttering therapy. J Speech Hear Disord 1985; 50:261–281.

Ingham RJ, Onslow M. Generalization and maintenance of treatment benefits for children who stutter. Semin Speech Lang 1987; 8:303–326.

Ingham RJ, Packman A. Treatment and generalization effects in an experimental treatment for a stutterer using contingency management and speech rate control. J Speech Hear Disord 1977; 42:394–407.

James JE. Behavioral self-control of stuttering using time-out from speaking. J Appl Behav Anal 1981; 14:25–37.

Kent RD. Facts about stuttering: neuropsychologic perspectives. J Speech Hear Disord 1983; 48:249–255.

Kent RD. Stuttering as a temporal programming disorder. In:

Curlee RF, Perkins WH, eds. Nature and treatment of stuttering: new directions. San Diego: College-Hill Press, 1984:283.

Kent RD, Lybolt JT. Techniques of therapy based on motor learning theory. In: Perkins WH, ed. Current therapy of communication disorders. General principles of therapy. New York: Thieme-Stratton, 1982:13.

Kidd KK. Stuttering as a genetic disorder. In: Curlee RF, Perkins WH, eds. Nature and treatment of stuttering: new directions. San Diego: College-Hill Press, 1984:149.

Koegel LK, Koegel RL, Ingham JC. Programming rapid generalization of correct articulation through self-monitoring procedures. J Speech Hear Disord 1986; 51:24–32.

Koegel RL, Rincover A. Research on the difference between generalization and maintenance in extra-therapy responding. J Appl Behav Anal 1977; 10:1–12.

LaCroix Z. Management of disfluent speech through self-recording procedures. J Speech Hear Disord 1973; 38:272–274.

MacDonald JD, Martin RR. Stuttering and disfluency as two reliable and unambiguous response classes. J Speech Hear Res 1973; 17:691–699.

MacKay DG, McDonald MC. Stuttering as a sequencing and timing disorder. In: Curlee RF, Perkins WH, eds. Nature and treatment of stuttering: new directions. San Diego: College-Hill Press, 1984:261.

Manning WH, Shirkey EA. Determining articulatory automatization of newly learned sounds. In: Lass NJ, ed. Speech and language: advances in basic research and practice. Vol. 7. New York: Academic Press, 1982:127.

Marshall RC, Starch SA. Behavioral treatment of acquired stuttering. Aust J Human Commun Disord 1984; 12:87–92.

Marteniuk RG. Information processing in motor skills. New York: Hold, Rinehart, & Winston, 1976a.

Marteniuk RG. Cognitive information processes in motor short-term memory and movement production. In: Stelmach GE, ed. Motor control: issues and trends. New York: Academic Press, 1976b:175.

Martin RR, Haroldson SK. Stuttering identification: standard definition and moment of stuttering. J Speech Hear Res 1981; 24:59–63.

Martin RR, Haroldson SK. Contingent self-stimulation for stuttering. J Speech Hear Disord 1982; 47:407–413.

Martin RR, Haroldson SK, Triden KA. Stuttering and speech naturalness. J Speech Hear Disord 1984; 49:53–58.

Martin RR, Kuhl P, Haroldson SK. An experimental treatment with two preschool stuttering children. J Speech Hear Res 1972; 15:743–752.

Martin RR, Lindamood LP. Stuttering and spontaneous recovery: implications for the speech-language pathologist. Language, Speech, and Hearing Services in Schools 1986; 17:207–218.

Martyn M, Sheehan J. Onset of stuttering and recovery. Behav Res Ther 1968; 6:295–307.

Moore WH Jr, Haynes WO. Alpha hemispheric asymmetry and stuttering: some support for a segmentation dysfunction hypothesis. J Speech Hear Res 1980; 23:229–248.

Perkins WH. Replacement of stuttering with normal speech: II. Clinical procedures. J Speech Hear Disord 1973; 38:295–303.

Perkins WH. Onset of stuttering: the case of the missing block. In: Prins D, Ingham RJ, eds. Treatment of stuttering in early childhood: methods and issues. San Diego: College-Hill Press, 1983a:1.

Perkins WH. The problem of definition. Commentary on "stuttering." J Speech Hear Disord 1983b; 48:246–249.

Perkins WH. Stuttering as a categorical event: barking up the wrong tree—reply to Wingate. J Speech Hear Disord 1984; 49:431–434.

Perkins WH, Bell J, Johnson L, Stocks J. Phone rate and the effective planning time hypothesis of stuttering. J Speech Hear Res 1979; 22:747–755.

Perkins WH, Rudas J, Johnson L, Bell J. Stuttering: discoordination of phonation with articulation and respiration. J Speech Hear Res 1976; 19:509–522.

Perkins WH, Rudas J, Johnson L, et al. Replacement of stuttering with normal speech: III. Clinical effectiveness. J Speech Hear Disord 1974; 39:416–428.

Peters AD. The effect of positive reinforcement on fluency: two case studies. Language, Speech, and Hearing Services in Schools 1977; 8:15–22.

Prins D. Improvement and regression in stutterers following short-term intensive therapy. J Speech Hear Disord 1970; 35:123–135.

Ramig PR, Wallace ML. Indirect and combined direct–indirect therapy in a disfluent child. J Fluency Disord 1987; 12:41–50.

Reed CG, Godden AL. An experimental treatment using verbal punishment with two preschool stutterers. J Fluency Disord 1977; 2:225–233.

Resick PA, Wendiggensen P, Ames S, Meyers V. Systematic slowed speech: a new treatment for stuttering. Behav Res and Ther 1978; 16:161–167.

Rickard HC, Mundy MB. Direct manipulation of stuttering behavior: an experimental clinical approach. In: Ullman LP, Krasner L, eds. Case studies in behavior modification. New York: Holt, Rinehart, & Winston, 1965:268.

Riley GD, Riley J. A component model for diagnosing and treating children who stutter. J Fluency Disord 1979; 4:279–293.

Riley GD, Riley J. Evaluation as a basis for treatment. In: Prins D, Ingham RJ, eds. Treatment of stuttering in early childhood: methods and issues. San Diego: College-Hill Press, 1983:43.

Riley GD, Riley J. A component model for treating stuttering in children. In: Peins M, ed. Contemporary approaches in stuttering therapy. Boston: Little, Brown, 1984:123.

Rockman BK, Elbert M. Generalization in articulation training. In: Winitz H, ed. Treating articulation disorders: for clinicians by clinicians. Baltimore: University Park Press, 1984:131.

Rotter JB. Generalized expectancies for internal versus external control of reinforcement. Psychol Monogr 1966; 80:1–28.

Ruscello DM. Motor learning as a model for articulation instruction. In: Costello JM, ed. Speech disorders in children: recent advances. San Diego: College-Hill Press, 1984:129.

Rustin L, Kuhr A. The treatment of stammering: a multi-modal approach in an in-patient setting. Br J Disord Commun 1983; 18:91–98.

Ryan BP. Operant procedures applied to stuttering therapy for children. J Speech Hear Disord 1971; 36:264–280.

Ryan BP. Programmed therapy for stuttering children and adults. Springfield:CV Thomas, 1974.

Ryan BP. Stuttering therapy in a framework of operant conditioning and programmed learning. In: Gregory HH, ed. Controversies about stuttering therapy. Baltimore: University Park Press, 1979:129.

Ryan BP, Van Kirk B. The establishment, transfer, and maintenance of fluent speech in 50 stutterers using delayed auditory feedback and operant procedures. J Speech Hear Disord 1974; 39:3–10.

Ryan BP, Van Kirk B. Programmed stuttering therapy for children: comparison of four establishment programs. J Fluency Disord 1983; 8:291–321.

Schmidt RA. Motor skills. New York: Harper & Row, 1975a.

Schmidt RA. A schema theory of discrete motor skill learning. Psychol Rev 1975b; 82:225–260.

Schmidt RA. The schema as a solution to some persistent problems in motor learning theory. In: Stelmach G, ed. Motor control: issues and trends. New York: Academic Press, 1976:41.

Shaw C, Shrum W. The effects of response-contingent reward on the connected speech of children who stutter. J Speech Hear Disord 1972; 37:75–88.

Shearer W, Williams J. Self-recovery from stuttering. J Speech Hear Disord 1965; 30:288–290.

Sheehan J. Current issues on stuttering and recovery. In: Gregory HH, ed. Controversies about stuttering therapy. Baltimore: University Park Press, 1979:175.

Shine R. Direct management of the beginning stutterer. Semin Speech Lang Hear 1980; 1:339–350.

Small MM. Treatment of stuttering: a case history. Percept Mot Skills 1975; 41:812.

Stokes TF, Baer DM. An implicit technology of generalization. J Appl Behav Anal 1977; 10:349–367.

Turnbaugh KR, Guitar BE. Short-term intensive stuttering treatment in a public school setting. Language, Speech, and Hearing Services in Schools 1981; 12:107–114.

Wakaba YY. Group play therapy for Japanese children who stutter. J Fluency Disord 1983; 8:93–118.

Webster RL. A behavioral analysis of stuttering: treatment and theory. In: Calhoun KS, Adams HE, Mitchell KM, eds. Innovative treatment methods in psychopathology. New York: John Wiley & Sons, 1974:17.

Webster RL. Empirical considerations regarding stuttering therapy. In: Gregory HH, ed. Controversies about stuttering therapy. Baltimore: University Park Press, 1979:209.

Webster RL. Evolution of a target-based behavioral therapy for stuttering. J Fluency Disord 1980; 5:303–320.

Wingate ME. Recovery from stuttering. J Speech Hear Disord 1964a; 29:312–321.

Wingate ME. A standard definition of stuttering. J Speech Hear Disord 1964b; 29:484–489.

Wolf MM. Social validity: the case for subjective measurement or how applied behavior analysis is finding its heart. J Appl Behav Anal 1978; 11:203–214.

Wright V, Shelton R, Arndt W. A task for evaluation of articulation change. III. Imitative task scores compared with scores for more spontaneous tasks. J Speech Hear Res 1969; 12:875–884.

Young MA. Observer agreement: cumulative effects of repeated ratings of the same samples and of knowledge of group results. J Speech Hear Res 1969; 12:144–155.

Young MA. Onset, prevalence, and recovery from stuttering. J Speech Hear Disord 1975; 40:49–58.

Zimmermann GN. Articulatory behavior associated with stuttering: a cineradiographic analysis. J Speech Hear Disord 1980; 23:108–121.

Chapter Six

GENERALIZATION IN THE TREATMENT OF APHASIA

CYNTHIA K. THOMPSON, Ph.D.

This chapter addresses generalization issues relevant to the treatment of aphasia. It provides a brief definition of aphasia and presents a framework for discussing the language problems and deficit patterns that are seen in the disorder. The importance of generalization in treatment of aphasia is also addressed, and based on a review of treatment research in aphasia, problems and variables related to facilitating both response generalization and stimulus generalization are discussed. Finally, suggestions for facilitating generalization in treatment of aphasia are presented, along with examples from relevant clinical research studies.

THE DISORDER

Aphasia is a complex disorder that has been defined and described from a variety of viewpoints (Benson, 1975, 1979; Benson and Geschwind, 1971; Berndt and Caramazza, 1981; Darley, 1982; Davis, 1983; Jackson, 1958; Lesser, 1979; Sidman, 1971; Sidman, Stoddard, Mohr, and Leicester, 1971; Wertz, 1985). Although it is beyond the scope of this chapter to provide more than a rudimentary understanding of aphasia and behaviors characterizing the disorder, most authorities, regardless of their theoretical orientation, are in agreement that a definition of aphasia comprises at least three basic components. First, aphasia is an acquired disorder; i.e., it occurs after language has been learned. Second, aphasia is a result of brain damage affecting areas of the brain that are involved in language. Third, aphasia is a language disorder resulting in impairment in speaking, writing, listening, or reading; in some cases, a diminishment of nonverbal communicative behaviors such as pantomime (Duffy and Duffy, 1981) is also evident.

Theorists attempting to explain the nature of the language disorder or the language disruption seen in aphasia have discussed aphasia as a loss of aspects of language and a disruption in processing linguistic units. Observations that language functioning is variable in aphasic persons, and that language expression and comprehension can be enhanced by using cues or other stimulation techniques have served to substantiate the belief that language elements remain stored within the brain in aphasic individuals; that is, they appear not to be "lost." These and other observations, coupled with knowledge that the aphasic individual mastered language prior to brain damage, have led many aphasiologists to believe that aphasia is a disorder reflecting a disruption (interference) or a reduction in efficiency of processing or "accessing" language elements, which is caused by alteration in language access mechanisms.

According to this conception, recovery from aphasia requires repair of language processing and retrieval mechanisms, and with this repair linguistic behaviors would be recovered. Accordingly, generalization would be expected as a natural outcome of treatment. This is a very simplistic explanation of a very complex subject, but this thinking, as pointed out by Kearns (1980), has had a major influence on our approach to language rehabilitation and treatment of aphasia. Many treatments for aphasia focus on decreasing language processing interference or on circumvention of disordered mechanisms through stimulation, facilitation, and other techniques intended to improve access to language. Because generalization is an expected by-product of these types of aphasia treatment, direct measurement of the generalization effects of intervention has not often been addressed.

Aphasic Behaviors

Numerous behaviors or symptoms of aphasia have been described in detail elsewhere (David, 1983; Johns, 1985; McNeil, in press; Sarno, 1981). These behaviors are traditionally discussed in terms of modality-specific deficits: spoken language, written language, auditory comprehension, and reading.

Spoken language deficiencies seen in aphasic individuals range from naming deficits to difficulty in production of sentences. Naming or word retrieval deficits may take many forms. These include literal, verbal, and neologistic *paraphasias* or word substitutions, and circumlocution in which the patient talks around a particular word, providing descriptions, definitions, and other information about the word he is attempting to say. In addition, word retrieval difficulty may be manifest by lengthy pauses between words, self-corrections, and other behaviors. Problems pertaining to production of morphological structures and sentences include agrammatism and paragrammatism. *Agrammatism* refers to sentence productions described as nonfluent, in which nouns and main verbs are preserved while functor words, such as articles and prepositions, and morphological structures are missing. Conversely, *paragrammatic sentence production* is fluent and complete but often unintelligible because sentence elements are incorrect and paraphasic. There are many other spoken language problems seen in aphasic patients, such as *stereotypic utterances* (production of strings of nonsensical words or repeated production of real words or phrases), *"perseverative" responding* (e.g., production of the same word over and over in naming a set of pictures), and others.

Aphasic writing problems are often similar to problems seen in spoken language and are referred to as *agraphia* or *dysgraphia*. Writing errors may be evident in single words or sentences and include grapheme errors called *literal paragraphias* and semantic errors called *verbal paragraphias*. As with agrammatism and paragrammatism of spoken language, writing responses may be laboriously executed and reduced in length and complexity, or they may be fluent and illegible or jargonistic, referred to as *jargonagraphia* (Lecours and Rouillon, 1976).

Auditory and reading comprehension deficits are also seen in aphasic patients and are somewhat more difficult to describe, because they cannot be directly observed. These deficits are inferred by observations of inappropriate or inaccurate responses to verbal or written words, sentences, or paragraphs. For example, aphasic patients may have difficulty following commands or responding to questions presented auditorily or in written form. Through careful presentation of stimuli that vary in content, length, and complexity, auditory and reading comprehension problems are identified. Specific auditory comprehension problems such as slow rise time (inferred when the initial portions of an auditory stimulus are responded to inaccurately), noise buildup (inferred when later portions of an auditory message are responded to inaccurately), and others may be identified (Brookshire, 1974, 1978). Reading comprehension problems (acquired dyslexia) may also be noted, such as *surface dyslexia* or *deep dyslexia*. For example, when asked to select a word that goes with a picture, the aphasic patient who selects a word that sounds like the target has made a surface dyslexic error, whereas the aphasic patient who selects a word that is semantically similar to the target has made a deep dyslexic error. Reading deficits may also be noted in oral reading. These errors are referred to as *paralexias* and are so labeled when either phonemic or semantic errors or both are noted in oral reading tasks.

As can be seen, a number of behaviors are symptomatic of aphasia. Readers interested in an in-depth understanding of behaviors characteristic of aphasia may consult any of a number of excellent texts (Brown, 1981; Davis, 1983; Johns, 1985; Kean, 1985; McNeil, 1988: Sarno, 1981). However, it is important to note here that the occurrence of aphasic behaviors is strongly related to the conditions under which they are observed and that variability both within and among patients is common. For example, an aphasic patient may produce certain words when presented with picture stimuli but may not produce these words in conversation, and vice versa. In addition, the aphasic patient may produce certain language elements or give evidence of good auditory comprehension on some days but not others. He may also have trouble understanding or talking to some people but not to others. Head pointed out the following in 1926, and it remains true: "It is a common observation in the best observed cases that on certain days tasks could be executed with ease, which were otherwise quite impossible. Familiar surroundings, friendly people...and the mode of examination have a profound effect on the results obtained." (p. 83). Finally, the pattern of communication deficit and the severity of aphasia vary from individual to individual, and aphasic patients often present with a variety of associated problems, such as apraxia of speech, which add to the complexity of the aphasic syndrome.

IMPORTANCE OF GENERALIZATION

Generalization is an important and often overlooked aspect of aphasia treatment. As pointed out by Warren, Rogers-Warren, Baer, and Guess (1980), effective treatment entails two processes: first, establishing the behaviors; and second, ensuring generalization and maintenance of trained behaviors. Two forms of generalization are important in the treatment of aphasia: response generalization and stimulus generalization. *Response generalization* refers to the occurrence of untrained language responses as a result of training other responses. For example, when an aphasic patient, trained to produce a set of question responses, begins to produce untrained questions, then response generalization has occurred. *Stimulus generalizaton* refers to the transfer of trained behaviors to stimulus conditions that differ from those in which training takes place (Guess, Keogh, and Sailor, 1978). When a patient, trained to produce question responses in the language clinic, begins to produce question responses outside the clinic environment, then stimulus generalization has occurred. Generalization is an essential component of treatment. If response generalization does not occur as a result of treatment, then, in theory, we must endeavor to train all responses that the aphasic patient will ever use. If stimulus generalization does not occur, our treatment may be deemed unsatisfactory, because it is this carry-over of responding from the clinic to natural settings that is the goal of treatment.

APHASIA GENERALIZATION RESEARCH

Basic Requirements for Investigation of Generalization

There are several requirements for investigation of generalization. As in all treatment research, it is necessary that well-controlled experimental research designs be employed, that subject variables, behaviors under study, and treatment methods employed be precisely described, and that interobserver reliability be calculated and reported (McReynolds and Kearns, 1983; McReynolds and Thompson, 1986). Further, in investigations of generalization, testing conditions or probes need to be designed to measure the extent of generalization, and the measures need to be administered throughout treatment so that generalization can be evaluated on a continuous basis.

The generalization probe measures used depend on whether response generalization or stimulus generalization is being investigated, although it is sometimes difficult to separate these aspects of generalization. That is, when response generalization is tested, auditory or visual stimuli not used in treatment are often employed. For example, when the response generalization effects of naming training are assessed, a set of untrained pictures may be selected to elicit untrained naming responses. In a strict sense, this practice provides a measure of stimulus generalization, because nontraining stimuli are used to assess responding. Similar confusion occurs when stimulus generalization is assessed. For example, in testing production of trained responses across settings, responses produced that are similar, but not identical, to those trained (e.g., incomplete) may be considered as evidence of stimulus generalization.

Response generalization probes should be designed to sample a number of responses similar to those trained. Studies in aphasia have examined response generalization by training behaviors such as specific naming responses (Helmick and Wipplinger, 1975; Thompson and Kearns, 1981; Weigel-Crump and Koenigsknecht, 1973) or production of particular sentence types (Doyle, Goldstein, and Bourgeois, 1987; Holland and Levy, 1971; Kearns and Salmon, 1984; Shewan, 1976; Thompson and McReynolds, 1986; Wambaugh and Thompson, in press; Weigel-Crump, 1976), while testing responses to untrained items within or across defined parameters. For example, Weigel-Crump and Koenigsknecht (1973) trained anomic aphasic subjects to name selected items in four superordinate categories: household items, clothing, living things, and action words. Generalization to untrained items in these categories and to items in another category (foods) was tested, with results indicating generalization to items within and across categories.

Aphasia studies examining stimulus generalization have selected behaviors for training such as sentence production (Doyle, Goldstein, and Bourgeois, 1987; Kearns and Salmon, 1984; Thompson and McReynolds, 1986), auditory comprehension (Burger and Wertz, 1984), or situation-specific responses including food requests and social conventions (Thompson and Byrne, 1984; Thompson and Warner, 1987); and measured generalization in nontreatment conditions in which the responses might be expected to occur. For example, Doyle, Goldstein, and Bourgeois (1987) trained agrammatic aphasic patients to produce specific sentence types from the Helm Elicited Language Program for Syntax Stimulation (HELPSS; Helm-Estabrooks, 1981), while measuring generalization of trained forms in novel stimulus conditions. That is, after comparative sentence training, subjects were presented with pairs of objects such as two boxes and told "this one is big (pointing to the smaller of the two); tell me about this one" (pointing to the larger of the two)" (p. 155).

Published Aphasia Generalization Studies

Studies in the aphasia literature in which at least two basic requirements for generalization research have been demonstrated are listed in Table 6–1. Those included were identified by reviewing reports published since 1970 in several journals including the *Journal of Speech and Hearing Disorders, Journal of Speech and Hearing Research, Journal of Communication Disorders, Cortex, Brain and Language, Brain, and the Archives of Neurology. In addition, studies published in Clinical Aphasiology*, a compilation of papers reported at the Clinical Aphasiology Conferences, were reviewed. Studies reviewed met at least the following two criteria: the behaviors under study were clearly specified, and generalization was tested using well-defined measures or probes other than standardized tests. Studies using standardized aphasia test batteries or other tests to evaluate treatment effects (Basso, Capitani, and Vignolo, 1979; Helm-Estabrooks, Fitzpatrick, and Barresi, 1981; Wertz and associates, 1981, 1986) were excluded from this review, because such tests do not adequately evaluate response generalization patterns and they do not address stimulus generalization, particularly to natural settings. In addition, only studies in which acquisition of target behaviors was demonstrated or reported were included, because without this demonstration, generalization could not be evaluated.

Selected studies were examined in several areas. The number of subjects included in each was noted and evaluated to determine whether this number met requirements of the experimental design chosen. Further, it was noted whether or not minimal subject data (the type of aphasia and months past onset of stroke) were reported. The behaviors selected for study and treatment methods utilized were also reviewed, as was the research design selected. With regard to experimental design, particular attention was given to whether internal validity was demonstrated. That is, the extent to which treatment effects could be attributed to the treatment applied was examined. Methods for measuring response generalization or stimulus generalization, generalization findings, and studies in which treatment was implemented to facilitate generalization were surveyed. Similarly, each study was evaluated with regard to measurement and establishment of maintenance. Finally, the review documented whether interobserver reliability was reported and continuous measurement was accomplished.

Review of Table 6–1 indicates that generalization research in aphasia is in an embryonic state. Given the number of published studies reviewed, a very small number (n = 35) have addressed generalization. In addition, methodological problems were found in many, further reducing the number of studies in which reliable generalization findings have been reported. In terms of the number of subjects studied, many studies included an inadequate number to satisfy experimental design requirements; in 37 percent, only one subject was studied. Further, incomplete subject data were reported in 20 percent; that is, the type of aphasia and months after onset of infarction were reported in only 28 studies. Given the importance of these and other subject variables in aphasia research (Brookshire, 1983), the lack of such minimal subject data was surprising. Of further interest is that Broca's aphasia was the most often studied, with 54 percent of the studies involving Broca's aphasic patients.

Other methodological problems were also found in this review. Although continuous measurement of dependent variables was accomplished in 77 percent of the

TABLE 6-1 Generalization Research in Aphasia

	Subject Data						Response Generalization		Stimulus Generalization		Maintenance				
Author	*No. of Patients*	*MPO**	*Type*	*Behavior Trained*	*Treatment Method*	*Design*	*Measured*	*Observed*	*Measured*	*Observed*	*Measured*	*Observed*	*Trained to Generalize*	*Reliability Data Reported*	*Continuous Measurement*
Doyle, Goldstein, Bourgeois, and Nakles (in press)	4	29+	Broca's	Topic-specific verbal requests	Loose training: specific question types or structures not trained, a variety reinforced	Multiple baseline across behaviors and subjects	Probes across topics	No	Probes in novel social dyads	Yes	Yes; within-session, 1 follow-up probe, 6 wks post-treatment	Yes	No; but treatment was designed to facilitate generalization	Yes	Yes
Wambaugh and Thompson (in press)	4	11+	Broca's	Production of *what* and *where* + *is* + *nominative* and *what* and *where* + *transposed noun phrase* sentences	Modeling, forward chaining, and feedback	Multiple baseline across behaviors and subjects	Probes of untrained exemplars of trained and un-trained question types and structures	Obtained to untrained question types only	Probes in three conditions: prompted interview, novel social dyad, and mealtime conversation	In prompted interview only	Yes; within-session, 2 follow-up probes, 1 to 4 wk post-treatment	Yes	Yes; sequential modification resulted in generalization to novel social dyad	Yes	Yes
Coelho and Duffy (1987)	12	6+	Nonfluent	Manual sign production	3 training steps: sign imitation, sign recognition, and sign production	Group study; no control group	No		Probes of trained signs with nontraining pictures	Yes	No		No	No	No
Davis and Tan (1987)	1	6	Broca's	Oral sentence production	Three-level stimulation procedure	Multiple baseline across behaviors	Probes of untrained sentences	No	No		Yes; within-session, 2 follow-up probes (time posttreatment unspecified)	Yes	No	Not on dependent measure	Yes
Bernstein-Ellis, Wertz, and Shubitowski (1987)	1	4	NR†	Decreased rate of speech production during picture description task	Pacing board and clinican feedback	ABA	Probes to untrained pictures; rate, content units, and accuracy/syntax measured	Decreased rate obtained	No	No	No		No	Yes	Yes
Doyle, Goldstein, and Bourgeois (1987)	4	30+	Broca's	Production of 5 sentence types	Helm Elicited Language Program for Syntax Stimulation (HELPS)	Multiple baseline across behaviors	Probes to untrained exemplars of trained and un-trained sentence types	To untrained exemplars of trained sentence types only	Probes in non-treatment conditions for each sentence type	For some sentence types but not others	Yes; within-session, no follow-up probes	Yes	No	Yes	Yes
Simmons, Kearns, and Potechin (1987)	1	48	Broca's + spouse	Trained spouse to decrease interruptions and use of convergent questions	Recognition training using video-taped dyads between aphasic patient and spouse	Multiple baseline across behaviors	To untrained spouse behavior: negative teaching	Yes	In three un-trained conditions: spouse/patient discussions, T.V. sports show conversations, and T.V. talk show conversations	In all conditions	Yes; within-session; 1 month follow-up	Yes	No; but treatment method was designed to facilitate maintenance	Yes	Yes
Thompson and Warner (1987)	6	7+	Broca's	Production of food request responses	Modeling, forward chaining, and feed-back	Multiple baseline across subjects	No		Probed trained responses in simulated restaurant and real restaurant	To both conditions for 3 to 6 subjects	No		Yes: programming a common stimulus and training sufficient stimulus exemplars	Yes	Yes
Cannito and Vogel (1987)	1	2	Agram-matic	Production of regular plural nouns	Closure procedure and clinician feedback	AB	Probes to untrained regular and irregular plurals	To regular but not irregular plurals	No		Yes; 1 follow-up probe, time post-treatment not specified	Yes	No	Yes	Yes

TABLE 6–1 Generalization Research in Aphasia (continued)

	Subject Data						*Response Generalization*		*Stimulus Generalization*		*Maintenance*				
Author	*No. of Patients*	*MPO**	*Type*	*Behavior Trained*	*Treatment Method*	*Design*	*Measured*	*Observed*	*Measured*	*Observed*	*Measured*	*Observed*	*Trained to Generalize*	*Reliability Data Reported*	*Continuous Measurement*
Steele, Weinrich, Kleczewska, Carlson, and Wertz (1987)	1	48+	Global	Naming of gestures using computer	Computer-aided visual communication system (C-VIC)	Multiple baseline across behaviors	To untrained sets of objects	Yes	No		Yes; within session; no follow-up	Yes	No	No	Yes
Hillis and Caramazza (1987)	1	3	Anomic, with dysgraphia and dyslexia	Spelling of single words	Teaching correct spelling and search strategies	Multiple baseline	To untrained set of spelling words	Yes	No		Yes; within session; no follow-up	Yes	No	No	Yes
Thompson and McReynolds (1986)	4	15+	Broca's	Production of *What, Where, Who,* and *Why* questions	Two treatments: auditory–visual stimulation and direct-production treatment	Combined alternating treatments design, multiple baseline across behaviors and subjects	Probes of untrained exemplars of trained and untrained question types	To untrained exemplars of trained question types, but not to untrained question types	Probes in picture description task	No	Yes; within session, no follow-up	Yes	No	Yes	Yes
Thompson, Hall, and Sisson (1986)	3	12+	Broca's	Object naming	Imagery and hypnosis	Multiple baseline across subjects	Probes to untrained items	For 1 of 3 subjects	No		No		No	Yes	Yes
Kearns (1985)	1	36	Broca's	Increased content units in picture description	Response Elaboration Treatment (RET)	Multiple baseline across behaviors	To untrained pictures	Increased content units with untrained pictures	No		Yes; within session, no follow-up probes	Yes	No	Yes	Yes
Salvatore (1985)	3	3+	2 nonfluent 1 fluent	Production of sentences	HELPSS program	Multiple baseline across behaviors	To untrained exemplars of trained and untrained sentence types	Little to untrained exemplars of trained or untrained sentences	No		Yes; within session, no follow-up probes	1 of 3 subjects	No	Yes	Yes
Johannsen-Horbach, Cegla, Mager and Schempp (1985)	4	6+	Global	Comprehension and production of Bliss Symbols	Nonspecific comprehension and production training	Case study	No		Observation in home environment	For 2 of 4 subjects	No		No	No	No
Howard, Patterson, Franklin, Orchard-Lisle, and Morton (1985)	12	6+	5 Broca's, 4 conduction 2 anomic	Naming pictures	Two methods: semantic treatment and phonologic treatment	Group study (ABC)	Probes to untrained items	Yes	Probes to untrained pictures of trained words	Yes	Yes; within session, follow-up at 1 and 6 wk	No	No	No	Yes
Kearns and Salmon (1984)	2	24	Broca's	Production of third person auxiliary *is* in sentences	Imitation followed by spontaneous production	ABAB	Probes of copula *is* + predicate adjective, locative, nominative, and plural auxiliary *are*	To copula *is* + predicate adjective; variability across subjects on other structures	Probes in spontaneous speech	Yes	Yes; follow-up probes 2 and 6 wk	Yes	No	Yes	Yes
Thompson and Byrne (1984)	3	14+	Broca's	Production of social conventions: greetings, self-disclosures, and questions	Loose training: 4 training steps in which stimuli and feedback progressively loosened	Multiple baseline across subjects	No		Probes in novel social dyads	For greetings and self-disclosures but not questions	Yes; follow-up probes 3 months following treatment	Yes	No; but treatment designed to facilitate generalization	Yes	Yes
Hoodin and Thompson (1983)	3	NR	Broca's	Verbal, gestural, and verbal + gestural production of nouns	Three treatments: verbal, gestural, and verbal + gestural training	Alternating-treatments design	Probes to verbal labels (cross modal)	With verbal + gestural training only	No		No		No	Yes	Yes

TABLE 6–1 Generalization Research in Aphasia (*Continued*)

	Subject Data						*Response Generalization*		*Stimulus Generalization*		*Maintenance*				
Author	*No. of Patients*	*MPO**	*Type*	*Behavior Trained*	*Treatment Method*	*Design*	*Measured*	*Observed*	*Measured*	*Observed*	*Measured*	*Observed*	*Trained to Generalize*	*Reliability Data Reported*	*Continuous Measurement*
Royall and Horner (1983)	1	60	Fluent	Reading comprehension with cued speech	Cued speech practice and clinician feedback	AB	Probes to untrained word list using cued speech	Yes	Probes with auditory stimulus only and auditory + lip posture stimulus	No	No		No	No	Yes
Thompson, McReynolds, and Vance (1982)	2	19+	Broca's	Production of NP + is + PP sentences containing locatives behind and beside	Modeling, forward chaining, and feedback	Multiple baseline across behaviors	Probes to untrained sentences within and across locatives	To sentences containing trained locatives only	Spontaneous speech probes using picture description	For 1 of 2 subjects	Yes; within-sessions, follow-up at 4 and 6 mo	Yes	No	Yes	Yes
Tonkovich and Loverso (1982)	4	26+	Broca's	Verb + noun gestural combinations	Matrix training	AB	Probes to untrained intramatrix and extramatrix combinations	To intramatrix and extramatrix combinations	No		Yes; follow-up probes at 2 and 3 mo	Yes	No; but treatment was designed to facilitate generalization	Yes	Yes
Prescott, Selinger, and Loverso (1982)	1	48	NR	Verbal and graphic productions of subject + action utterances	Verb center treatment: auditory + visual verbal prompt, *wh* question cues and clinician feedback	Multiple baseline across behaviors	Probes to untrained verbs	Yes	No		Yes; follow-up probes at 2 and 3 mo	Yes	No	No	Yes
Kearns, Simmons, and Sisterhen (1982)	2	6	NR	Gestural production, verbal + gestural production	Two treatments: gestural training, verbal + gestural training	Multiple baseline across behaviors	Probes of verbal production of items trained gesturally (cross modal)	No	No		Yes: within-session, no follow-up probes	Yes	No	Yes	Yes
Thompson and Kearns (1981)	1	48	Anomic	Naming pictured nouns	Cuing hierarchy	Multiple baseline across behaviors	Probes to untrained semantically paired nouns	No	No		Yes; within-session, no follow-up probes	Yes	No	Yes	Yes
Linebaugh and Lehner (1979)	5	12	Broca's	Naming nouns	Cuing hierarchy	Case study	Probes to untrained word lists of low and high frequency nouns using cuing hierarchy	Yes	No		No		No	No	Yes
Seron, Deloche, Bastard, Chassin, and Hermand (1979)	8		5 Anomic 2 Wernicke's 1 Broca's	Naming pictured objects and actions belonging in four categories	Two methods: unspecified "traditional language therapy" and nonspecific stimulation of access mechanisms	Group; control group received traditional treatment; experimental group received stimulation	To untrained items within trained and untrained categories	Yes, for 3 of 4 experimental subjects	No		No		No	No	No
Salvatore (1976)	1	112	NR	Auditory comprehensions of part III level items of Token Test (TT)	Gradual reduction of interstimulus pause duration in auditory commands	Case Study	Probes of untrained items on parts III and V of TT	Yes to part III but not to part V items	No		Yes; follow-up probes on part III of TT at 12 weeks	Yes	No	Yes	Not on all measures
Weigel-Crump (1976)	6	3	Broca's	Production of three sentence types: noun phrase + to be predicate, noun phrase + present progressive verb + object, noun phrase + intransitive verb + prepositional modifier	Two methods: programmed treatment and nonspecific stimulation	Group; three subjects per group; no control group	Probes to untrained exemplars of each sentence type	Yes, with programmed instruction	No		No		No	No	No

TABLE 6–1 Generalization Research in Aphasia (continued)

	Subject Data						*Response Generalization*		*Stimulus Generalization*		*Maintenance*				
Author	*No. of Patients*	*MPO**	*Type*	*Behavior Trained*	*Treatment Method*	*Design*	*Measured*	*Observed*	*Measured*	*Observed*	*Measured*	*Observed*	*Trained to Generalize*	*Reliability Data Reported*	*Continuous Measurement*
Shewan (1976)	1	21	Broca's	Production of two sentence types: subject + verb + object, and subject + verb + prepositional phrase	Two treatments: sequencing of all components of sentences and modeling of verb phrase only	Case study	Probes to untrained sentences of trained form	No	No		No		No	No	No
Helmick and Wipplinger (1975)	2	2	Anomic	Naming of nouns and verbs	Two treatments: maximum and minimum stimulations	Alternating-treatments design	Probes of untrained items	Yes	No		No		No	No	No
Kushner (1875)	1	1	NR	Auditory comprehension of nouns	Repetition and modeling	ABAB	Probes to production of trained nouns (cross modal)	Yes	No		Yes; 2 follow-up probes at 1 and 2 mo	Yes	No	No	Yes
Weigel-Crump and Koenigsknecht (1973)	4	3	Anomic	Naming items in four categories: household items, clothing, living things, action words	Nonspecific stimulation	Case study	Probes to untrained items in trained and untrained categories	Yes	No		No		No	No	No
Holland and Levy (1971)	7	NR	NR	Production of an active sentence (The man opened the door)	Reading, repetition, writing, and verbal production focused on one or two words in a sentence at a time	Case study	Probes to reading, writing, repetition and production of trained sentence (cross modal); to interrogative, negative, and passive forms of trained sentence; to untrained active sentences	To writing only (cross modal); to interrogative form; no change in negative or passive forms; to untrained active sentences	No		No		No	No	Yes

* MPO = months post onset
† NR = not reported

studies, interobserver reliability data were reported in only 54 percent. Further, it was noted that several generalization studies are lacking in experimental control, thus resulting in questionable findings (McReynolds and Thompson, 1986). Some reports of generalization have been based on case study investigations that are inherently lacking in internal validity; and although investigators have begun to use controlled single subjet experimental designs (Barlow and Hersen, 1986; Barlow, Hayes and Nelson, 1984; Hersen and Barlow, 1976; Kazdin, 1982; McReynolds and Kearns, 1983) for studying generalization, several investigators have used them inappropriately by overlooking important design requirements such as replication, counterbalancing, and so on. Interestingly, no controlled group studies investigating generalization were identified.

Table 6–1 also indicates that few aphasic behaviors have been studied and, relative to the number of treatments that have been designed for treating aphasic behaviors (Chapey, 1986), few have been investigated for generalization. In terms of investigation of response generalization, stimulus generalization and maintenance, most studies in the literature have addressed response generalization (n = 31; 88 percent), and far fewer have investigated stimulus generalization (n = 13; 37 percent). Further, it is interesting to note that only three studies were identified in which stimulus generalization to the natural environment was measured, and only six studies have focused on identification of methods for facilitating generalization when it was not observed as a natural outcome of treatment.

Based on this review, it is evident that a need for generalization research in aphasia exists. Limitations in the number and type of aphasic behaviors studied are evident, as are limitations in treatment variables investigated. Conditions for measuring generalization have varied across studies, and little research has been directed at identification of methods for facilitating generalization. Perhaps most importantly, several generalization studies are procedurally problematic and lacking in experimental control. Given these problems, it is not surprising that equivocal findings have been reported. Only recently have treatment studies begun to focus directly on generalization, using well-controlled research designs.

A growing interest in generalization and increasing recognition of its importance in understanding aphasia, treating the disorder, and evaluating the effects of treatment are evident (LaPointe, 1978). Influenced by Darley's (1972) observation that a need existed for data-based investigations of aphasia treatment, and by Stokes and Baer's (1977) discussion of generalization, aphasiologists are carefully reexamining effects of aphasia interventions. Also, observations that language recovery is sometimes limited and that recovered language is not always used in functional situations have influenced research and raised questions about existing theories of aphasia (Thompson and Kearns, 1981; Thompson and McReynolds, 1986). We have begun to take a more functional approach (Holland, 1982) to research and language training, investigating the extent to which recovered language is used by aphasic patients to communicate.

FACILITATING GENERALIZATION IN APHASIA

Given the limitations that are inherent in research pertaining to generalization in aphasia, it is difficult to discuss principles for facilitating generalization. However, from the research, problems encountered in obtaining or facilitating generalization in aphasia and considerations for solving or avoiding those problems in research and clinical practice may be identified. In this section, pertinent variables, including selection of behaviors for training, measurement of generalization, and the influence of subject and environmental variables on generalization, are discussed. Selection of treatment for facilitating generalization and maintenance of trained responses are also addressed.

Selection of Behaviors for Training

The generalization effects of training only a few language behaviors (relative to the many language deficits seen in aphasic individuals) have been studied. As indicated in Table 6–1, research has focused largely on syntax and naming, with a few studies addressing aspects of auditory comprehension and gestural production. Further, results indicate that response generalization is often limited and that stimulus generalization occurs some, but not all, of the time. Therefore, clinicians may be unable to rely heavily on published research findings when selecting intervention targets that will result in generalization.

That generalization does not always occur as a result of treatment has been noted by several researchers investigating acquisition and generalization of behaviors such as naming and production of phrases and sentences in aphasic subjects (Davis and Tan, 1987; Doyle, Goldstein, and Bourgeois, 1987; Holland and Levy, 1971; Kearns and Salmon, 1984; Shewan, 1976; Thompson and Kearns, 1981; Thompson and McReynolds, 1986; Thompson, McReynolds, and Vance, 1982). That is, even when acquisition of selected behaviors or a clear treatment effect has been demonstrated, a lack of generalization has been documented. This lack of generalization has been noted for both response generalization and stimulus generalization.

One study, demonstrating a lack of response generalization, was reported by Thompson and Kearns (1981). In this study, a multiple baseline design across behaviors (Barlow and Hersen, 1986; Kazdin, 1982; McReynolds and Kearns, 1983) was used to investigate the effects of a treatment, using a cuing hierarchy, on the acquisition and generalization of naming in an anomic aphasic subject. Four lists of ten pictured items were selected for study, with the items on list one being semantically paired with those on list three and the items on list two being paired with those on list four. Prior to the study, it was postulated that training naming responses from list one might facilitate generalized naming of semantically paired items on list three and that, similarly, training list two might facilitate generalization to items in list four. However, results of the study indicated no such generalization. As each word list was trained, the subject acquired the ability to name only trained items, and continual probing of untrained items indicated failure (Fig. 6–1).

Similar generalization effects were noted by Kearns and Salmon (1984) in a study evaluating the effects of training aphasic subjects to produce sentences. In this study, both response and stimulus generalization were examined following sentence production treatment. Findings indicated that response generalization was obtained to a limited number of sentence types, and no stimulus generalization was noted. Two Broca's aphasic subjects demonstrating telegraphic verbal output were trained to produce third person auxiliary *is* constructions in sentence contexts (e.g., *The man is eating*); generalization was assessed in copula *is* + predicate nominative, predicate adjective, and predicate locative contexts and in plural auxiliary *are* sentences. In addition, stimulus generalization was tested in conversational contexts between the examiner and the subject. Results indicated consistent response generalization limited to copula *is* + predicate adjective contexts, and stimulus generalization was not observed in spontaneous speech samples. Findings corroborating these have also been reported by Thompson and McReynolds (1986), Wambaugh and Thompson (in press), and others.

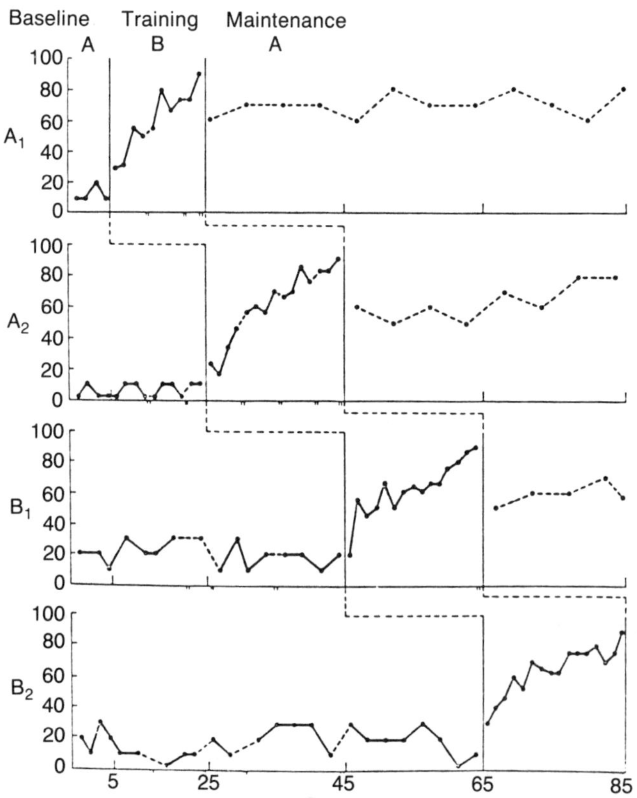

Figure 6–1 Percent correct naming across four word lists (A_1, A_2, B_1, B_2) in an anomic aphasic subject. Lists A_1 and B_1 contained semantically paired items, as did lists A_2 and B_2. Data indicate a lack of response generalization across word lists. (Reprinted with permission. Thompson CK, Kearns KP. Clinical aphasiology conference proceedings. Minneapolis, MN: BRK Publishers, 1981:39.)

Results of these and other studies indicate that some trained behaviors may not generalize either to untrained responses or to untrained stimulus conditions. A number of reasons for this lack of generalization may be advanced, including the behavior selected for training, the treatment method used, and subject variables. The point is that without generalization research indicating the effects of training a number of specific aphasic behaviors, selection of targets for training is difficult; even when responses trained are based on presenting deficits of individual patients, generalization may not occur. Therefore, other considerations may be necessary in selecting behaviors to promote generalization.

Suggestions for Choosing Treatment Targets

Two major considerations in selecting treatment targets that may influence generalization have been highlighted in the literature. These concern the relationship between trained responses and (1) responses tested for generalization and (2) context or stimulus conditions in which the trained responses are tested for generalization. In general, research has shown that generalization often occurs across responses that are structurally related to each other, and that stimulus generalization occurs when trained responses are tested in environments in which they are likely to be used naturally or functionally. That is, responses that are functionally significant to the stimulus generalization environment may generalize more readily than those that are not. Consideration of response structure and function is important for the enhancement of response generalization, whereas consideration of the functional significance of responses trained is important for promoting stimulus generalization.

Response Form or Function

In facilitating response generalization, it is important to consider the topographical or structural similarity between trained responses and those responses to which generalization is desired. Topographical similarity generally refers to responses that are similar in surface form (Hughes, 1985; Warren, 1985). For example, responses may be similar in syntactic form (e.g., noun-verb-object) or morphological form (e.g., regular plurals, regular past tense). That is, exemplars of a particular structural form may be selected for training and generalized use of the trained form can be tested in untrained utterances. This type of generalization was noted by Cannito and Vogel (1987) when their training of an agrammatic aphasic subject to produce plural markers on a set of nouns resulted in generalized use of plurality in untrained nouns. Response generalization of this type has been referred to as *substitution generalization* by Hegde (1985) because grammatical rules are used with untrained or substituted vocabulary.

Generalization may also be evaluated across structural forms (e.g., from present tense to past tense or from one type of sentence to another). However, as trained responses become less similar in surface structure to those tested for generalization, less generalization may be observed. For example, Doyle, Goldstein, and Bourgeois, (1987) found little generalization across sentence types in aphasic subjects.

Responses may also be related in terms of function: pragmatic function (e.g., requests), linguistic function (e.g., verbs, pronouns), and so on. Generalization may be tested to untrained members of a linguistic class (e.g., nouns, prepositions, verbs) or across pragmatic functions after training a few members of a particular class. For example, a set of verbs (Prescott, Selinger, and Loverso, 1982) or prepositions (Thompson, McReynolds, and Vance, 1982) may be trained, and generalization may be tested to untrained verbs or prepositions. Thompson, McReynolds, and Vance (1982) trained agrammatic aphasic patients to produce locative prepositions in noun phrase (NP) + *is* + prepositional phrase (PP) sentences and tested generalization to untrained locatives, finding limited generalization.

Research in aphasia has shown that generalization occurs most often across responses that are similar in surface form and that generalization across forms is rare. Further, research has indicated that generalization to untrained members of a particular linguistic class often does not occur. Studies of syntax training provide the best examples of these response generalization patterns in aphasic subjects (Doyle, Goldstein, and Bourgeois, 1987; Holland and Levy, 1971; Kearns and Salmon, 1984; Shewan, 1976; Thompson and McReynolds, 1986; Thompson, McReynolds, and Vance, 1982; Wambaugh and Thompson, in press). In these studies, responses to selected exemplars belonging to a particular linguistic class have been trained in a specific sentence form with subsequent measurement of response generalization to untrained members of the trained linguistic classes or to untrained sentence forms.

Thompson and McReynolds (1986) investigated the acquisition and generalization effects of training *wh* questions in four neurologically stable agrammatic aphasic subjects. The purpose of the study was to determine whether response generalization would occur to untrained exemplars within or across trained question types. Four questions were selected for investigation, including *where* questions, *what* questions, *who* questions, and *why* questions. Using a multiple baseline design across behaviors (McReynolds and Kearns, 1983), each question type was trained in selected sentence contexts, and daily, following each treatment session, probes were administered to test generalization to untrained sentences containing both trained and untrained question types. Results of the study for one subject are shown in Figure 6–2, indicating that generalization within but not across question types was seen. That is, following baseline, when *what* questions were trained, improved responding was noted on untrained *what* questions, but no change in producton of *where, who,* or *why* questions was noted. Similarly, training of *where* questions resulted in improved production of untrained *where* question responses, but no change was noted in production of *who* or *why* questions. These data indicate that generalization to untrained members of the linguistic class, questions, did not occur. However, generalization of the trained grammatical structure was noted.

In a follow-up study investigating *wh* question production in agrammatic aphasic subjects, Wambaugh and Thompson (in press) found similiar results. In this study, *wh* questions were defined and studied in smaller units. That is, *what* and *where* questions were studied in several structural contexts including *wh + is + nominative* sentences, *wh + is + transposed noun phrase* sentences, and others. One question type was trained in one sentence context as generalization to untrained exemplars of trained and untrained sentence structures and to untrained question types was tested. Figure 6–3 illustrates results for one subject trained (following baseline, *A*) to produce exemplars of *where + is + nominative* questions (during the treatment phase, *B*), indicating no generalization across sentence structures or types. That is, no change in *what* questions was noted during *where* training, and further, no change in structurally different *where* questions (*where + is + transposed noun phrase*) was noted. However, all but one subject evidenced generalization to untrained examples of trained sentence structures using the trained question type.

Similar patterns of response generalization have also been noted when aphasic subjects are trained to produce other sentence structures. Doyle, Goldstein, and Bourgeois (1987) and Salvatore (1985) trained aphasic subjects to produce declarative transitive, declarative intransitive, *wh* interrogatives, and other sentence structures. Selected examples of each structure were trained, one at a time, while generalization was tested to untrained exemplars of trained and untrained structures. Results indicated generalization within but not across trained structures. Holland and Levy (1971) reported similar results; when aphasic subjects were trained to produce active sentences, generalization to negative or passive sentences was not observed.

Results of these and other studies involving syntax training indicate that generalization to the same type of sentence occurs in some aphasic subjects, once they are trained to produce a particular syntactic structure. Only one study in the literature has indicated a lack of such generalization (Shewan, 1976). However, most studies have indicated that generalization to different sentence structures may not occur, although there are exceptions here as well (Kearns and Salmon, 1984; Weigel-Crump, 1976). It should be pointed out that response generalization has not been extensively studied when training other aphasic language behaviors. Therefore, it is possible that patterns of generalization may vary, depending on what behaviors are trained. What is important, clinically, is that responses for training be selected to maximize the potential for generalization. Items belonging to a particular class should be selected for training while response generalization is

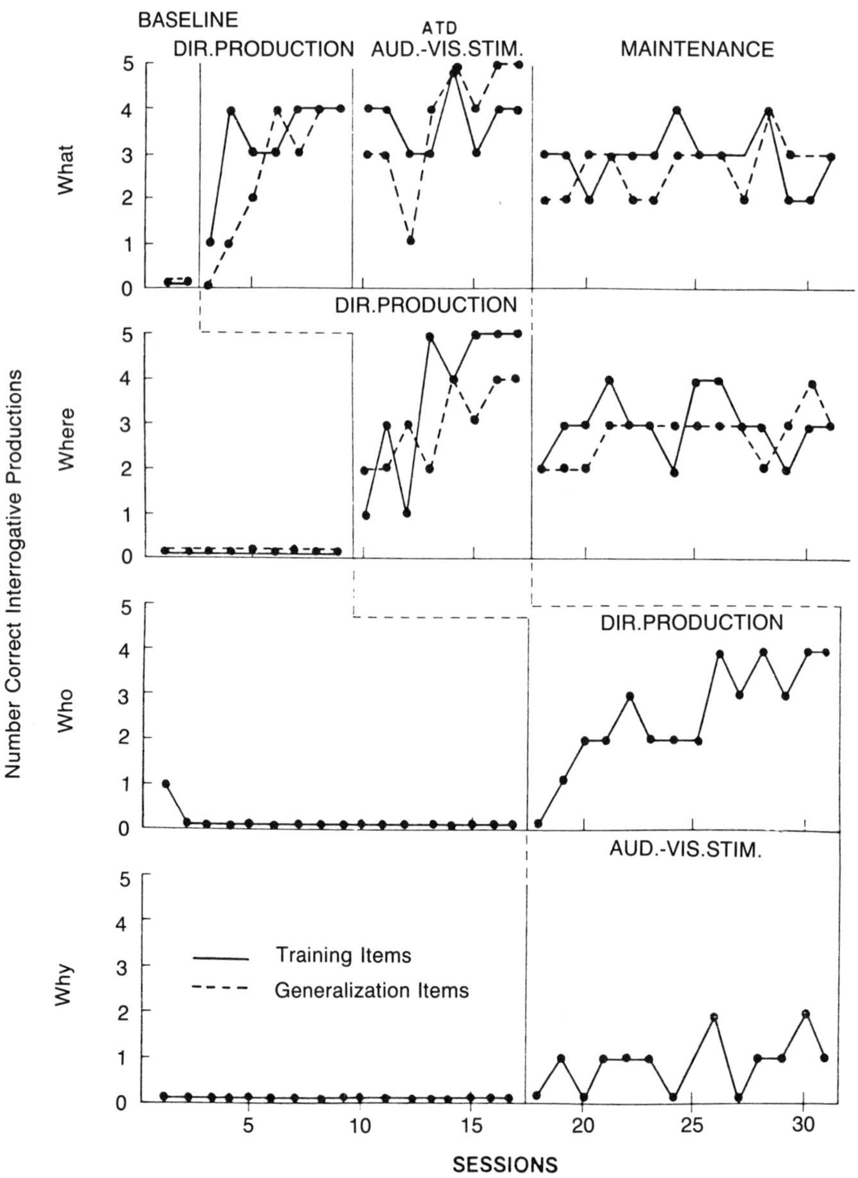

Figure 6–2 Acquisition, response generalization, and maintenance effects of training *wh* question types using direct-production treatment and auditory–visual stimulation treatment in an agrammatic aphasic patient. (Reprinted with permission. Thompson CK, McReynolds LV. J Speech Hear Res 1986; 29:200.

tested within or across classes or structures. When generalization to untrained responses does not occur, training may be extended systematically across responses until generalization is noted.

Functional Significance

Another consideration in choosing behaviors for training to facilitate generalization is the functional significance of chosen targets. Functionally significant behavior or responses can be defined as those used in the natural environment. When aphasic patients are trained to produce responses of functional significance for communication in functional situations or conditions, stimulus generalization is enhanced, perhaps because the patient's communicative attempts result in potentially reinforcing responses from the environment (Guess, Sailor, and Baer, 1978). This principle, that we "choose functional targets" in our treatment, has also been suggested by Hughes (1985), and is evident in aphasia research focused on stimulus generalization.

Table 6–1 indicates that stimulus generalization studies in aphasia have resulted in equivocal findings. That is, some studies have shown a lack of stimulus generalization (Doyle, Goldstein, and Bourgeois, 1987; Egolf and Chester, 1977; Kearns and Salmon, 1984; Thompson and McReynolds, 1986; Thompson, McReynolds, and Vance, 1982; Wambaugh and Thompson, in press), whereas others have found positive stimulus generalization effects (Doyle, Goldstein, Bourgeois, and Nakles, in press; Thompson and Byrne, 1984: Thompson and Warner, 1987). These equivocal findings might, in part, be ex-

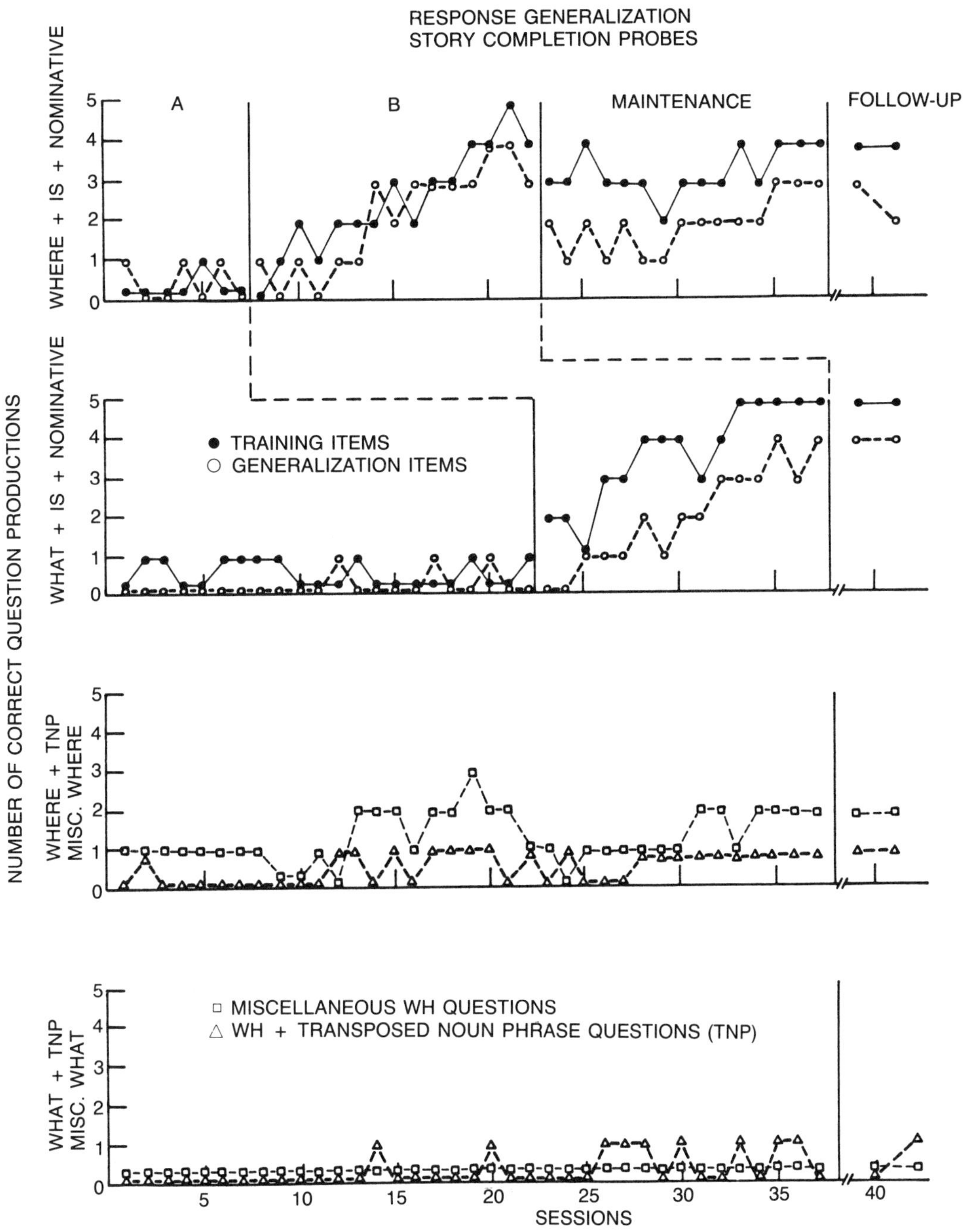

Figure 6–3 Acquisition, response generalization, and maintenance data for one agrammatic aphasic subject, indicating successful generalization from trained *where* and *what + is + nominative* questions to untrained *where* and *what + is + nominative* exemplars, but not across *wh* types (*where* to *what*) or structures (*what + nominative* to *what + transposed noun phrase*). (Reprinted with permission. Wambaugh JL, Thompson CK. J Speech Hear Disord, in press.)

plained by relationships between the behaviors were trained and the stimulus generalization probe conditions were used to assess generalization. Kearns and Salmon (1984) and Thompson and McReynolds (1986), for example, did not find stimulus generalization of trained syntactic forms in picture description tasks, perhaps because responses trained were not functional in these probe conditions. Thompson and McReynolds (1986) tested stimulus generalization of trained question responses by instructing subjects to ask questions about pictures such as the "Cookie Theft" (Goodglass and Kaplan, 1983). As pointed out by Hart (1980), responses such as questions may only be used functionally by children if they "want to know the answer." Certainly, in an artificial probe condition such as asking questions about pictures, aphasic patients may not want to know the answer and may, therefore, not ask questions. Whether or not the lack of generalization observed by Thompson and McReynolds (1986) occurred because stimulus generalization was tested in a nonfunctional situation is unknown. That is, the subject may not have evidenced generalized production of questions even in a more functional testing context. However, more positive stimulus generalization has been reported when aphasic subjects are trained to produce responses needed or likely to be used in the generalization condition (Doyle, Goldstein, Bourgeois, and Nakles, in press; Snyder, 1984; Thompson and Byrne, 1984; Thompson and Warner, 1987).

Snyder (1984) trained a nonverbal aphasic woman to use gestures to communicate in functional situations in a nursing home in which she lived. Gestures were selected after observations of the patient in her living environment indicated two situations in which she communicated unsuccessfully. One was a coffee hour; the other was when a hospitality cart was brought into her room. Therefore, two sets of gestures were selected for training, one for use during the coffee hour and the other for requesting items from the hospitality cart.

One set of gestures was trained at a time, and throughout treatment the patient's ability to use the trained gestures in the corresponding functional situation was assessed. Results of the study are presented in Figure 6–4. Following baseline, when the subject did not produce gestures from either set, set 1 (coffee hour gestures) was trained, resulting in rapid acquisition and subsequent generalized use of gestures during coffee hour to request sugar and cream, a spoon, coffee or tea, and so on. Similarly, when set 2 was trained, the patient began using gestures to request items from the hospitality cart.

Another example of training functionally significant responses was reported by Thompson and Warner (1987). Six Broca's aphasic subjects were trained to produce food requests (individually selected for each subject), as stimulus generalization probes were conducted in two naturalistic settings: a simulated restaurant in a speech and hearing clinic and a real restaurant. Results indicated that three of the six subjects readily evidenced generalization both to the simulated restaurant condition and to the natural environment. Data for one of the subjects for whom successful generalization was noted are shown in Figure 6–5. The lack of generalization for the other three subjects is discussed in later sections in this chapter (see "Training Sufficient Stimulus Exemplars" and "Programming Common Stimuli" below).

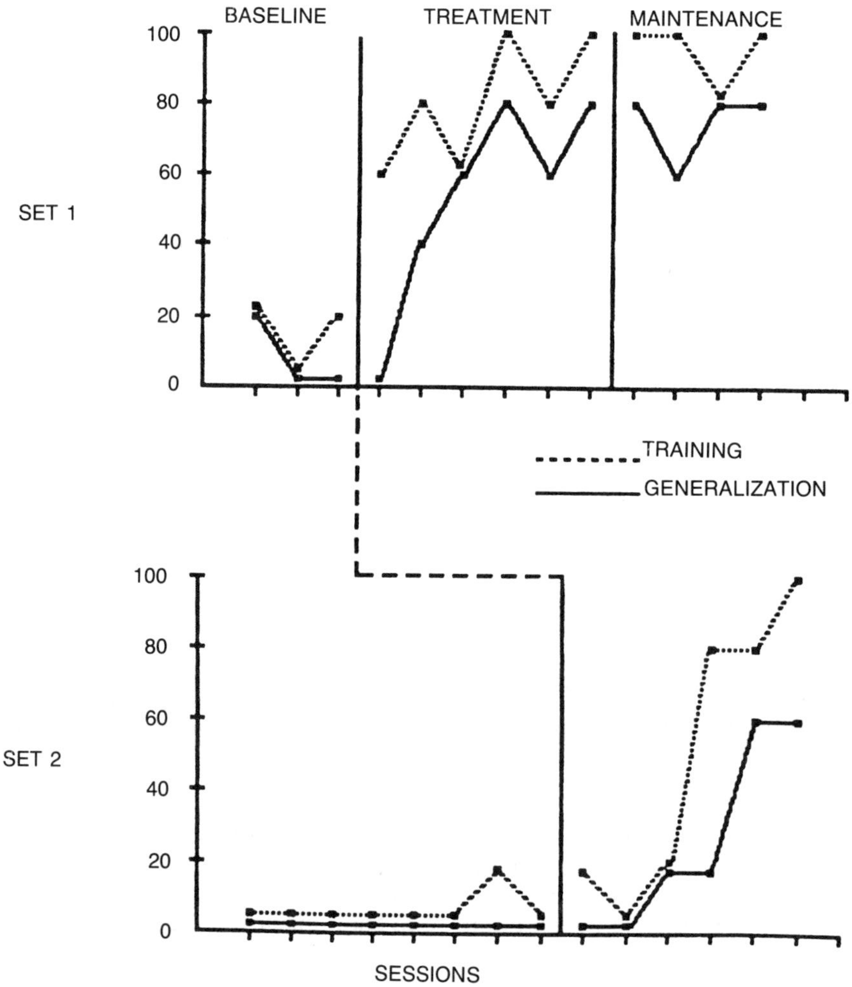

Figure 6–4 Acquisition and stimulus generalization effects of training functional gestural responses in a nonverbal Broca's aphasic subject, indicating successful acquisition and generalization of two sets of gestures across settings (*set 1*: coffee hour gestures; *set 2*: hospitality cart gestures). (Reprinted with permission. Snyder A. Masters thesis, The Pennsylvania State University, 1984.)

Several other stimulus generalization studies in aphasia have indicated that generalization to naturalistic situations may occur when responses likely to be used in those situations are trained. Therefore, in clinical practice it is advisable to choose responses for training by observation of the aphasic patient in his or her living environment or by interviewing the patient's family members or other caregivers. As pointed out by Hughes (1985), observation may help in identification of language targets that would be useful in various environments, and talking to people who frequently interact with the patient may provide insight into what language targets would be most helpful for the patient. Once functional targets are selected and training has begun, it is important to assess generalization periodically in the natural environment or in simulated environmental probes to evaluate treatment effects. If stimulus generalization is not observed, treatment should be implemented to facilitate such generalization.

Measurement of Generalization

Another consideration in obtaining or facilitating generalization is the question of how to test for generalization. Many aphasia clinicians are trained to use standardized tests to measure treatment effects. Although this activity is important for determining general progress and changes in overall language status, as pointed out earlier, standardized tests or other tests for aphasia may not adequately address the generalization effects of treatment. Therefore, clinicians need to design special probes for this purpose, which means considering salient responses and stimulus conditions to which generalization is desired. Table 6–1 indicates that studies of generalization in aphasia have utilized probes designed to test generalization to responses similar to those trained and to conditions different from training conditions. This seems simple and straightforward; however, the problem in both research and clinical practice lies in defining "similar responses" for testing response generalization and in deciding what components of the training condition to alter in testing stimulus generalization.

Defining "similar responses" is a difficult task. Because covariance among different language responses is not well understood and patterns of response recovery have not been extensively studied, deciding what responses to test for generalization may be somewhat arbitrary. A general rule in response generalization testing is to probe untrained members of a particular response class. However, response classes are defined by observing generalization across responses. That is, if training a particular response results in generalization to another response, then we consider the trained response and the generalized responses to belong to the same response class. Because response generalization in aphasic individuals is not well understood, we can only guess, when setting up probes, that certain responses belong to the same class, using plausible response dimensions in making these guesses. For example, when training word retrieval or lexical responses, response generalization may be tested across semantically, functionally, or phonologically related responses, and so on. Similarly, in training syntax, generalization probes may be designed to test untrained exemplars of trained structures or other structures that are related in some way.

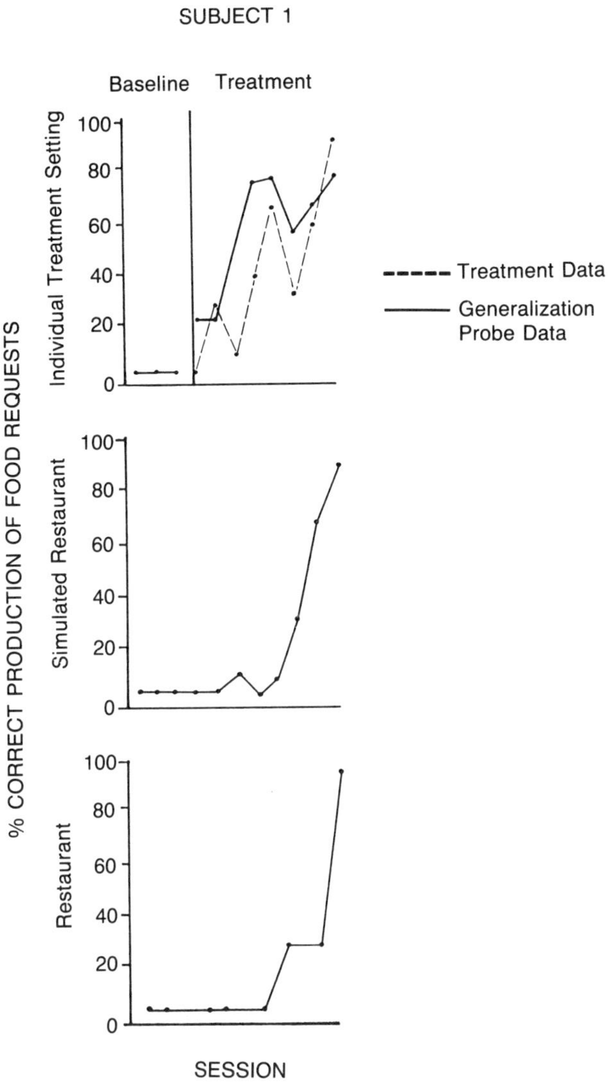

Figure 6–5 Acquisition and generalization of functional food request responses from an individual clinical treatment setting to a simulated restaurant and to a real restaurant for one Broca's aphasic patient. (Reprinted with permission. Thompson CK, Warner E. Paper presented at American Speech-Language-Hearing Association Convention: New Orleans, LA: 1987.)

Setting up stimulus generalization probes is perhaps more straightforward, although this also may be difficult. Stimulus generalization testing may be expensive, requiring time, equipment, and sometimes other professionals or family members. Of course, the amount of time and equipment and the number of participants required depend on the dimensions of stimulus generalization being tested. Stimulus generalization can be examined across a number of variables including other people or environments, or novel visual or auditory stimuli (e.g., pictures or verbal instructions not used in treatment).

Deciding what stimulus condition inherent in the treatment condition should be changed in order to assess stimulus generalization is a major concern in probing. Of course, the ultimate goal is to facilitate use of trained responses in functional communicative situations. However, some studies have shown that this generalization may not occur, perhaps because stimulus conditions in the functional environment differ too greatly from those in the training environment. For example, Thompson and Byrne (1984) trained aphasic patients to produce social conventions that are often used when meeting people for the first time. Eight responses, including greetings, self-disclosures, and questions, were trained, and stimulus generalization was tested in 5-minute conversational dyads (novel social dyads) between the aphasic subjects and an unfamiliar person. In the initial phase of the study, the subjects learned to produce all desired responses using a modeling and feedback procedure. However, the subjects did not use the trained responses in the novel social dyad condition, therefore training was continued in an attempt to facilitate generalization. The initial lack of generalization was not surprising, because the stimulus generalization probe condition and the training condition differed in many ways. The place was different (generalization probes were administered in a nontreatment room), the people were different (trainer versus unfamiliar person), and the stimuli to elicit a response were different. Clearly, it may be too much to expect that generalization would immediately occur in the natural environment. In designing stimulus generalization probes, the clinician may want at first to choose only a few variables of the natural environment to include in generalization probing, and then later may include others.

Types of Generalization Probes

Several methods have been used to evaluate generalization in aphasia research, including the use of questionnaires and anecdotal reporting (Goodkin, Diller, and Shah, 1972; Jenning and Lubinski, 1981; Schlanger and Schlanger, 1970). Other more objective measures or probes utilized, have included stimulus-specific probes (Doyle, Goldstein, and Bourgeois, 1987; Kearns and Salmon, 1984; Thompson and McReynolds, 1986), simulated environmental probes (Doyle, Goldstein, Bourgeois, and Nakles, in press; Thompson and Byrne, 1984; Thompson and Warner, 1987; Wambaugh and Thompson, in press), and naturalistic sampling (Wambaugh and Thompson, in press). The type of probe chosen for assessment of generalization may influence generalization results. That is, stimulus-specific probes may result in very different findings from those derived from naturalistic sampling procedures. Therefore, it is important to choose and design measures so that results of probing reflect desired aspects of generalization.

Stimulus–Specific Probes. Stimulus-specific probes are distinct tests for generalization in which certain training variables are altered systematically to assess response generalization, stimulus generalization, or both. For example, a set of stimuli such as pictures, written cue cards, or verbal instruction not used in training may constitute a generalization probe; or, different persons or settings may be included. Stimulus-specific probes are often desirable, because the clinician can control the stimuli presented and, therefore, responding can be controlled to a certain degree. That is, there are a limited number of responses that may be produced under the specific stimulus conditions. However, this control over responding is also the major limitation of stimulus-specific probes; such probe procedures preclude evaluation of any generalization that may have occurred beyond that which is appropriate for production under the specified probe condition. For example, if an aphasic patient were trained to produce a set of naming responses, and generalization to another untrained set was measured for generalization, the clinician would only know about generalization to items tested and nothing more. Similarly, in this example, nothing can be said about naming in response to questions, or about naming in other environments. Of course, stimulus-specific probes could be designed to test such generalization.

Another limitation of stimulus-specific probes is that, in some cases, stimuli presented may not provide obligatory contexts for production of responses of interest. For example, a clinician interested in an aphasic patient's use of prepositions in connected discourse may choose to use picture stimuli depicting a variety of people or objects in particular spatial relationships (e.g., a person *behind* a tree; a cloud *in* the sky) and may instruct the patient to describe the picture. However, the patient may adequately "describe" the picture without using any prepositions; even when prompted by the clinician's question, "Where is the man standing?", the patient may appropriately respond by pointing to the man and saying, "Right there." This example highlights the problem of ability versus demonstration of ability. That is, it is unknown whether the patient *could* not have used prepositions in connected speech or whether he just *did* not.

Simulated Environmental Probes. Simulated environmental probes are useful for determining the extent to which trained responses will be used across settings. Such probes are carefully designed to provide stimulus characteristics that are common in the natural environment. For example, the simulated restaurant probe used by Thompson and Warner (1987) included stimuli found in restaurants (e.g., tablecloths on tables and menus). Other simulated probes may also be designed using roleplaying (Aten, Caliguiri, and Holland, 1982; Schlanger and Schlanger, 1970), dyads (Doyle, Goldstein, Bourgeois, and Nakles, in press; Simmons, Kearns, and Potechin, 1987; Thompson and Byrne, 1984), and props (Prinz, 1980). Whether simulated environmental probes accurately estimate the extent to which generalization to natural environments will occur is an empirical question. However, when observation of the patient in naturalistic settings is not possible, simulated environmental probes may be useful. Simulated environmental probes also do not circumvent the problem discussed above regarding ability versus demonstration of ability. That is, if a given aphasic patient *does* not use trained or desired language responses in simulated probes, it does not necessarily mean that the patient *cannot* use them.

Naturalistic Sampling. Naturalistic sampling probes have not been used extensively in aphasia generalization research. Naturalistic probes differ from other probes described, in that no specific stimuli are arranged to elicit target responses. Instead, observations of the patient in his or her natural environment are made, indicating the extent to which he or she uses trained language responses in actual communication. Of course, generalization to the natural environment is the ultimate goal of treatment, so it seems that naturalistic probes might be the best method for assessment of generalization. Two experimental studies in aphasia have systematically assessed and reported generalization using naturalistic sampling (Thompson and Warner, 1987; Wambaugh and Thompson, in press). Wambaugh and Thompson tested aphasic patients' use of questions in mealtime conversations, and Thompson and Warner (1987) tested aphasic patients' use of trained food request responses in a restaurant. This type of sampling is necessary in order to determine the efficacy of treatment and the need for further training.

Clearly, there are several types of generalization probes, all of which require time and thought in terms of design and administration. Further research in this area is needed to identify and standardize procedures for efficient probing. Until such procedures have been developed, clinicians might begin designing stimulus-specific probe procedures for testing across particular responses, persons, and settings; simulated environmental probes; and routine naturalistic sampling procedures that can be realistically administered given the constraints of the work setting.

Social Validity

Another concern relative to generalization testing is social validity. Kazdin (1982) identifies two types of social validity: social comparison and subjective evaluation. Social comparison refers to measurement of target behaviors in normal populations. That is, the use of certain language behaviors in certain situations by normal peers of the aphasic patient are measured to determine expected levels of production. In evaluation of generalization, these levels of normal performance can then be used to provide a range of normal responding with which aphasic responding can be compared.

Thompson and Byrne (1984) gathered social comparison data in the study described earlier in which aphasic patients were trained to produce responses for use in novel conversational dyads. Specifically, the number of target social conventions produced by non-brain-damaged adults meeting each other for the first time was measured, providing levels of normal responding. These normative data were very helpful for evaluating the effects of treatment (see Fig. 6–15). Without the normative data, it might have been concluded that treatment did not result in high levels of performance. However, when compared to the normal data, the effects of treatment could be seen clearly. Prior to treatment, the aphasic subjects' performance was below the normal range; upon completion of treatment, performance was within the normal range.

Subjective evaluation, the second method of social validation described by Kazdin (1982), is generally discussed with regard to selecting behaviors for treatment. However, it is also important in measurement of generalization. This method involves "soliciting the opinions of others who by expertise, consensus, or familiarity with the client are in a position to judge or evaluate" (Kazdin, 1982, p. 21). In appraising generalization, subjective evaluation may be useful; by gathering information from persons who interact with the aphasic patient, the generalization effects of treatment may be estimated. For example, nurses, physical therapists, occupational therapists, or other professionals who are in contact with patients in a hospital setting, the patient's spouse, or family members might be involved. As with other types of generalization testing, when subjective evaluation is used, it is necessary to obtain data prior to, during, and after completion of the treatment. Further, it is essential that procedures or observational conditions be specified as much as possible. That is, opinions such as "the patient seems to be doing better," are insufficient for evaluating generalization. Instead, the clinician may wish to provide observers with suggested times and activities during which the patient can be observed, as well as with a set of responses or types of responses to identify. Although data collected in this manner are "subjective," they can provide helpful information about the extent of generalization across situations and can point out needs and directions for generalization training.

Criteria for Generalization

Specifying criteria for generalization is another measurement consideration. Decisions must be made about how many untrained responses need to be observed in order to say that response generalization has occurred, or how many trained responses need to be observed across stimulus conditions in order to say that stimulus generalization has occurred. In addition, acceptable forms of responses need to be considered. A few guidelines for making these decisions are offered here.

Based on findings from response generalization research in aphasia, successful generalization is considered to have occurred with correct responding between 50 percent (Tonkovich and Loverso, 1982) and 80 percent (Thompson and McReynolds, 1986) on response generalization probes consisting of a specified number of items (between 20 and 40). Response generalization below the 50-percent level on such probes has been considered "limited" (Wambaugh and Thompson, in press), but still offers evidence of generalization when levels are above those observed during baseline. Clinically, when low levels of responding are evidenced on response generalization probes (e.g., 30 percent of trained responses produced correctly), it is advisable to continue treatment until responding reaches at least a 50-percent level or higher. Similar levels of responding are also appropriate when deciding whether stimulus generalization has occurred. For example, if a set of ten responses (e.g., requests for clothing and personal items) was trained in a speech-language clinic and generalized use of these responses was tested with another examiner (e.g, rehabilitation nurse) in the speech-language clinic, production at a 30-percent level (three correct of ten items trained) would be considered insufficient; in such a case, treatment would be continued until higher levels of responding were observed.

Setting generalization criteria also involves consideration of the context in which responses are measured because, as pointed out, some testing conditions may not provide obligatory contexts for responses of interest to be produced. This consideration is particularly important when measuring stimulus generalization. Using the above example (training requests for clothing and personal items), suppose that stimulus generalization probes were also administered during dressing activities with an occupational therapist who was given instruction to require the aphasic patient to request items verbally that he or she wanted to wear. Using this context for measuring generalization, not all trained responses would be expected to be produced. That is, the aphasic patient may appropriately request some trained items (e.g., shirt, pants, shoes, and socks) and not others (e.g., glasses or coat). Therefore, in this example, a 40- or 50-percent criterion for correct responding may be considered sufficient.

Another consideration in setting criteria for generalization concerns the operational definition of a generalized response. Clinicians need to define carefully what responses during generalization probes are considered evidence of generalization. For example, variations in trained responses such as response time, self-correction, or grammaticality may occur during generalization probes. The extent to which response variation is allowed in measurement of generalization is an important issue. If no variation is allowed, some generalization effects may not be revealed during probing.

For example, in the Wambaugh and Thompson (in press) study in which aphasic subjects were trained to produce *what* and *where* questions, the original operational definition of a generalized response served to mask generalization effects. During training that involved a story completion task (Goodglass, Gleason, Bernholtz, and Hyde, 1972), subjects were required to produce question morphemes in the context of grammatically complete sentences; during generalization probes, subjects' use of trained question morphemes in complete sentences was measured using untrained story completion items. Because the study involved syntax training and generalization across syntactic structures, grammatically correct responses on generalization probes were expected. However, when the generalization data were analyzed closely, positive changes in some of the aphasic subjects' responses were noted, but could not be considered generalization according to the established response criterion. One subject, for example, after receiving treatment on production of *what* questions, was presented with the following stimulus: "Jim has a problem. Mary wants to know what the problem is. So she asks Jim..." The subject responded, "Problem?...Yes, what?" The response produced by the subject was considered incorrect, although it was clearly superior to responses produced during baseline. A question morpheme was produced and, in a functional sense, the response was communicative; therefore, it could have been considered evidence of generalizaton. To describe generalization better, an error analysis was conducted in which grammatically incomplete questions, appropriate alternative questions, and other question responses were tallied, revealing patterns of generalization that would have been overlooked given the original operational response definition.

Influence of Subject and Environmental Variables

Variability among subjects regarding the pattern of generalization noted following training has been pointed out by several researchers (Doyle, Goldstein, Bourgeois, and Nakles, in press; Kearns and Salmon, 1984; Thompson and McReynolds, 1986). In part, this variability may be explained by subject or environmental variables such as severity and pattern of language deficits, associated or complicating neurobehavioral deficits, personality factors, and factors related to the patient's living or communicative environments. The problem is that research has not clearly delineated which of these variables affect generalization or how generalization is affected by them.

Different generalization patterns were noted among the Broca's aphasic subjects studied by Doyle, Goldstein, Bourgeois, and Nakles (in press). When trained to produce requests for information about specific topics, generalized use of trained responses occurred for three of four subjects studied; the fourth subject required specialized training before generalization similar to that observed for the others was noted. Similarly, Wambaugh and Thompson (in press) and Thompson and Warner (1987) noted variability in subjects' use of trained question forms and food request responses, respectively, across stimulus generalization conditions. Although there are many reasons for the variability, Thompson and Warner (1987) reported that severity of apraxia of speech may have contributed to the lack of generalization noted in three of six subjects studied. Interestingly, the subject who was most resistant to generalization in the Doyle, Goldstein, Bourgeois, and Nakles (in press) study also evidenced severe apraxia of speech.

Another subject variable that may well be related to generalization is motivation. Tullos (1985), for example, found differences in generalization patterns of two aphasic patients that may have been explained by differences in motivation or desire to use trained responses. In this study, nonverbal Broca's aphasic subjects were trained to request food from a menu using a synthesized speech device, and generalized use of trained responses was tested in a restaurant. Results indicated that one subject readily generalized across settings, but the other did not, refusing to use the communication device during the restaurant probes. Not until the examiner explained that he should do so only to demonstrate his ability, was generalization seen. A similar problem was noted by Thompson and Byrne (1984) when subjects were trained to produce responses used while conversing with unfamiliar people. The second subject in the study required more training than the first, and levels of generalization were lower in the second than in the first subject (see Fig. 6–15). Although not scientifically tested, one explanation for these differences may have been the premorbid personality of the second subject. The individual's wife reported that he had "never talked much, especially to strangers," even before his stroke.

Another set of variables that may influence generalization is environmental. Included in this set of variables are aspects of the physical environments in which an aphasic patient may be communicating and the people in these environments with whom he or she is communicating. For example, unfamiliar, noisy environments may interfere with generalized use of language and, similarly, unfamiliar people or even a patient's spouse, family member, or other caregiver's style of communicative interaction may influence generalization. It is common, for example, to observe an aphasic subject interacting with a spouse or other person outside of the speech-language clinic using less language or less sophisticated language structure than the patient demonstrates in clinical training. One reason for this may be that the spouse or caregiver (e.g., nurse in a nursing home) may anticipate the needs of the aphasic individual and, therefore, may not provide opportunity for him or her to use language. Persons communicating with the aphasic individual may also interrupt or not provide sufficient time for him or her to respond. Clearly, these situations and many others may preclude generalization. A few studies in the aphasia literature have provided insight here. Simmons, Kearns, and Potechin (1987), Goodkin, Diller, and Shah (1972), and others have included spouses of aphasic patients in their training protocol, finding that modifications in spouse behaviors (such as decreasing interruptions) increase aphasic patients' use of language, sometimes without training the aphasic individual (Simmons, Kearns, and Potechin, 1987).

Controlling subject and environmental variables in facilitating generalization is perhaps the most difficult task for clinicians. It is suggested that for all patients, regardless of variables such as severity, time after onset, or other factors that may influence generalization, clinicians carefully select treatment targets based on the patient's level and pattern of language deficit, that they continually test generalization across salient responses and in salient stimulus conditions, that they use treatment strategies to promote generalization, when possible, and that they implement treatment to facilitate generalization when it does not occur. The effects of treatment can then be evaluated on an individual basis, and adjustments may be made when necessary. Until research is conducted that demonstrates generalization profiles for patients with certain behavioral patterns, clinicians must rely on their clinical skills in determining the influence of certain variables on generalization.

In consideration of environmental factors affecting generalization, observation of the aphasic patient interacting in various communicative situations may reveal needs for altering physical aspects of these environments or for involving caregivers or spouses in treatment. Involvement of persons with whom the patient communicates outside the training environment may enhance generalization, because caregivers, familiar both with the patient's language skills and with behaviors that are detrimental to the patient's use of language, may encourage and provide opportunities for the use of trained language skills.

Selection of Treatment Methods

Other considerations regarding generalization pertain to selection of a treatment method. Many treatments for aphasia have been described in the literature (Chapey, 1986). However, only a few existing methods have been investigated for their effect on generalization, and controlled comparisons of treatments are limited. For example, very few methods have been studied for training syntax, a major area in which generalization research has focused; only one study evaluating the relative effectiveness of more than one method has been published (Thompson and McReynolds, 1986). Further, research has shown that some treatments do not result in generalization. As has been pointed out throughout this chapter, generalization sometimes does not occur when treatment is provided for aphasic patients. Many variables may be related to this observation, but the treatment strategy may be one of the most important. Naming studies, for example, utilizing a variety of treatments including cuing (Linebaugh and Lehner, 1979; Thompson and Kearns, 1981), nonspecific stimulation techniques (Seron and co-workers, 1979; Weigel-Crump and Koenigsknecht, 1973), specific auditory–visual stimulation (Helmick and Wipplinger, 1975), semantically and phonologically based treatments (Howard and co-workers, 1985), and "verb as core" training (Prescott, Selinger, and Loverso, 1982) have resulted in equivocal findings. Unfortunately, the studies cannot be compared, because methods of investigation varied across them. Further, there are many methods for training these behaviors that have not been studied. Therefore, even though generalization is a major goal when treating syntactic deficits, naming deficits, and other aphasic behaviors, selecting treatments to meet this end may be difficult.

Research is needed to determine the generalization effects of treatments and treatment components that have not been studied. Also, research on the relative effectiveness of various treatments for specific neurolinguistic behaviors is necessary. The main point here is that clinicians may not be able to rely on their favorite treatment methods when generalization is their goal, because the generalization effects of these methods may not be known. Instead, new treatment methods or combinations of old ones may be more appropriate.

Methodologies for Promoting Generalization

Because some treatment methods do not result in generalization, research in aphasia has recently begun to investigate the effects of treatment methods designed specifically to facilitate generalization so that treatment efforts may be economized and promote the most generalization possible. Researchers have moved a step beyond "train and hope" studies (Stokes and Baer, 1977), in which a treatment method is applied and generalization is merely measured with no attempt made to facilitate it when it does not occur. Based on principles advanced by Stokes and Baer (1977) and others, methods for facilitating both response and stimulus generalization have been investigated, including training sufficient exemplars, programming common stimuli, sequential modification, and loose training. These strategies are discussed below in some detail, along with examples from clinical research in aphasia to demonstrate their application.

Training Sufficient Exemplars

Training sufficient exemplars is a technique for programming generalization, as discussed by Stokes and Baer (1977). It refers to the number of examples that need to be trained before generalization occurs to untrained members of a trained response class or across a number of stimulus conditions. The number of examples that need to be trained may vary depending upon the particular behaviors trained, the stimulus conditions involved, and the patient's level of language involvement. However, this strategy is important to keep in mind when designing treatment programs to facilitate generalization. When response generalization is the desired outcome of treatment, a few responses of a particular type (e.g., production of a morphological structure, sentence type, pragmatic behavior, and so on) can be trained while untrained members of that response type are measured. When generalization does not occur, new training responses can be selected from the pool of untrained items until generalization is noted. Similarly, when stimulus generalization across settings is of interest, responses first may be trained in one setting or stimulus exemplar (e.g., treatment room) and may be measured across a variety of others, such as the waiting room and the cafeteria in a hospital. If generalization is not seen across settings, it is programmed by training production of responses across a sufficient number of settings until generalization to others occurs.

Training Sufficient Response Exemplars. Studies in the aphasia literature have not investigated specifically the effects of training sufficient exemplars for facilitating response generalization. Several studies have simultaneously trained a number of exemplars from a particular response class and measured generalization to untrained members of that class. However, in only one study has training of additional exemplars been attempted when response generalization was lacking (Doyle, Goldstein, and Bourgeois, 1987). Further research is needed in order to evaluate the effects of this method for training a variety of language behaviors in aphasic patients.

One method of systematically training and measuring the generalization effects of training sufficient response exemplars is matrix training. Matrix training is most useful for training comprehension or production of two or more word combinations. By training selected word combinations, generalization to untrained word combinations, referred to as *recombinative generalization* by Goldstein (1985), may be observed. In addition, when generalization does not occur, additional combinations may be trained until generalization is seen.

Designing a matrix for training requires, first, identification of components to be trained such as noun + verb combinations or spatial preposition + object combinations; and, second, arrangement of these components in a matrix with one component (e.g., nouns) in rows and the other (e.g., verbs) in columns, as shown in Figure 6–6. Once the matrix has been designed, selected cells within the matrix are trained while generalization to untrained cells is measured. Figure 6–6 provides an example of a 4 × 4 matrix in which the first noun (*N1*) is trained in combination with all verbs (*V1, V2, V3,* and *V4*), and the first verb (*V1*) is trained in combination with all nouns (*N1, N2, N3,* and *N4*). These cells are marked with a T in the figure. Throughout this training, generalization is assessed in the remaining cells marked with a G. There are several possible arrangements for training cells within matrices, such as a diagonal training (Foss, 1968) and diagonal step-wise arrangements (Karlan and co-workers, 1982). In reference to Figure 6–6, diagonal training would require training of N1 + V1, N2 + V2, N3 + V3, and N4 + V4, whereas diagonal stepwise training would require training of N1 + V1, N1 + V2, N2 + V2, N2 + V3, N3 + V3, N3 + V4, and N4 + V4. In each of these arrangements, generalization to the remaining cells is assessed.

Two studies in the aphasia literature have investigated response generalization using a matrix training procedure. Tonkovich and Loverso (1982) trained gestural production in four Broca's aphasic patients using a 4 × 8 matrix consisting of verbs on one axis of the matrix and objects on the other. By dividing the 4 × 8 matrix into two 4 × 4 matrices, one matrix could be used for training and analysis of intramatrix generalization and the other could be used to examine extramatrix generalization (Fig. 6–7). Prior to treatment, all subjects evidenced ability to produce target gestures in isolation; therefore, the goal of treatment was to facilitate combined gestural use by training seven verb + object combinations. In Figure 6–7, items trained are marked with a T, intramatrix generalization items are marked with an I, and extramatrix generalization items are marked with an E.

Results of the study, shown in Figure 6–8, indicate

Nouns \ Verbs	V1	V2	V3	V4
N1	T	T	T	T
N2	T	G	G	G
N3	T	G	G	G
N4	T	G	G	G

Figure 6–6 A 4 × 4 matrix designed for training and measuring generalization of *noun + verb* combinations. *T*, trained combinations; *G*, combinations tested for generalization.

that after a stable baseline, all subjects readily acquired ability to produce trained gestural combinations and, at the same time, both intramatrix and extramatrix generalization was seen. Unfortunately, experimental control was not demonstrated in this study. As pointed out by Tonkovich and Loverso (1982), staggering the length of baseline phases among subjects would have provided the necessary experimental control. However, this study nicely demonstrates application of matrix training to aphasia treatment.

The second study in which a matrix training approach was employed was completed by Thompson, McReynolds, and Vance (1982). In this study, two Broca's aphasic subjects with agrammatism were trained to produce noun phrase (NP) + prepositional phrase (PP) combinations. Four 3 × 3 matrices were designed, two containing the preposition *behind* and two the preposition *beside*. Using a multiple baseline design across behaviors, responses from one matrix for each preposition were diagonally trained, while generalization was assessed to responses within and across matrices. Data for one subject involved in the study are shown in Figure 6–9, indicating generalization to untrained NP + PP combinations within and across matrices containing trained prepositions. However, generalization across matrices containing untrained prepositions was not seen.

Findings from these studies are similar to those reported with normal children and adults (Esper, 1925; Goldstein, 1983) and with language-delayed children (Striefel, Wetherby, and Karlan, 1976). Aphasic patients evidence generalized ability to sequence stimuli from two classes following training of only a few exemplars in which members of one class are combined with those of the second. The number of exemplars necessary for training may vary among aphasic patients. However, a matrix training approach provides a systematic mechanism for training responses and for measuring generalization.

Training Sufficient Stimulus Exemplars. Training sufficient stimulus exemplars for programming generalization may be accomplished by extending training across persons or across settings. This method requires selection of a response or responses for training, measurement of responses in desired stimulus conditions, and training across conditions when generalization is lacking.

One report in the aphasia literature by Egolf and Chester (1977) demonstrates how training sufficient stimulus exemplars might be accomplished in a rehabilitation center, although the study was not focused on investigating the effects of this methodology. The purpose of the study was to examine the extent to which language structures trained by a speech-language pathologist were used by aphasic subjects in other settings and with other rehabilitation professionals. Using a questionnaire, nurses, physical therapists, occupational therapists, and others commented on subjects' use of language in various conditions. Results of the study indicated that the aphasic subjects used more complex and varied language structures

	MILK	COKE	TEA	COFFEE	JUICE	WATER	BEER	WINE
SPILL	SPILL MILK T	SPILL COKE T	SPILL TEA T	SPILL COFFEE T	SPILL JUICE E	SPILL WATER E	SPILL BEER E	SPILL WINE E
DRINK	DRINK MILK T	DRINK COKE I	DRINK TEA I	DRINK COFFEE I	DRINK JUICE E	DRINK WATER E	DRINK BEER E	DRINK WINE E
BUY	BUY MILK T	BUY COKE I	BUY TEA I	BUY COFFEE I	BUY JUICE E	BUY WATER E	BUY BEER E	BUY WINE E
POUR	POUR MILK T	POUR COKE I	POUR TEA I	POUR COFFEE I	POUR JUICE E	POUR WATER E	POUR BEER E	POUR WINE E

T = Training Items (7)
I = Intramztrix Generalization Items (9)
E = Extramatrix Generalization (16)

Figure 6–7 A 4 × 8 matrix designed for training gestural *verb + object* combinations. (Reprinted with permission. Tonkovich J, Loverso F. Clinical aphasiology conference proceedings. Minneapolis, MN: BRK Publishers, 1982:284.)

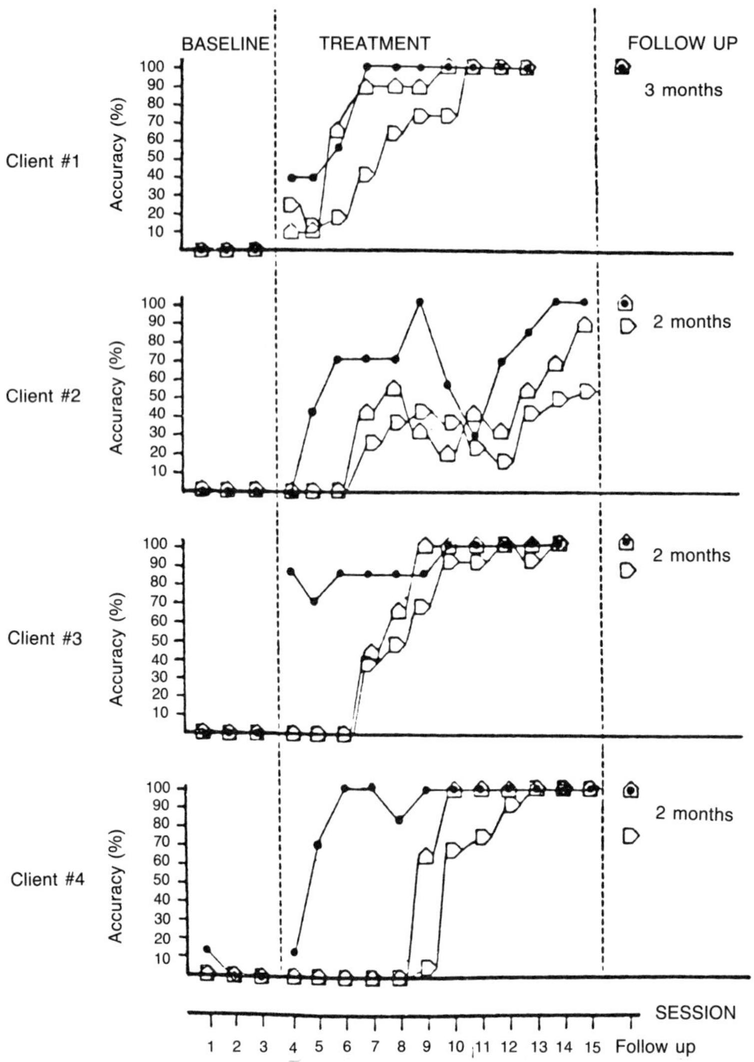

Figure 6–8 *Verb + object* gestural combinations produced by Broca's aphasic subjects during baseline, treatment, and follow-up phases. ●–●, training data; ⌂–⌂, intramatrix generalization items; ▷–▷, extramatrix generalization items. (Reprinted with permission. Tonkovich J, Loverso F. Clinical aphasiology conference proceedings. Minneapolis, MN: BRK Publishers, 1982:286.)

in the speech clinic with the speech-language pathologist than in other settings with other professionals, indicating a need for programming generalization. For example, training sufficient exemplars across settings or people might have facilitated generalization.

Using professionals or settings in a rehabilitation center, the method of training sufficient exemplars could be easily practiced. However, a few alterations in the methodology used by Egolf and Chester (1977) would be required. In using such a method, it is necessary to specify target responses and to probe these responses continually either across persons (e.g., by rehabilitation staff members eliciting trained responses in the training setting) or across settings (e.g., by the trainer eliciting responses in nontraining settings). It is advisable to manipulate either persons *or* settings for generalization testing and programming, because generalization may be less likely to occur if both variables are altered. Guidelines for training sufficient exemplars across settings are listed below. Using this approach, the number of settings (stimulus exemplars) required (sufficient) for generalization to occur could easily be examined.

1. Select a specific target response or responses.
2. Design stimulus generalization probes to measure responses across settings (e.g., specify times and situations in which the examiner will test the patient's use of target responses).
3. Train target responses in the speech-language clinic.
4. Periodically (e.g., daily or weekly) readminister stimulus generalization probes across settings.
5. If no generalization occurs, extend training to the

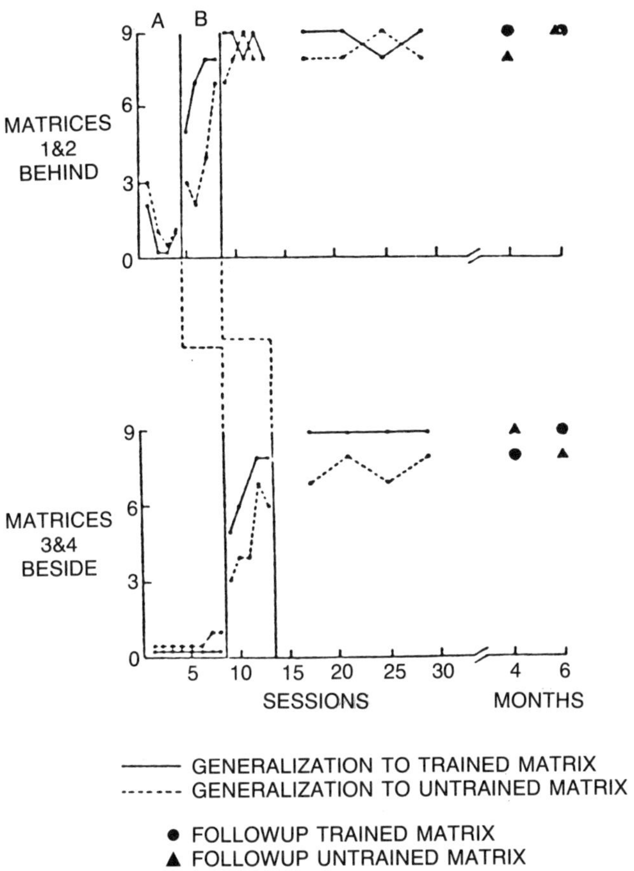

Figure 6–9 Number of correct *noun phrase + is + prepositional phrase* utterances produced within trained and untrained matrices by one Broca's aphasic subject during baseline (*A*), treatment (*B*), and follow-up phases of the study. (Reprinted with permission. Thompson CK, McReynolds LV, Vance C. Clinical aphasiology conference proceedings. Minneapolis, MN: BRK Publishers, 1982:294.)

generalization settings, one at a time.

6. Continue to administer generalization probes in untrained settings.
7. Continue to extend treatment across settings until generalization is noted.

One study in the aphasia literature, designed specifically to investigate the effects of training sufficient stimulus (setting) exemplars, was completed by Thompson and Warner (1987). This study is discussed in detail with regard to programming common stimuli, because Thompson and Warner (1987) attempted to facilitate stimulus generalization both by programming a common stimulus and by training sufficient stimulus exemplars.

Programming Common Stimuli

Another method discussed by Stokes and Baer (1977) that may be very useful for programming generalization in aphasia treatment is programming common stimuli. This method operates on the premise that generalization is more likely to occur when there are one or more stimulus components in common between the training environment and the generalization environment. In practice, common stimuli may be selected from the generalization environment and incorporated into the training environment, or they may be selected from the training environment and incorporated into the generalization environment. For example, an aphasic patient trained to produce language targets in the presence of someone with whom he will communicate in the natural environment (e.g., a family member, a caregiver in a nursing home) may be more likely to use trained responses in the natural environment when that someone is present. In this example, the common stimulus (family member or other caregiver) is taken from the generalization environment and incorporated into treatment. When the common stimulus is selected from stimulus components in the training environment, stimulus pictures or other items used in treatment may be displayed in the generalization environment. So, if an aphasic patient were trained to retrieve names of family members using photographs, then displaying the training photographs in the patient's room might result in generalized word retrieval in this setting.

The literature about aphasia indicates only one study in which the generalization effects of programming a common stimulus were examined. Thompson and Warner (1987), as discussed previously with regard to training functionally significant responses, trained aphasic subjects to produce food requests for ordering food in a restaurant. Language responses were trained in a traditional therapy room by one examiner (examiner 1), and the patient's use of trained responses in more naturalistic contexts, a simulated restaurant and a real restaurant, was examined. The simulated restaurant condition took place in a group therapy room arranged with three tables for two, tablecloths, and other items found on tables in a restaurant. Aphasic subjects, seated with an adult volunteer, ordered food from a menu when examiner 2, acting as a waitress, asked to take their order. In the real restaurant, aphasic subjects were individually escorted to lunch by unfamiliar volunteers. Results of the study, as pointed out earlier, indicated that three of the six subjects generalized across both stimulus generalization conditions, but the other three did not. Therefore, further training to facilitate generalization was implemented.

Two techniques were used. First a common stimulus, selected from the original training environment, was introduced into the simulated restaurant. Specifically, after subjects and volunteers were seated in the simulated restaurant, examiner 1 entered, sat in a corner chair, and observed as examiner 2 elicited responses as usual. Results of this procedure are shown in Figure 6–10 for one subject. As can be seen, programming a common stimulus (examiner 1) had no effect on use of food requests either in the simulated probe condition or in the real restaurant probe. Therefore, a second technique was employed. After a return to baseline procedures, when examiner 1 was removed from simulated restaurant probes, a second stimulus exemplar was trained. That is, food requests were trained in the simulated restaurant condition by examiner

1 using procedures identical to those used during the original training, while simulated restaurant probes with examiner 2 and real restaurant probes were continued. As can be seen in Figure 6–10, training an additional stimulus exemplar resulted in generalization to both generalization conditions. Similar results were noted for all three subjects who required generalization training.

Results reported by Thompson and Warner (1987) indicate that, in some cases, programming a common stimulus may not facilitate generalization in aphasic patients. However, it should be kept in mind that there are numerous stimulus components that may be selected for programming generalization that have not yet been tested. For example, the generalization effects of including people and items from the patient's living environment in the training environment have not been tested; in addition, many components used in training, such as objects and pictures, have not been incorporated systematically into the generalization environment. These strategies are in need of investigation.

Sequential Modification

Sequential modification is a method of facilitating stimulus generalization that is similar to training sufficiént stimulus exemplars. In this, a particular behavior is trained, as generalization is assessed across a number of salient stimulus conditions (e.g., settings or experimenters). If generalization is absent or incomplete, treatment is sequentially extended to nongeneralized conditions. The major difference between training sufficient stimulus exemplars and sequential modification is the number of stimulus condi-

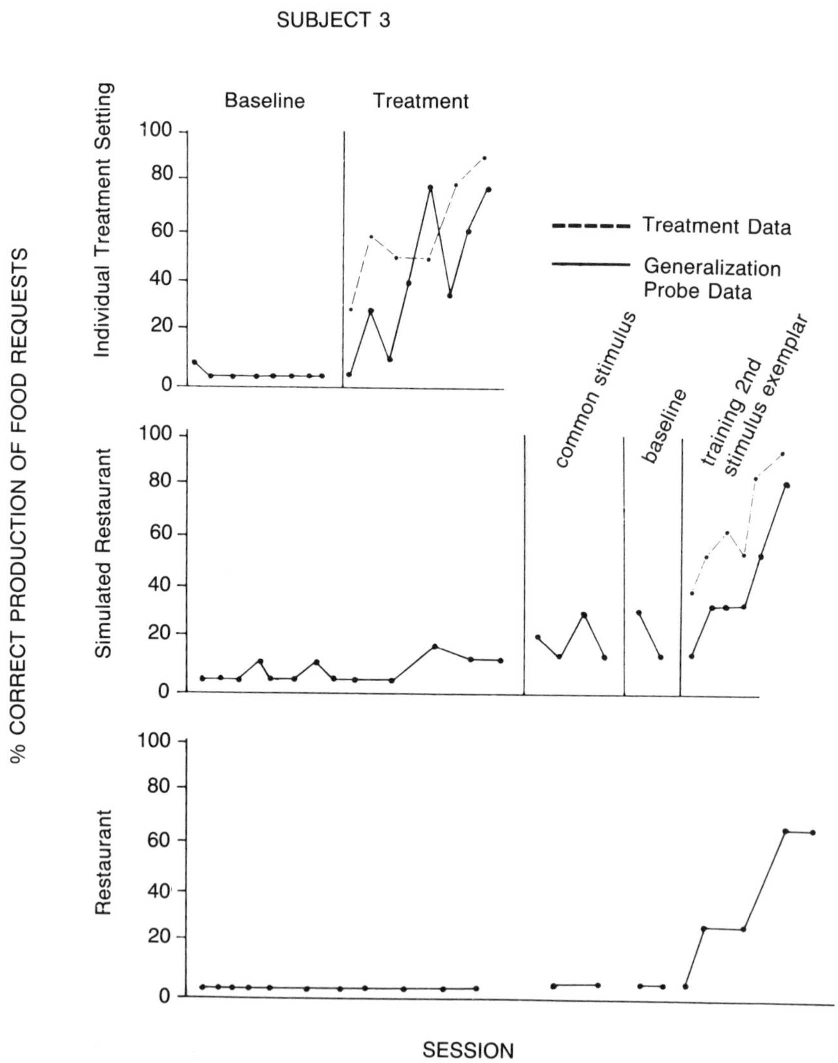

Figure 6–10 Effects of two generalization facilitation methods, programming a common stimulus and training sufficient stimulus exemplars, on production of food request responses in two stimulus generalization environments (a simulated restaurant setting and a real restaurant setting) in a Broca's aphasic subject. (Reprinted with permission. Thompson CK, Warner E. Paper presented at American Speech-Language-Hearing Association Convention: New Orleans, LA, 1987.

tions across which treatment is extended. Sequential modification requires training in "every nongeneralized condition"* (Stokes and Baer, 1977; p. 352), whereas, training sufficient stimulus exemplars requires training in only a "sufficient" number of stimulus conditions. Requirements for using both generalization procedures are the same. Responses are selected and measured prior to training in all stimulus conditions of interest. Treatment is then initiated in one stimulus condition while stimulus generalization probes in all others are administered. When generalization does not occur, treatment is extended to a second stimulus condition, and generalization probing is continued. If generalization occurs to untrained conditions, as in the Thompson and Warner (1987) study, then sufficient stimulus exemplars were trained. On the other hand, if training was required in every stimulus generalization condition, then sequential modification was necessary. In both of these procedures, the researcher or practitioner works to effect changes across conditions as a part of the treatment program.

Wambaugh and Thompson (in press) demonstrated the use of sequential modification in facilitating aphasic subjects' use of questions across stimulus conditions. As discussed previously with regard to response topography, this study focused on evaluating the response generalization effects of treatment across untrained *wh* questions. In addition, the study was designed to evaluate and program stimulus generalization. That is, throughout training, subjects' ability to produce trained question responses was measured in three conditions:

1. An interview in which the use of trained questions was prompted using written cue cards.
2. A novel social dyad in which subjects were engaged in 5-minute conversations with an unknown person.
3. Mealtime conversations with a family member.

Figure 6–11 shows the number of questions produced by one subject in these stimulus conditions during training of *where* and *what* questions (*arrows* at the top of each graph indicate the initiation of *where* and *what* training, respectively). As can be seen, training resulted in use of trained question forms in the prompted interview but not in the novel social dyads or in the conversational condition. Therefore, sequential modification was initiated. That is, the examiner trained subjects to produce *where* and *what* questions in the social dyad condition as generalization probing was continued in the novel social dyads and in mealtime conversations. Results indicated improved responding in novel social dyads but not in conversation, as shown in Figure 6–12.

These data indicate that sequential modification was successful and necessary for effecting generalization across conditions. Because generalization did not occur to conversation, it may be inferred that such generalization might have been facilitated if treatment had been extended to this condition. Of course, this remains an empirical question. However, if similar results were obtained in clinical practice, sequential modification might be a useful method for programming further generalization.

The technique of sequential modification is also salient for facilitating response generalization. Using such a method, responses to which generalization does not occur are sequentially trained until all desired responses have been trained. Examples of sequential modification across responses in aphasia treatment have not been published. As pointed out earlier, response generalization studies generally have focused on measurement and not on facilitation of generalization. Of course, practitioners would hope that sequential response modification would not be required. However, when the desired result of treatment is for an aphasic patient to produce a set of responses and generalization does not occur to untrained responses within the set, sequential training of all responses may be necessary.

Loose Training

Loose training is a concept for promoting generalization, advanced by Stokes and Baer (1977), which has received perhaps more attention in the aphasia literature than other methods. This concept operates on the premise that generalization may occur when the treatment environment approximates stimulus conditions and response variations found in the environment to which generalization is desired. Loose training, not to be confused with unstructured training, is designed to "avoid restricted stimulus control...by introducing a rich and varied set of stimuli and conditions that sample relevant dimensions of the subject's natural environment and by allowing for variation in response topography" (Doyle, Goldstein, Bourgeois, and Nakles, in press). Three general components that may be loosened or varied in loose training procedures include: (1) dimensions of the stimuli used in treatment, such as clinicians, treatment rooms, tone of voice, instructions, pictures, and objects; (2) the responses trained, for example, training a variety of responses within and across response classes; and (3) the feedback employed in treatment, for example, varying the type or frequency of feedback.

Studies in aphasia that have investigated loose training have focused on facilitating both response (Kearns, 1985) and stimulus generalization (Doyle, Goldstein, Bourgeois, and Nakles, in press; Thompson and Byrne, 1984) and have manipulated one or more components of loose training procedures. For example, Kearns (1985) developed a loose training technique for facilitating response generalization called *response elaboration training* (RET) in which the stimuli and feedback used in training were controlled while the response criteria were loosened. Specifically, treatment incorporated incidental teaching procedures (Hart and Risley, 1974) in which responses were

* Because sequential modification requires training across "every nongeneralized environment," it does not qualify as a generalization facilitation method per se. According to the definition of generalization advanced by Stokes and Baer (1977) as "the occurrence of relevant behavior under different, nontraining conditions...*without the scheduling of the same events in those conditions as had been scheduled in the training condition*" (p. 350), listing sequential modification as a technique for programming generalization (as indicated by Stokes and Baer on page 350) is a contradiction to the authors' definition.

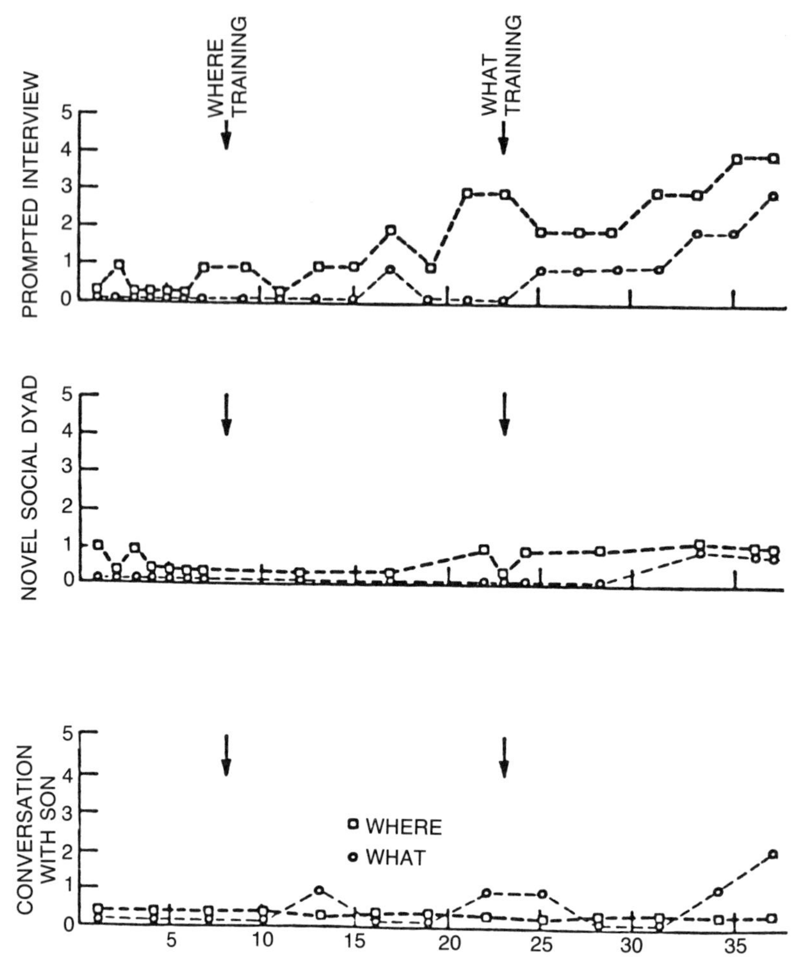

Figure 6–11 Number of *where* and *what* questions produced in stimulus generalization probes across three conditions for one agrammatic aphasic patient: (1) a prompted interview, (2) a novel social dyad, and (3) mealtime conversations with a family member. Arrows indicate sessions in which training of *where* and *what* questions, respectively, was begun. (Reprinted with permission. Wambaugh JL, Thompson CK. J Speech Hear Disord, in press.)

not restricted with regard to structure, content, or other criteria; instead, all subject-initiated responses were reinforced, modeled, and expanded.

Kearns (1985) demonstrated the effectiveness of this procedure for increasing the number of content units produced in a picture description task in one chronic Broca's aphasic patient. Treatment was extended across two sets of training pictures, and response generalization probes were administered using a third, untrained set. Results of treatment are shown in Figures 6–13 and 6–14, indicating the number of content units produced to training and generalization pictures, respectively, during baseline and treatment phases of the study. As can be seen, loose training in which a variety of responses (as opposed to a restricted set of responses) were reinforced and expanded upon resulted in an increase in production of content units on both training and generalization items. These findings suggest that response generalization may be enhanced when variations in response are encouraged.

Loose training procedures have also been utilized to promote stimulus generalization. Instead of focusing on responses produced, as in the Kearns (1985) study, Thompson and Byrne (1984) designed a loose training procedure in which a variety of naturalistic stimuli were progressively introduced into treatment to elicit responses of interest, and the feedback provided was progressively loosened. The purpose of the study, discussed in the section of this chapter addressing measurement of generalization, was to train aphasic patients to produce a set of social conventions including greetings, self-disclosures, and questions that could be used when meeting people for the first time. In addition, the study was designed to facilitate generalized use of trained responses in novel conversational dyads.

Treatment involved four levels of training. At each level, stimuli and feedback used in treatment were progres-

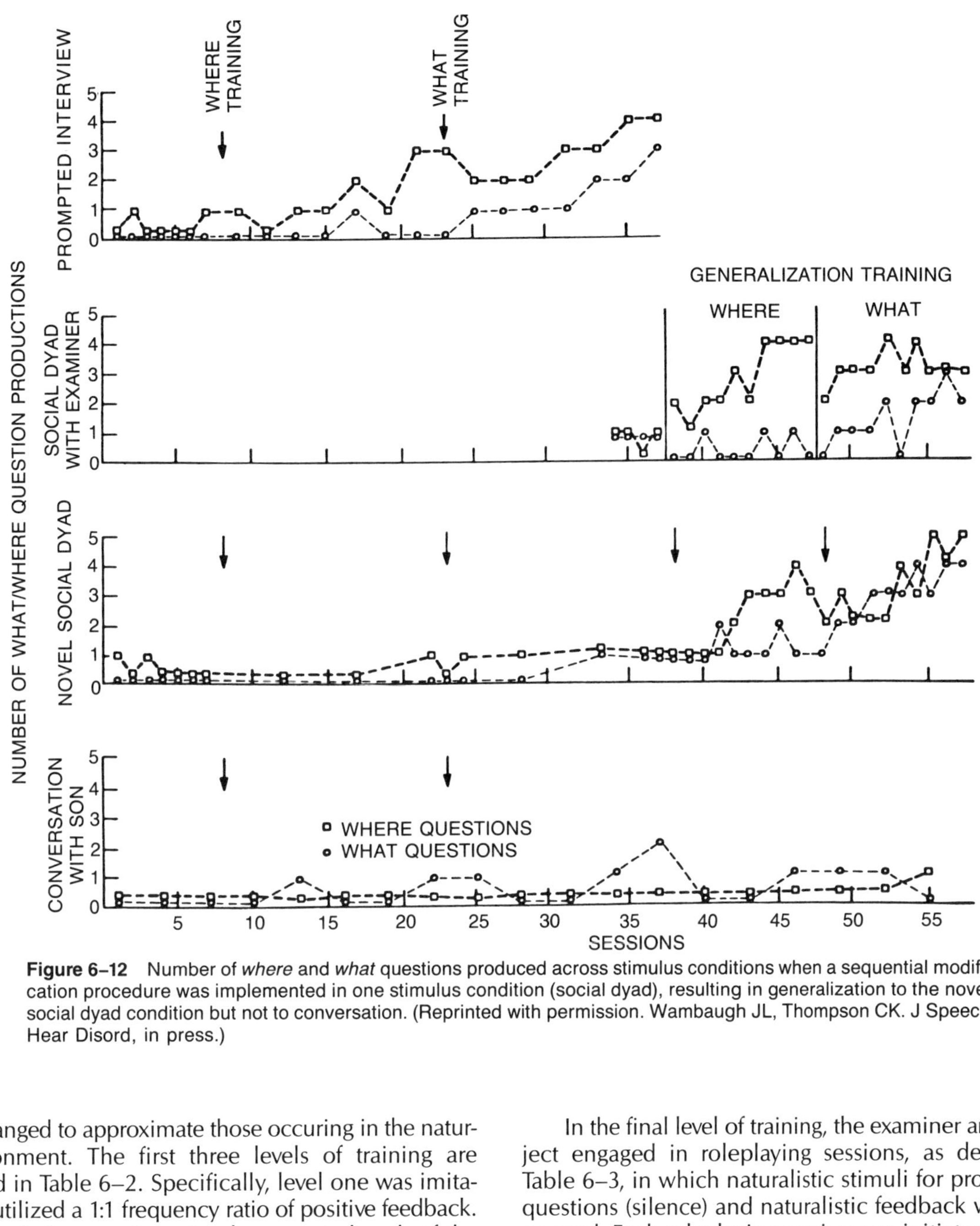

Figure 6–12 Number of *where* and *what* questions produced across stimulus conditions when a sequential modification procedure was implemented in one stimulus condition (social dyad), resulting in generalization to the novel social dyad condition but not to conversation. (Reprinted with permission. Wambaugh JL, Thompson CK. J Speech Hear Disord, in press.)

sively changed to approximate those occuring in the natural environment. The first three levels of training are described in Table 6–2. Specifically, level one was imitative and utilized a 1:1 frequency ratio of positive feedback. At this level, the examiner simply presented each of the target responses for the subject to repeat. At level two, stimuli used to elicit responding were modified, and the frequency of feedback was changed to a 1:2 ratio. The subject was expected to produce the target responses when the examiner provided instructions to do so (e.g., the examiner said, "Tell me your name," to elicit the subject's name). At the third level of training, the stimuli used to elicit responding were further "loosened" for greetings and self-disclosures, and feedback was provided on a variable schedule. Greetings and self-disclosures were elicited using a variety of statements and questions commonly used to elicit these responses in the natural environment.

In the final level of training, the examiner and the subject engaged in roleplaying sessions, as described in Table 6–3, in which naturalistic stimuli for production of questions (silence) and naturalistic feedback were incorporated. Each roleplaying session was initiated by the examiner saying, "Hi," or, "Hello." The subject was then expected to respond with a greeting and to produce a question within a 30-second delay time, which served as a stimulus for question production. If a question was not produced within the 30-second response interval, prompts and modeling procedures identical to those used at level three were implemented. The examiner then answered each question (providing natural feedback) and asked a new question.

Figure 6–15 illustrates the results of the study, indicating percent correct production of target responses during conversational dyads. The arrows at the top of the graph

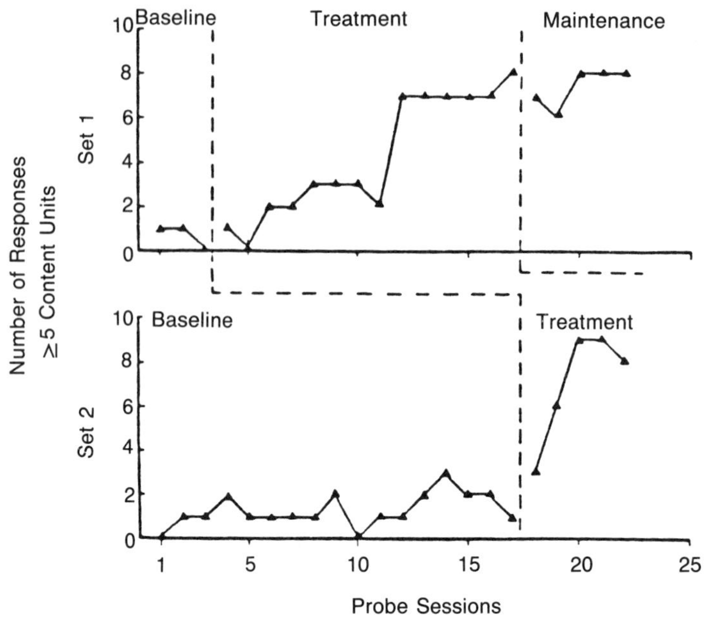

Figure 6–13 Number of responses produced by a Broca's aphasic subject containing five or more content units across two sets of training pictures during baseline, treatment, and maintenance phases. These data indicate successful response acquisition using a loose training procedure (RET). (Reprinted with permission. Kearns KP. Clinical aphasiology conference proceedings. Minneapolis, MN: BRK Publishers, 1985:199.)

indicate when levels of treatment were changed, and the horizontal lines depict the mean and standard deviation of a normal comparison group, reflecting the number of target responses produced by normal individuals in the dyad condition. These data indicate that during treatment, the aphasic subjects began using target responses in conversational dyads with unfamiliar people, and that by the end of the study, the aphasic subjects' performance was within the range of normal.

The third loose training technique was described by Doyle, Goldstein, Bourgeois, and Nakles (in press) in a study designed to investigate both stimulus and response generalization. Four Broca's aphasic subjects participated in the study, and were trained to produce questions about three topics: personal information, health, and leisure activities.

The loose training procedure (Doyle, Goldstein, Bourgeois, and Nakles, in press) incorporated loosening of stimuli, responses, and feedback. Each treatment session was conducted by one of three randomly assigned speech-language pathologists (representing a loosening of training stimuli). The responses trained were loosened by allowing production of several question types (e.g., *wh* questions, *do* questions, *is* and *are* questions), requiring

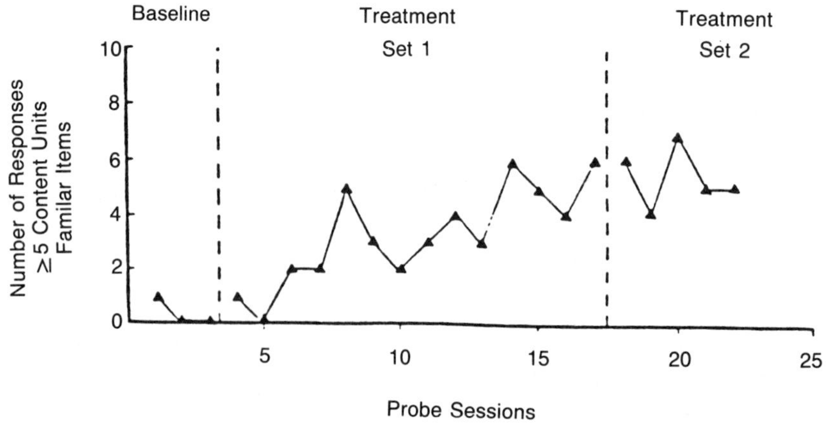

Figure 6–14 Response generalization (number of responses produced containing five or more content units to untrained picture stimuli), occurring during loose training of picture sets 1 and 2 (see Fig. 6–13) for one Broca's aphasic subject. (Reprinted with permission. Kearns KP. Clinical aphasiology conference proceedings. Minneapolis, MN: BRK Publishers, 1985:201.)

TABLE 6–2 Expected Responses, Discriminative Stimuli and Feedback Schedule used at Levels 1, 2, and 3 of Training

	Discriminative Stimuli		
Expected Responses	*Level 1*	*Level 2*	*Level 3*
Hello	"Hello."	"Tell me hello."	"Hello." "Hi."
How are you? I am fine.	"How are you?" "I am fine."	"Ask me how I am." "Tell me how you are."	"Ask me how I am." "How are you?" "How are you doing?" "How are you feeling?"
What is your name? My name is _____.	"What is your name?" "My name is _____."	"Ask me my name," "Tell me your name."	"Ask me my name." "What is your name." "Who are you?" "Your name is?"
Where do you live? I live in _____.	"Where do you live?" "I live in _____."	"Ask me where I live." "Tell me where you live."	"Ask me where I live." "Where do you live?" "Where are you living?" "You live where?"
Goodbye.	"Goodbye."	"Tell me goodbye."	"Goodbye." "Bye."

Feedback schedule: Level 1, Frequency ratio (FR) 1:1; Level 2, FR 1:2; Level 3, FR 1:4. From Thompson CK, Byrne ME (1984).

production of no particular structure (e.g., questions were considered to be "adequate" if they were intelligible, contained a question morpheme and a content word, or ended with rising inflection), and requiring no specific content other than being on the topic in training. Finally, naturalistic feedback was provided for adequate subject responses, and inadequate responses were followed by a procedure in which a variety of responses were prompted or modeled. When intelligible, on-topic questions were produced, the trainer responded with verbal feedback such as, "That's a good question," and provided the solicited information. When inadequate question responses were produced, a modeling procedure was implemented in which the subject-initiated topic was modeled in question form for the subject to repeat or a question prompt was randomly selected from a prepared list consisting of a variety of questions pertaining to the training topic.

During baseline and throughout training phases, subjects participated in conversational dyads with trainers and volunteers, in which subjects were expected to ask as many questions as possible about a specified topic. The number of questions produced about topics in training served to evaluate the stimulus generalization effects of treatment, whereas questions produced about untrained topics served as a means for evaluating response generalization. Results of the study for one subject are shown in Figure 6–16. As can be seen, during baseline, this subject produced few questions during any of the probes, regardless of topic. However, when treatment was applied to health questions, an increase in the number of such questions during health probes with both the trainers and volunteers was noted, but stable baselines were maintained in leisure and personal information probes. Similarly, when treatment was focused on production of questions pertaining to leisure activities, increased production of leisure activity questions was noted, with no change seen in production of questions about personal information. Finally, when personal information questions were

TABLE 6–3 Treatment Level 4: Structured Roleplaying

E. Initiates conversation: "Hi," or, "Hello."

S. Replies, "Hello," and asks question, "How are you?" within 30-second response time (incorrect responses were prompted).

E. Replies, "I am fine," and asks, "How are you?"

S. Replies, "I am fine," and asks, "What is your name?" within 30-second response time (incorrect responses were prompted).

E. Replies, "My name is __________," and asks, "Who are you?"

S. Replies, "My name is _______," and asks, "Where do you live?" within 30-second response time (incorrect responses were prompted).

E. Replies, "I live in ________," and asks, "Where do you live?"

S. Replies "I live in ________." Goodbye," within 30-second response time (incorrect responses were prompted).

From Thompson CK, Byrne ME (1984).

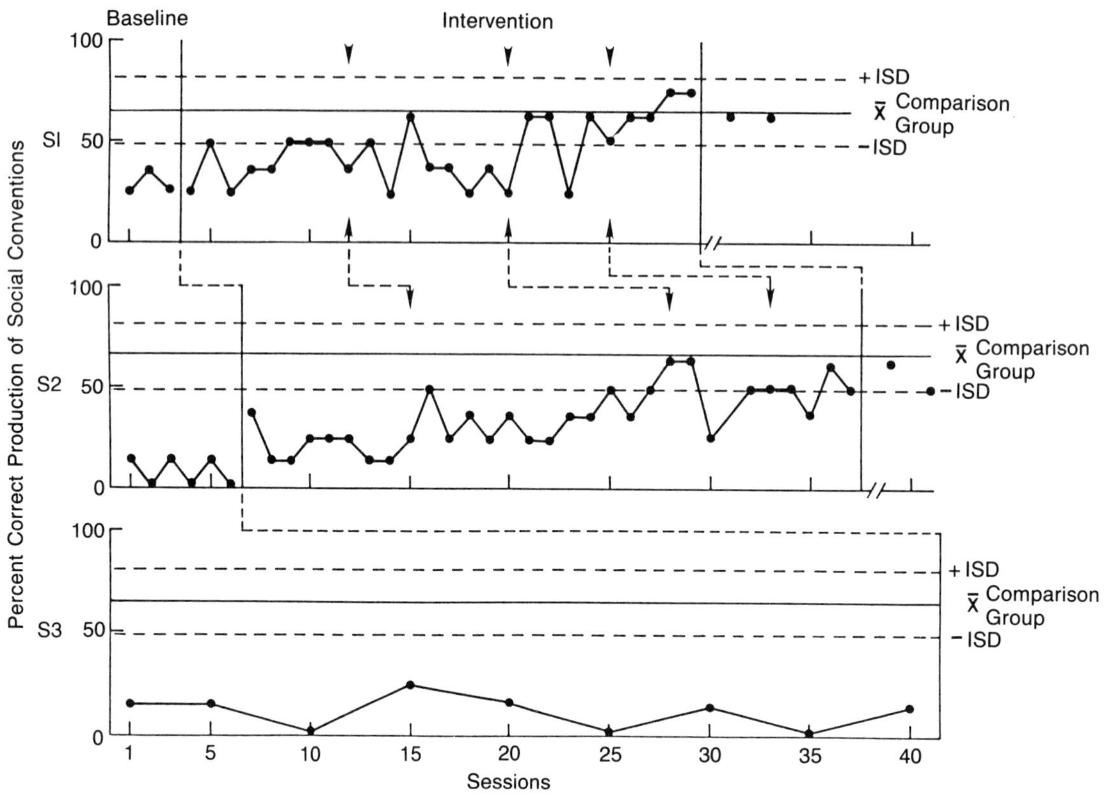

Figure 6–15 Percent correct production of social conventions (greetings, self-disclosures, and questions), trained using a loose training procedure, during stimulus generalization probes (novel social dyads) for two Broca's aphasic subjects. Arrows indicate sessions in which new levels of the loose training procedure were introduced. Horizontal lines represent the mean and one standard deviation about the mean for a normal comparison group, providing social validity data. (Reprinted with permission. Thompson CK, Byrne ME. Clinical aphasiology conference proceedings. Minneapolis, MN: BRK Publishers, 1984:137.)

trained, increased usage of questions was noted during personal information probes. These data indicate that the loose training procedure was useful for promoting stimulus generalization, in that improved responding was noted in stimulus generalization probes (dyads) corresponding to training topics. However, response generalization was less apparent, in that use of questioning did not generalize across topics.

Results of clinical training studies utilizing loose training procedures indicate that such procedures may be useful for facilitating response generalization, stimulus generalization, or both, in aphasic patients. In using a loose training method, it is suggested that clinicians:

1. Decide which component or components of training are to be loosened: the stimuli used to evoke responding, the responses trained, or the feedback and training procedure.
2. Decide and specify how these components are to be loosened, perhaps using the studies described in this section as a guideline.
3. Design probes for measuring stimulus generalization, or response generalization, or both.
4. Administer probe procedures periodically, and
5. When generalization does not occur, incorporate other generalization facilitation techniques.

Maintenance and Trained Behavior

Maintenance of trained behavior or the durability of responding, evaluated after treatment has been completed, is an important aspect of intervention, sometimes referred to as *generalization over time* (Ingham, this volume). Research in aphasia in which the maintenance of treatment effects has been measured has indicated that trained behavior is often maintained, although variable results have been reported (see Table 6–1) and a lack of maintenance is often observed in clinical practice. For example, aphasic patients, discharged from treatment temporarily during semester breaks in a university setting or for various reasons in a hospital setting, sometimes return without the behaviors that had previously been demonstrated. A few possible reasons for discrepancies between what has been reported in the literature and what is often noted in clinical practice are addressed in the following discussion of measurement and facilitation of maintenance.

Measurement of Maintenance

There are at least three aspects that need to be considered in measurement of the maintenance effects of

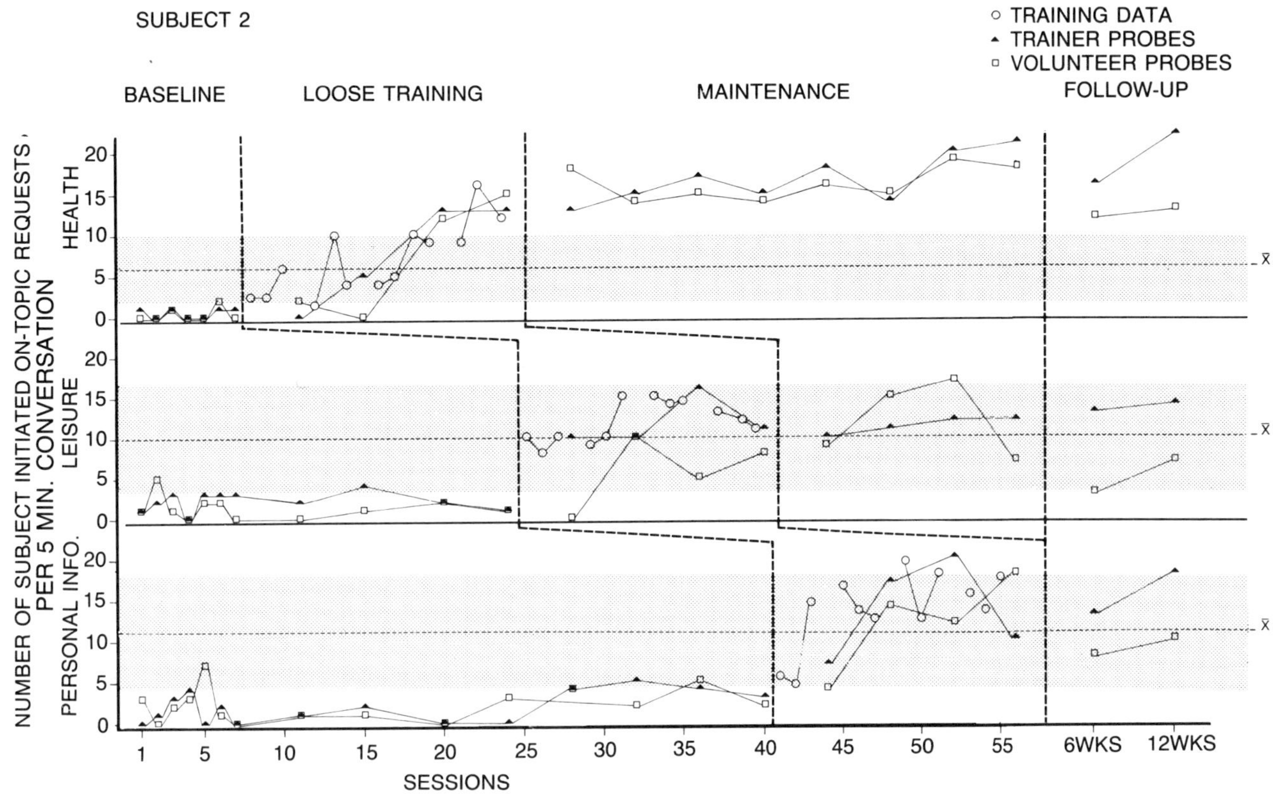

Figure 6–16 Number of requests produced during health, leisure, and personal information dyads conducted during baseline, treatment, and maintenance phases with trainers and volunteers, indicating the generalization effects of a loose training procedure. Social validity data depicted by shaded area, showing the mean and one standard deviation about the mean for a normal comparison group. (Reprinted with permission. Doyle P, Goldstein H, Bourgeois M, Nakles K. J Appl Behav Anal, in press.)

treatment: the amount of time between treatment and measurement of maintenance, the number of probes administered to demonstrate that maintenance has or has not occurred, and the conditions for evaluating maintenance. Research in aphasia has not systematically addressed these aspects of maintenance. As can be seen in Table 6–1, some treatment studies have not measured maintenance at all and in studies in which maintenance has been measured, there appears to be little agreement regarding the length of time required between the end of treatment and administration of probes to evaluate maintenance. That is, some researchers have administered maintenance probes of trained behaviors while other behaviors are still being trained (Kearns and Salmon, 1984; Thompson and Kearns, 1981; Thompson and McReynolds, 1986), illustrating maintenance effects of treatment for as long as 20 sessions after training. This type of maintenance testing, referred to as *within-session probing*, is an inherent property of multiple baseline designs across behaviors (McReynolds and Kearns, 1983; McReynolds and Thompson, 1986). After criterion level responding is reached on the first behavior or set of language responses, treatment is extended to a new set, as maintenance probes on the first set are initiated. This type of maintenance testing also may be practiced by randomly interspersing a few previously trained items within each training session, or by testing all trained responses for maintenance on a weekly or monthly basis.

Maintenance testing may also be accomplished after all treatment has ended, in *follow-up maintenance probes* administered a week, a month, or several months following treatment. Some maintenance or follow-up probes in aphasia research have been conducted as soon as 1 week following treatment, whereas others have been administered several months after completion of treatment. Generalization research in aphasia has not provided information regarding when maintenance testing should be accomplished. Therefore, it is possible that different schedules of maintenance testing may result in different findings.

The number of maintenance probes administered is another important factor that may influence results. Several treatment studies in aphasia have administered only one or two maintenance probes, which may not adequately demonstrate the maintenance effect of treatment. According to Hughes (1985), "a rigorous measure of maintenance should be repeated several times to determine stability" (p. 128). The frequency of maintenance probing may vary depending upon the clinical setting, time, subject availability, and other considerations. However, as a guideline, it is suggested that within-session maintenance probes be administered weekly and that follow-up maintenance probes be administered at least once within a 2- to

3-month period, and at 6 months and 1 year following discharge from treatment, if possible. Research comparing within-session to follow-up maintenance data, or comparing follow-up data, for example at 3 months and 1 year after treatment, is needed. However, until such data are available, when to administer maintenance probes remains a clinical decision.

Another aspect of maintenance testing concerns the conditions of the probe measure used. As with other forms of generalization testing, it is important to measure maintenance using consistent procedures across all probes. That is, the stimulus conditions for measuring maintenance should not be changed from those in which the behaviors of interest were measured during training, and responses tested should be identical to those trained. For example, if maintenance of word retrieval is important, then it is necessary to elicit trained responses using the same set of stimuli that were used in training, the same examiner, the same room, the same auditory or verbal stimuli, and so on. If the stimuli are varied, the clinician is measuring stimulus generalization rather than maintenance; likewise, if untrained responses are tested during maintenance probes, then response generalization is being measured. Of course, if measuring maintenance of stimulus or response generalizaton patterns established during treatment is desired, then maintenance probes would be designed to test the previously demonstrated generalization. What is important to note here is that, if the maintenance measurement conditions or responses tested are different from those trained, it is possible for maintenance effects to be obscured.

Facilitating Maintenance

Programming maintenance, in the event that it is not observed during within-session or follow-up probes, has not been addressed in aphasia research. Two suggestions for promoting maintenance are to retrain desired responses using the same procedures used to train responses initially, or to provide new training. Retraining provides additional practice in producing desired responses using the original training procedures; this may be all that is required in some cases. For example, retraining may be the method of choice when maintenance is not observed during within-session maintenance probes. When treatment is extended to new behavior, it is common for a decrease in performance to be noted on the old behavior. Additional training on the old behavior while the new behavior is in training often serves to establish both behaviors (Lovaas, 1977).

When maintenance is not observed during follow-up probes, new training may be necessary, because retraining would most likely result, again, in a lack of maintenance. When follow-up testing indicates a lack of maintenance, it becomes necessary to investigate potential reasons for this, so that the type of new training to use can be determined. For example, the clinician may find clues in the patient's communicative environment. Often, a lack of maintenance can be explained by examining the differences between the patient's communicative environment and the training environment. The opportunity to use trained responses in the patient's communicative environment may be lacking, which would extinguish trained responses. One way to facilitate maintenance is to incorporate aspects of the patient's environment into training or to incorporate aspects of training into the patient's communicative environment, using principles of programming common stimuli. Loose training procedures might also be beneficial for promoting maintenance. In some cases, even sequential modification might be necessary. That is, for certain responses to be maintained, it may be necessary to train and to test maintenance in environments in which the patient communicates. Other guidelines for facilitating maintenance are described by Kazdin and Esveldt-Dawson (1981) and summarized by Hughes (1985).

SUMMARY AND CONCLUSIONS

This chapter has discussed the importance of generalization in treatment for aphasia, addressed problems and variables related to facilitating generalization, and provided suggestions and considerations for planning treatment to promote generalization. It has pointed out that research in aphasia is limited and that variability exists with regard to generalization patterns noted in these patients. Some general points pertaining to facilitation of generalization in treatment are as follows:

1. To select functional treatment targets and plan to program response generalization, if necessary, across structurally or functionally different responses.
2. To design probes carefully for measuring generalization across responses and stimulus conditions and to administer them periodically throughout treatment.
3. To establish criteria for generalization and to look closely at error responses.
4. To introduce aspects of the generalization environment into treatment or to introduce aspects of the training environment into the generalization environment in early stages of treatment.
5. To use treatment methods, such as loose training, that have resulted in generalization, when possible.
6. To extend treatment across settings or persons, when required.

The need for further research in generalization has been addressed. In order to understand and facilitate generalization in treatment of aphasia, the following areas are in need of investigation:

1. Research investigating the generalization effects of training focused on a number of aphasic behaviors, identifying response class phenomena in aphasia.
2. Research identifying efficient testing or probing procedures for both response generalization and stimulus generalization.
3. Research identifying the validity of various generalization testing methods such as simulated environmental probes versus naturalistic sampling methods.

4. Research identifying the relationship between specific subject variables such as severity of aphasia, patterns of language involvement, time after onset, personality factors, and generalization.
5. Research investigating the generalization effects of treatment variables that have not been studied.
6. Research comparing the generalization effects of various treatments.
7. Research investigating the maintenance effects of treatment.
8. Research investigating treatment methods for facilitating generalization and maintenance.
9. Research identifying and evaluating the effects of language training packages with built-in generalization measurement and facilitation procedures.

Research focused on these and many other issues relative to generalization in aphasia is needed, in order to provide optimal treatment for aphasic patients. At the present time, we have only rudimentary information for making recommendations about facilitation of generalization in aphasia. The future of generalization research in aphasia is exciting; results of which may greatly influence future approaches to aphasia rehabilitation.

Acknowledgment. The author wishes to express thanks to Jill B. Georges and Julie L. Wambaugh for their assistance in reviewing the aphasia treatment literature.

REFERENCES

Aten JL, Caliguiri MP, Holland AL. The efficacy of functional communication therapy for chronic aphasic patients. J Speech Hear Disord 1982; 41:93–96.

Barlow DH, Hersen M. Single case experimental designs. Strategies for studying behavioral change. 2nd ed. New York: Pergamon Press, 1986.

Barlow DH, Hayes SC, Nelson RD. The research practitioner. Research and accountability in clinical and educational settings. New York: Pergamon Press, 1984.

Basso W, Capitani E, Vignolo LA. Influence of rehabilitation on language skills in aphasic patients. Arch Neurol 1979; 36:190–196.

Benson DF. Disorders of verbal expression. In: Benson DF, Blumer L, eds. Psychiatric aspects of neurologic disorders. New York: Grune & Stratton, 1975.

Benson DF. Aphasia, alexia, and agraphia. New York: Churchill Livingstone, 1979.

Benson DF, Geschwind N. Aphasia and related cortical disturbances. In: Baker AB, Baker LH, eds. Clinical neurology. New York: Harper & Row, 1971.

Berndt RS, Caramazza A. Syntactic aspects of aphasia. In: Sarno MT, ed. Acquired aphasia. New York: Academic Press, 1981:157.

Bernstein-Ellis E, Wertz RT, Shubitowski Y. More pace, less fillers: a verbal strategy for a high-level aphasic patient. In: Brookshire RH, ed. Clinical Aphasiology, Vol 17. Minneapolis, MN: BRK Publishers, 1987:12.

Brookshire RH. Differences in responding to auditory verbal materials among aphasic patients. Acta Symbolica 1974; 5:1–18.

Brookshire RH. Auditory comprehension and aphasia. In: Johns DF, ed. Clinical management of neurogenic communicative disorders. Boston: Little, Brown, 1978:103.

Brookshire RH. Subject descriptions and generality of results in experiments with aphasic adults. J Speech Hear Disord 1983; 48:342–346.

Brown JW, ed. Jargonaphasia. New York: Academic Press, 1981.

Burger LH, Wertz RT. The effects of a token training program on auditory comprehension in a case of Wernicke's aphasia. In: Brookshire RH, ed. Clinical aphasiology conference proceedings. Minneapolis, MN: BRK Publishers, 1984:173.

Cannito MP, Vogel D. Treatment can facilitate reacquisition of a morphological rule. In: Brookshire RH, ed. Clinical aphasiology, Vol 17. Minneapolis, MN: BRK Publishers, 1987:23.

Chapey R, ed. Language intervention strategies in adult aphasia, 2nd ed. Baltimore: Williams and Wilkins, 1986.

Coelho CA, Duffy RJ. The relationship of the acquisition of manual signs to severity of aphasia. A training study. Brain Lang 1987; 31:328–345.

Darley FL. The efficacy of language rehabilitation in aphasia. J Speech Hear Disord 1972; 37:3–21.

Darley FL. Aphasia. Philadelphia: WB Saunders, 1982.

Davis GA, Tan LL. Stimulation of sentence production in a case with agrammatism. J Commun Disord 1987; 20:447–457.

Davis GQ. A survey of aphasia. Englewood Cliffs, NJ: Prentice Hall, 1983.

Doyle P, Goldstein H, Bourgeois MS. Experimental analysis of syntax training in Broca's aphasia: a generalization and social validation study. J Speech Hear Disord 1987; 52:143–155.

Doyle P, Goldstein H, Bourgeois M, Nakles K. Programming "loose training" as a strategy to facilitate generalization of questioning in Broca's aphasic subjects. J Appl Behav Anal (in press).

Duffy RJ, Duffy JR. Three studies of deficits in pantomimic expression and pantomimic recognition in aphasia. J Speech Hear Res 1981; 24:70–84.

Egolf DB, Chester SC. A comparison of aphasics' verbal performance in the language clinic with their verbal performance in other program areas in a comprehensive rehabilitation center. Rehabil Lit 1977; 38:9–12.

Esper E. A technique for the experimental investigation of associative interference in artificial linguistic materials. Language Monograph I. 1925.

Foss D. Learning and discovery in the acquisition of structured material: effects of number of items and their sequence. J Exp Psychol 1968; 77:341–344.

Goldstein H. Training generative repertoires within agent-action-object miniature linguistic systems with children. J Speech Hear Res 1983; 26:76–89.

Goldstein H. Matrix and stimulus equivalence training. In: Warren SF, Rogers-Warren A, eds. Teaching functional language. Baltimore: University Park Press, 1985:225.

Goodglass H, Gleason JB, Bernholtz NA, Hyde MR. Some linguistic structures in the speech of Broca's aphasia. Cortex 1972; 8:191–212.

Goodglass H, Kaplan E. The assessment of aphasia and related disorders. Philadelphia: Lea & Febiger, 1983.

Goodkin R, Diller L, Shah N. Training spouses to improve the functional speech of aphasic patients. In: Lahey B, ed. The modification of language behavior. Springfield, IL: CC Thomas, 1972:218.

Guess E, Keogh W, Sailor W. Generalization of speech and language behavior: measurement and training tactics. In: Schiefelbusch RL, ed. Basis of language intervention. Baltimore: University Park Press, 1978:373.

Guess D, Sailor W, Baer D. Functional speech and language training for the severely handicapped. Lawrence, KS: H and H Enterprises, 1978.
Hart B. Pragmatics and generalization. In: Lahey BB, Kazdin AE, eds. Advances in clinical child psychology, Vol 3. New York: Plenum Press, 1980.
Hart B, Risley TR. Using preschool materials to modify the language of disadvantaged children. J Appl Behav Anal 1974; 7:243–256.
Head H. Aphasia and kindred disorders of speech, Vol 1. New York: Hafner Publishing Co, 1926.
Hegde MN. Treatment principles and procedures in communicative disorders. San Diego: College-Hill Press, 1985.
Helm-Estabrooks N. Helm's elicited language program for syntax stimulation. Austin, TX: Exceptional Resources, 1981.
Helm-Estabrooks N. Fitzpatrick PM, Barresi B. Response of an agrammatic patient to a syntax stimulation program for aphasia. J Speech Hear Disord 1981; 46:422–427.
Helmick JW, Wipplinger M. Effects of stimulus repetition on the naming behavior of an aphasic adult: a clinical report. J Commun Disord 1975; 8:23–29.
Hersen M, Barlow DH. Single case experimental designs, strategies for studying behavior change. New York: Pergamon Press, 1976.
Holland AL. Observing functional communication of aphasic adults. J Speech Hear Disord 1982; 47:50–56.
Holland AL, Harris AB. Aphasia rehabilitation using programmed instruction: an intensive case study. In: Sloane HN, MacCauley DB, eds. Operant training procedures in remedial speech and language training. Boston: Houghton Mifflin, 1969:197.
Holland AL, Levy CB. Syntactic generalizaton in aphasics as a function of relearning an active sentence. Acta Symbolica 1971; 2:34–41.
Holland AL, Sonderman TC. Effects of a program based on the token test for teaching comprehension skills to aphasics. J Speech Hear Disord 1974; 17:589–598.
Hoodin R, Thompson CK. Facilitation of verbal labeling in adult aphasia by gestural, verbal, or verbal plus gestural training. In: Brookshire RH, ed. Clinical aphasiology conference proceedings. Minneapolis, MN: BRK Publishers, 1983:62.
Howard D, Patterson K, Franklin S, et al. Treatment of word retrieval deficits in aphasia. Brain 1985; 108:817–829.
Hughes DL. Language treatment and generalization. A clinician's handbook. San Diego: College-Hill Press, 1985.
Jackson JH. Selected writings of John Hughlings Jackson. In: Taylor J, ed. London: Hodder & Stoughton, 1958.
Jenning EA, Lubinski RB. Strategies for improving productive thinking in the language impaired adult. J Commun Disord 1981; 14:255–271.
Johannsen-Horback H, Cegla B, Mager U, Schempp B. Treatment of chronic global aphasia with a nonverbal communication system. Brain Lang 1985; 24:74–82.
Johns DF, ed. Clinical management of neurogenic communicative disorders. Boston: Little, Brown, 1985.
Karlan G, Brenn-White B, Lentz A, et al. Establishing generalized, productive verb-noun phrase usage in a manual language system with moderately handicapped children. J Speech Hear Disord 1982; 47:31–42.
Kazdin AE. Single-case research designs: methods for clinical and applied settings. New York: Oxford University Press, 1982.
Kazdin A, Esveldt-Dawson K. How to maintain behavior. Lawrence, KS: H and H Enterprises, 1981.
Kean ML, ed. Agrammatism. New York: Academic Press, 1985.
Kearns KP. Approaches to language rehabilitation in aphasia: a perspective on generalization. Paper presented at the University of Kansas Symposium: Current Trends and Recent Developments in Speech/Language Pathology and Audiology, Kansas City, 1980.
Kearns KP. Response elaboration training for patient initiated utterances. In: Brookshire RH, ed. Clinical aphasiology, Vol 15. Minneapolis, MN: BRK Publishers, 1985:196.
Kearns KP, Salmon SJ. An experimental analysis of auxiliary and copula verb generalization in aphasia. J Speech Hear Disord 1984; 49:152–163.
Kearns KP, Simmons N, Sisterhen C. Gestural sign (Amer-Ind) as a facilitator of verbalization in patients with aphasia. In: Brookshire RH, ed. Clinical aphasiology conference proceedings. Minneapolis, MN: BRK Publishers, 1982:183.
Kushner D. Extended comprehension training leading to improved verbal production: a treatment program for an aphasic patient. In: Brookshire RH, ed. Clinical aphasiology conference proceedings. Minneapolis, MN: BRK Publishers, 1975:79.
LaPointe LL. Multiple baseline designs. In: Brookshire RH, ed. Clinical aphasiology conference proceedings. Minneapolis, MN: BRK Publishers, 1978:20.
Lecours AR, Rouillon F. Neurolinguistic analysis of jargonaphasia and jargonagraphia. In: Whitaker H, Whitaker HA, eds. Studies in neurolinguistics, Vol. 2. New York: Academic Press, 1976:95.
Lesser R. Linguistic investigations of aphasia. New York: Elsevier, 1979.
Linebaugh C, Lehner L. Cueing hierarchies and word retrieval: a therapy program. In: Brookshire RH, ed. Clinical aphasiology conference proceedings. Minneapolis, MN: BRK Publishers, 1979:19.
Lovaas OI. The autistic child, language development through behavior modification. New York: Irvington Publishers, 1977.
McNeil M. Aphasia. In: Lass NJ, McReynolds LV, Yoder DE, Northern JL, eds. Handbook of speech-language pathology and audiology. Toronto: BC Decker, 1988.
McReynolds LV, Kearns KP. Single-subject experimental designs in communicative disorders. Austin, TX: Pro-ed, 1983.
McReynolds LV, Thompson CK. Flexibility of single-subject experimental designs. Part I. Review of the basics of single-subject designs. J Speech Hear Disord 1986; 51:194–203.
Prinz PM. A note on requesting strategies in adult aphasics. J Commun Disord 1980; 13:65–73.
Prescott T, Selinger M, Loverso F. An analysis of learning, generalization, and maintenance of verbs by an aphasic patient. In: Brookshire RH, ed. Clinical aphasiology conference proceedings. Minneapolis, MN: BRK Publishers, 1982:178.
Royall J, Horner J. Acquisition and generalization of cued speech by a chronically aphasic adult. In: Brookshire RH, ed. Clinical aphasiology conference proceedings. Minneapolis, MN: BRK Publishers, 1983:85.
Salvatore AP. Training an aphasic adult to respond appropriately to spoken commands by fading pause duration within commands. In: Brookshire RH, ed. Clinical aphasiology conference proceedings. Minneapolis, MN: BRK Publishers, 1976:172.
Salvatore AP. Experimental analysis of a syntax stimulation training procedure. In: Brookshire RH, ed. Clinical aphasiology Vol. 15. Minneapolis, MN: BRK Publications, 1985:214.
Sarno MT, ed. Acquired aphasia. New York: Academic Press, 1981.
Schlanger PH, Schlanger BB. Adapting role playing activities with aphasic patients. J Speech Hear Disord 1970; 35:229–235.
Seron X, Deloch G, Bastard V, et al. Word finding difficulties and learning transfer in aphasic patients. Cortex 1979; 15:149–155.
Shewan CM. Facilitating sentence formulation: a case study. J Commun Disord 1976; 9:191–197.

Sidman M. The behavior analysis of aphasia. J Psychiatr Res 1971; 8:4123–4422.

Sidman M, Stoddard LT, Mohr JP, Leicester J. Behavioral studies in aphasia: methods of investigation and analysis. Neuropsychologia 1971; 9:119–140.

Simmons NN, Kearns KP, Potechin G. Treatment of aphasia through family member training. In: Brookshire RH, ed. Clinical aphasiology, Vol. 17. Minneapolis, MN: BRK Publishers, 1987;106.

Snyder A. A study of the generative use of gestures across behaviors and across settings in a Broca's aphasic client. Master's thesis, The Pennsylvania State University, 1984.

Stokes T, Baer DM. An implicit technology of generalization. J Appl Behav Anal 1977; 10:349–367.

Striefel S, Wetherby B, Karlan G. Establishing generalized verb-noun instruction following skills in retarded children. J Exp Child Psychol 1976; 22:247–260.

Thompson CK, Byrne ME. Across setting generalization of social conventions in aphasia: an experimental analysis of "loose training." In: Brookshire RH, ed. Clinical aphasiology conference proceedings. Minneapolis, MN: BRK Publishers, 1984:132.

Thompson CK, Hall H, Sisson C. Effects of hypnosis and imagery training on naming behavior in aphasia. Brain Lang 1986; 28:141–153.

Thompson CK, Kearns KP. An experimental analysis of acquisition, generalization and maintenance in a patient with anomia. In: Brookshire RH, ed. Clinical aphasiology conference proceedings. Minneapolis, MN: BRK Publishers, 1981:35.

Thompson CK, McReynolds LV. *Wh* interrogative production in agrammatic aphasia: an experimental analysis of auditory–visual stimulation and direct-production treatment. J Speech Hear Res 1986; 29:193–206.

Thompson CK, McReynolds LV, Vance C. Generative use of locatives in multiword utterances in agrammatism: a matrix training approach. In: Brookshire RH, ed. Clinical aphasiology conference proceedings. Minneapolis, MN: BRK Publishers, 1982:289.

Thompson CK, Warner E. Stimulus generalization of functional responses in aphasic subjects. Paper presented at American Speech-Language-Hearing Association Convention, New Orleans, LA, 1987.

Tonkovich J, Loverso F. A training matrix approach to gestural acquisition by the agrammatic patient. In: Brookshire RH, ed. Clinical aphasiology conference proceedings. Minneapolis, MN: BRK Publishers, 1982:283.

Tullos D. Stimulus generalization: an experimental analysis using the touch talker. Doctoral research project, The Pennsylvania State University, 1985.

Wambaugh JL, Thompson CK. *Wh* interrogative production in agrammatic aphasia: an experimental analysis of stimulus and response generalization. J Speech Hear Disord (in press).

Warren SF. Clinical strategies for the management of language generalization. In: Warren SF, Rogers-Warren A, eds. Teaching functional language skills. Baltimore: University Park Press, 1985:197.

Warren S, Rogers-Warren A, Baer D, Guess D. Assessment and facilitation of language generalization. In: Sailor W, Wilcox B, Brown L, eds. Methods and instruction for severely handicapped students. Baltimore: Brooks, 1980:227.

Weigel-Crump C. Agrammatism and aphasia. In: Lebrum Y, Hoops R, eds. Neurolinguistics 4: recovery in aphasics. Amsterdam: Swets and Zeitlinger, 1976:243.

Weigel-Crump C. Koenigsknecht R. Tapping the lexical store of the adult aphasic: analysis of the improvement made in word retrieval skills. Cortex 1973; 9:411–418.

Wertz RT. Neuropathologies of speech and language: an introduction to patient management. In: Johns DF, ed. Clinical management of neurogenic communicative disorders. Boston: Little, Brown, 1985:1.

Wertz RT, Collin MJ, Weiss D, et al. Veterans Administration cooperative study on aphasia: a comparison of individual and group treatment. J Speech Hear Res 1981; 24:580–594.

Wertz RT, Weiss DG, Aten JL, et al. Comparison of clinical, home, and deferred language treatment for aphasia. A Veterans Administration cooperative study. Arch Neurol 1986; 43:653–658.

Chapter Seven

GENERALIZATION IN THE TREATMENT OF AUTISM

ROBERT L. KOEGEL, Ph.D.
LYNN KERN KOEGEL, M.A., CCC–SP
ROBERT E. O'NEILL, Ph.D.

Children with the syndrome of autism have presented a major challenge to educators, researchers, and therapists, with respect to producing generalized treatment gains. Early reports of the difficulties of providing treatment date back hundreds of years, and pessimism was prominent throughout many of the accounts (Lane, 1976). The last few decades have provided steadily increasing findings to indicate that such children are responsive to treatment and that major behavioral improvements can be obtained under intensive treatment conditions.

However, a continuing difficulty in treatment relates to the fact that the disorder represents a composite of behavioral excesses and deficits, and that altering each of these, one behavior at a time in one setting at a time, is an almost impossible task under any reasonable set of time constraints. Therefore, clinical researchers have been searching for pivotal target behaviors that, when altered, will also result in generalized changes in many other behaviors in many other settings over extended periods of time (Kazdin, 1982; Koegel and Koegel, 1988; Voeltz and Evans, 1982). This chapter discusses the characteristics of children with autism and concludes that such children exhibit severe deficiencies in responsiveness and stimulus control (O'Neill, 1987). Research findings demonstrate that the responsiveness and the stimulus control deficiencies can be remediated by training, and that when they are, there may be general and durable treatment gains. Following a description of the conceptual issues and empirical data, we present several case studies that illustrate various intervention strategies.

CHARACTERISTICS OF CHILDREN WITH AUTISM

An overview of the characteristics of children with autism points to a pervasive lack of responsivness to environmental stimuli as a central aspect of the disorder. As shall be seen below, we postulate that this lack of responsiveness to a variety of stimulus input may be at the heart of many of the generalization problems that need to be addressed.

The syndrome of autism was first described by Leo Kanner in a classic article in 1943. In that and subsequent papers (Kanner, 1971), Kanner described the inability to relate appropriately to people or objects as the cardinal characteristic of the disorder. The assessment and diagnosis of the syndrome have evolved since it was first described. An influential definition proposed by Ritvo and Freeman (1978) included these six characteristics: disturbances of developmental rate and sequence (motor, cognitive, and social); onset before 30 months; impaired language or communication abilities; *an insistence on sameness in the environment; inappropriate responses to sensory stimuli* (hypo- and hyperactivity to auditory and visual input); and a lack of appropriate relations with people, events, and objects. The diagnostic criteria from the *Diagnostic and Statistical Manual of Mental Disorders,* third edition, revised, (*DSM III-R;* APA, 1987) include the following: onset during infancy, qualitative impairment in reciprocal social interaction, qualitative impairment in verbal and nonverbal communication and in imaginative activity, and *markedly restricted repertoire of activities and interests*.

As is evident from these lists of characteristics, the impoverished environmental interactions of children with autism are a key feature of the disorder (Schopler, Reichler, Devellis, and Daly, 1980). Wenar, Ruttenberg, Kalish-Weiss, and Wolf (1986), using a behavior rating instrument, compared the behavior and development of 41 autistic children with that of 355 normal preschool-aged children. One rating category was concerned with the children's interactions with objects and environmental stimuli. The autistic children were most often characterized as displaying hesitant, fleeting engagement when presented with objects. Similarly, Siegel, Anders, Ciaranello, Bienenstock, and Kraemer (1986) presented results of a factor analysis of questionnaire and observational data on 46 autistic children, in order to identify subgroups with different behavioral characteristics. One identified factor was that of *bizarre play*, or unusual interactions with environmental stimuli. This factor was the one identified most in all four subgroups.

Research has attempted to delineate the prevalence and characteristics of this aspect of the syndrome. For example, Ornitz, Guthrie, and Farley (1977, 1978) conducted a retrospective study in which they gathered, from the parents of 74 children with autism, data regarding the children's development, particularly as it related to autistic symptomatology. They found object-relating disturbances and perceptual and motility disturbances reported for 50 percent or more of the children involved, indicating problematic development, especially in the area of environmental interactions. DeMyer (1979) discussed survey and questionnaire data obtained from parents. Ninety-six percent of the parents of 200 autistic children described their autistic children as being extremely uncurious in comparison with their normal children. The children were described as primarily interested in stimuli that could be used in a repetitive, manipulative manner, and not interested in exploring other aspects of the environment. In contrast, their normal children were characterized as being curious about everything and involved in constant exploration of environmental stimuli. Freeman (1984) reported data on the application of the Behavior Observation System (BOS) for autism to groups of autistic, retarded, and normal children. The major behavioral categories of the scale that differentiated children with autism from others included the purposeful and nonpurposeful use of objects (with the normal versus autistic children displaying more or less of these, respectively). Thus, it is possible that this category of behavior is related to some of the key deficits observed in children with autism which, if remedied, could produce widespread and durable response generalization, because many types of responses to many types of stimuli would be involved.

Stimulus Overselectivity

Stimulus overselectivity, a term first proposed by Lovaas, Schreibman, Koegel, and Rehm (1971), refers to the partial or restricted use of available cues or stimuli demonstrated by many children with autism. In the initial study, Lovaas and co-workers (1971) trained autistic, retarded, and normal children to respond to simultaneous stimuli, which included a light, a tone, and tactile stimulation from a blood pressure cuff. When control by the individual stimuli was separately assessed, it was found that the children with autism most often responded differentially to only one of the cues, in contrast to the normal children, who responded equally to all the cues. This finding has been replicated with various paradigms in both the auditory and visual modalities (see Dunlap, Koegel, and Burke, 1981, and Lovaas, Koegel, and Schreibman, 1979, for reviews). These and other authors have speculated that such restricted responding could contribute to deficits in many areas, such as speech and language, as well as various types of social and environmental interactional development. The problems would be especially likely to relate to generalization, because responses to only partial aspects of a stimulus (e.g., a person's hand instead of the entire person) would be likely to make consistency in responding across settings rather erratic (Rincover and Koegel, 1975). Past and current work has indicated that children who are overselective can be taught to respond to larger numbers of cues (Burke and Koegel, 1982; Koegel and Schreibman, 1977), but further work is necessary to delineate specifically how such a problem may contribute directly to the type of behavior often exhibited by children with autism.

Environmental Interactions of Children with Autism

The above mentioned characteristics of children with autism suggest that a pervasive lack of responding to the environment may be a pivotal deficit which, if remediated, might produce widespread behavioral changes across time and settings with a single treatment intervention. However, the assessment of this deficit is only beginning to provide a clear picture of the magnitude of the problem that clinicians might be facing. Most of the studies conducted to date have focused on assessing different types of play behavior of children with autism. An early comparison study of autistic, retarded, and normal children was conducted by Tilton and Ottinger (1964). They recorded the number of different toy uses demonstrated by the children, as well as the occurrence of combinational uses of the toys. The results indicated that the children with autism engaged in significantly fewer combinational and total uses, and significantly more repetitive manipulations and oral contacts with the toys. A later reanalysis of the data by Weiner, Ottinger, and Tilton (1969) indicated that the combinational variable was the most significant in differentiating the children with autism from the normal and retarded children.

A study by Black, Freeman, and Montgomery (1975) assessed the effects of four different environments on the interactional behavior of five children with autism. One setting was a bare room, two settings were indoor rooms with various play equipment and toys, and one setting was an outdoor play area. The results indicated that the children engaged in very low levels of object interactions (approximately 10 to 20 percent of the observation time), most of which were limited to simpler manipulative types of behavior.

Ungerer and Sigman (1981) and Sigman and Ungerer (1984) have assessed the interactional behavior of 16 children with autism in comparison with groups of normally developing children and children with retardation. Assessments were done under both structured and unstructured conditions (free play versus toy presentation). Under unstructured conditions the children with autism displayed significantly less functional manipulation and fewer sequences of relational behavior.

The studies above have primarily focused on assessing the level or quality of the interactions of children with autism. Other more quantitative aspects (number of stimuli, shifts, etc.), as well as the assessment of more general systematic patterns displayed by children with autism during environmental interactions were addressed in a study by O'Neill (1987). The following experimental questions were asked:

1. Do autistic and normal children differ in the number of available stimuli with which they interact?
2. Do autistic and normal children differ in the number of times they shift from one stimulus to another?
3. Do autistic and normal children differ in the percent of interactions in which they are engaged in various types of manipulative and relational types of behavior?
4. Do autistic and normal children differ in the types of stimuli with which they appear to prefer to interact?
5. Do autistic and normal children differ in the systematic patterns they exhibit in their repeated interactions with stimuli?

The results of the analyses indicated that, relative to the normal children, the children with autism interacted with fewer available stimuli; shifted less often among individual stimuli; engaged in appropriate relational and social-relational interactions less often, and did not show age-related decreases in simple manipulative behavior or increases in functional-relational behavior; appeared to prefer to interact relatively more with stimuli more suited to singular, repetitive activities; and displayed less systematic overall patterns in interacting across stimuli.

Related results were presented by Boucher (1977), who compared the performance of autistic and normal children on a maze-solving task. When two paths were available through the maze, significantly fewer alterations and shifting between routes were made by the children with autism. When a third route was made available, significantly fewer children with autism followed it, which is indicative of a lack of response to novel, multiple stimuli. More recently, Mullins and Rincover (1985) compared autistic and normal children on the dimensions of reinforcement maximization, stimulus sampling, and responsiveness to extinction. Using a laboratory-based choice paradigm, they found that the children with autism displayed deficits in their sampling of alternative stimuli and schedules.

Neurophysiologic Involvement

It is important to consider both organismic and environmental variables and their reciprocal influence, in attempting to understand the current expression of behavioral patterns (Baldwin and Baldwin, 1981; Bijou and Dunitz-Johnson, 1981). Early theories regarding the cause of autism often focused on the effects of a deviant and deficient social environment. For example, the parents of children with autism were often considered to be responsible for their children's withdrawal and bizarre behavior (Bettelheim, 1967). Since such early formulations were proposed, a great deal of empirical research has demonstrated that the parents of children with autism are not different from parents of normally developing children (DeMyer, 1979; Koegel, Schreibman, Britten, Burke, and O'Neill, 1982; Koegel, Schreibman, O'Neill, and Burke, 1983; McAdoo and DeMyer, 1978). The focus has since shifted to attempting to discover possible neurochemical or neurophysiological bases for the disorder (Ritvo, 1976; Rutter and Schopler, 1978; Wetherby, 1984). A number of areas and structures in the brain have been implicated as possibly being involved, including the lower brainstem, thalamus, and other subcortical structures, as well as areas of the frontal and temporal lobes of the cerebral cortex (Ornitz, 1983; Wetherby, 1984). It has been difficult to pinpoint specific areas, especially because some researchers have begun to provide evidence that similar characteristics of the autistic syndrome in different children may be caused by or related to very different underlying conditions or etiologies (Ciaranello, VandenBerg, and Anders, 1982; Rosenberger-Debiesse and Coleman, 1986).

Organisms and their environment are involved in mutually influential interactions, determined by the characteristics of each and their mutual past history (Kantor, 1959). In the case of children with autism, it appears that special organismic characteristics may have a powerful influence on their reciprocal interactional development. For example, interbehavioral and balanced biosocial theories both emphasize the role of sensory reinforcement effects in reinforcing and maintaining environmental interactions (Baldwin and Baldwin, 1981; Bijou, 1980). Due to habituation to certain levels of sensory input, and other behavioral effects, children's behavior is presumably shaped in the direction of greater complexity. More complex behavior typically produces more complex sensory stimulation, which may be necessary to maintain optimally reinforcing levels of arousal (Baldwin and Baldwin, 1978, 1981). Problematic organismic characteristics would be disruptive to such a process.

It is possible to see how such a learning or motivational process leads to more complex repertoires, as children are reinforced for interacting with many available social and nonsocial stimuli (breadth), and in more and different ways (level or type of interactions). For example, a child may attend and respond to a certain stimulus in the environment (e.g., a toy or object), and receive reinforcing stimulation for doing so. Through discrimination and generalization processes (Catania, 1984; Miller, 1980), the child may then interact with other similar available stimuli (breadth). Also, habituation processes function to shape the child's continued interactions with particular stimuli. More complex manipulations, or incorporation of other stimuli in a relational fashion, would be needed to maintain optimal levels of sensory input. This is a bidirectional process, because a lack of appropriate reciprocal child–environment interactions may also have physiological (e.g., lack of neuronal growth and complexity) as well as behavioral effects.

Lack of Curiosity and Normal Motivation

One can see how such processes may operate to produce generalized behavior changes considered representative of curiosity or creativity in children. As normal children come in contact with wider varieties of social and nonsocial stimuli, the breadth and depth of their interactive skills increase owing to reinforcement of behavioral variation. Also, as they come into contact with novel stimulus combinations, novel combinations of responses occur (Baldwin and Baldwin, 1981; Bijou, 1980; Cheyne and Rubin, 1983; Dansky and Silverman, 1973, 1975; Smith and Dutton, 1979; Goldstein 1984). That is, the opportunity to interact with particular materials may facilitate children's creative understanding and use of the materials. For example, Smith and Dutton (1979) found that the opportunity to interact with sets of blocks and sticks facilitated the children's use of such materials in solving an object retrieval task. Similar results have been reported in other studies (Cheyne and Rubin, 1983; Dansky and Silverman, 1973, 1975).

Such processes are presumably "driven" by the conditioning effects involved (e.g., reinforcement and punishment due to different levels of sensory stimulation). It has been hypothesized that interactive deficits seen in children with autism may be at least partially explained by their failure to develop responsiveness to conditioned, or secondary reinforcers, that is, stimuli that acquire reinforcing effects because of their association with other, more primary, reinforcing stimuli (Bijou and Baer, 1965; Fantino, 1977). Due to attentional and other problems, children with autism may be responding to a limited portion of available stimuli, and thus other stimuli (e.g., other persons or objects) are not acquiring their typical reinforcement functions (Ferster, 1961; Lovaas, Koegel, Simmons, and Long, 1973. Such a failure of conditioning may be reflected in the apparent preference for repetitive, stereotyped behavior often noted in children with autism (Dyer, 1985; Johnson and Koegel, 1982; Koegel and Covert, 1972; Koegel, Firestone, Kramme, and Dunlap, 1974). Such behavior may focus on a child's own body or involve simple repetitive manipulations of toys or objects. Such lack of appropriate attention and response to available stimuli can be conceptualized as a functional state of sensory deprivation (Koegel and Felsenfeld, 1977). The possible effects of a lack of environmental interactions and stimulation on neurologic development were mentioned above (Rosenzweig, 1971, 1976).

A related issue has to do with what might be called ability versus motivational factors (Koegel and Mentis, 1985). The preceding discussion mentioned factors that may interfere with the normal development of interactions with nonsocial and social environmental stimuli (e.g., disrupted neurophysiological functioning). However, it may be that such problematic development could result in what might be called preferential abnormalities, as opposed to a lack of an ability to respond. That is, children may be able to engage in some appropriate types of behaviors but may prefer to engage in other, possibly inappropriate behaviors.

For example, Dyer (1985, 1987) has recently proposed the concept of a reinforcer hierarchy existing in autistic children with regard to self-stimulatory behavior. Her data demonstrated that some children with autism are apparently able to suppress their self-stimulatory behavior in order to attempt tasks and receive typical extrinsic reinforcers. However, in order to obtain a similar result with other children, it was necessary to employ specially assessed reinforcers that appeared to be strongly preferred by those particular children. Similar results were reported by Pace, Ivancic, Edwards, Iwata, and Page (1985), in a study with severely retarded children. They found that levels of correct responding to tasks were consistently greater when preferred stimuli were presented contingently upon correct responding. Dyer speculated that self-stimulation (and its accompanying sensory effects) may be in different positions on a hierarchy for different children; that is, it may be more or less preferred over other activities or reinforcers. Such a viewpoint implies that the children may have some ability to access the more usual stimuli, but that they do not do so because of preference for other types of input. Such a conceptual approach would have implications for aspects of generalization treatment and intervention (see discussion below), because such children would be expected to revert continually to less appropriate (but preferred) types of responding when external treatments would be terminated.

IMPLICATIONS FOR TREATMENT AND INTERVENTION

Presumably, one of the most important functions of diagnostic or assessment procedures is to suggest the direction of treatment interventions for a particular client (Johnson and Koegel, 1982). The conceptual and empirical material reviewed above suggests two major avenues or approaches to remediating possible deficient environmental interactions of children with autism. One approach would be to attempt to change pivotal or key responses that may be involved in the deficits, (Koegel and Koegel, 1988), such as the lack of responding to multiple stimuli (e.g., stimulus overselectivity; Lovaas, Koegel, and Schreibman, 1979). Such a change may then have a widespread effect on a large variety of classes of behavior. Another pivotal approach would be to target response patterns of interest directly (such as shifting among stimuli, interacting with multiple stimuli in a relational fashion) with particular characteristics or topographies (Koegel and Koegel, 1988). Such response patterns could potentially be altered by appropriate antecedent and consequence manipulations. Both approaches have been used with children with autism. Relevant research and related issues are discussed below.

Targeting Pivotal Behaviors: Responsiveness

Discrimination Training

One approach to dealing with such problems has been to attempt directly to teach children with autism to respond on the basis of multiple cues. This has typically been done in the context of conditional discrimination training. For example, Koegel and Schreibman (1977) initially trained four children with autism to respond to single visual and auditory cues. The children were then reinforced for responding only when both components were presented. All of the children eventually learned to respond to this complex stimulus involving both auditory and visual cues, and one child demonstrated generalized responding to both trained and nontrained stimuli on the basis of multiple cues after training. Another study by Schreibman, Charlop, and Koegel (1982) demonstrated that such training to respond on the basis of multiple cues was effective in facilitating the children's generalized use of extrastimulus prompts to learn a complex task. That is, by learning to respond generally on the basis of multiple cues, the children began to utilize extra prompt stimuli (such as pointing), added to facilitate the learning task.

A study by Burke and Koegel (1982) attempted to measure even more generalized effects of conditional discrimination (multiple cue) training. Their data showed that such training resulted in generalized improvements in responses to nontrained multiple cue instructions from a standardized language test. The children also began to demonstrate widespread incidental vocabulary learning, based on nontrained stimuli in their environments. Further improvements in subjective ratings of social responsiveness to complex social stimuli occurred while the children were interacting with adults during unstructured play sessions. Such results indicate the potential for facilitating the children's attention and responding to complex social and nonsocial environmental stimuli, thus possibly improving the children's ability to respond to typical conditioned reinforcers, and so on. Further research is necessary to replicate and extend these findings.

The above, more indirect approaches hold promise, particularly as possible adjuncts to more directive approaches, which have focused on increasing particular types of behavior through the use of various prompting and reinforcement strategies.

Direct Training Approaches

As mentioned above, some studies have directly focused on training and reinforcing the desired topographies of behavior. For example, Romanczyk, Diament, Goren, Trunell, and Harris (1975) conducted two studies in which they alternately reinforced children with autism for either manipulating toys by themselves or being in contact with other children. The procedures were effective in increasing both types of interactions, but there was no maintenance of behavior once the contingencies were discontinued. A similar lack of generalization and maintenance effects was reported by Murphy, Callias, and Carr (1985).

A study by Eason, White, and Newsom (1982), involving six children with autism, assessed appropriate play responses and self-stimulatory behavior. Following baseline measures, the children were trained to perform specific responses with certain toys, through prompting and reinforcement procedures (e.g., praise or edibles). Following training, generalization and maintenance assessments were conducted in a variety of settings, with no contingencies in effect. All of the children displayed high rates of appropriate play and low rates of self-stimulatory behavior in all of the settings. The authors speculated that such positive results may have been because of the children being introduced to natural maintaining consequences, possibly involving sensory stimulation and reinforcement.

Such a position is supported by findings from other studies. Koegel, Firestone, Kramme, and Dunlap (1984) conducted a study involving two children with autism who engaged in high rates of self-stimulatory behavior. When such behavior was suppressed, the children engaged in high rates of appropriate interactions with available toys (Fig. 7–1). The authors hypothesized that the children may have engaged in play behavior in order to receive sensory input, which was lost when the self-stimulation was suppressed. Further evidence for this position was provided in a study by Rincover, Cook, Peoples, and Packard (1979). Using sensory extinction procedures, they systematically identified the sensory consequences that appeared to be maintaining the self-stimulatory behavior of four children with autism. The children were taught to play with toys that provided their preferred sensory consequence (e.g., auditory, visual, etc.). Such procedures were effective in eliminating the children's self-stimulatory behavior and increasing their appropriate play for a period of months, without other programmed contingencies. Other studies have also demonstrated the effectiveness of sensory reinforcement, or toys that provide sensory feedback, on maintaining responsiveness and interactions of children with autism and retardation (Bambara, Spiegel-McGill, Shores, and Fox, 1984; Murphy, Carr, and Callias, 1986; Rincover and Newsom, 1985).

Such results lend support to the idea discussed previously, that the children's deficits may often be at least partially related to motivational or reinforcement variables, along with other possible attentional difficulties. That is, although children may be able to be taught to respond to complex stimuli involving multiple cues, whether or not they actually do may be dependent on the types of stimulation and reinforcement available.

Implications for Increasing Environmental Interactions

The studies above suggest several avenues of exploration for increasing the generalized environmental interactions of children with autism. A great deal of research is needed to delineate the extent of effects that can be expected from particular interventions applied by themselves. For example, conditional discrimination training appears to hold promise for increasing the children's breadth of attention and responding to complex stimuli, in both more restricted and more naturalistic settings (Burke and Koegel, 1982). However, it is unclear what extent and type of generalized gains may occur with this approach. Similarly, although direct training of particular behavior appears to be effective, more research is necessary to assess carefully the variables that may contribute to the generalization and maintenance of such behavior (Eason, White, and Newsom, 1982).

At this point, it would seem important to focus on both aspects in order to have as much of an impact as possible, given the often severe deficits displayed by children with autism. Multiple cue training could be conducted in more clinical or analog types of settings, in order to influence the children's breadth of attention and response to complex stimuli, and possibly to induce broader changes as well. Direct training of behavioral characteristics could be applied to particular areas in which children appear to be deficient, based on results of an assessment procedure such as the one employed in O'Neill's (1987) study. It would be relatively easy to identify a number of settings in which prompting, reinforcement, and other techniques could be employed to increase the children's breadth of interactions (e.g., number of stimuli), their systematic sampling of such available stimuli, and the complexity or level of their interactions with particular stimuli. Such training could occur in classrooms, on playgrounds, and in

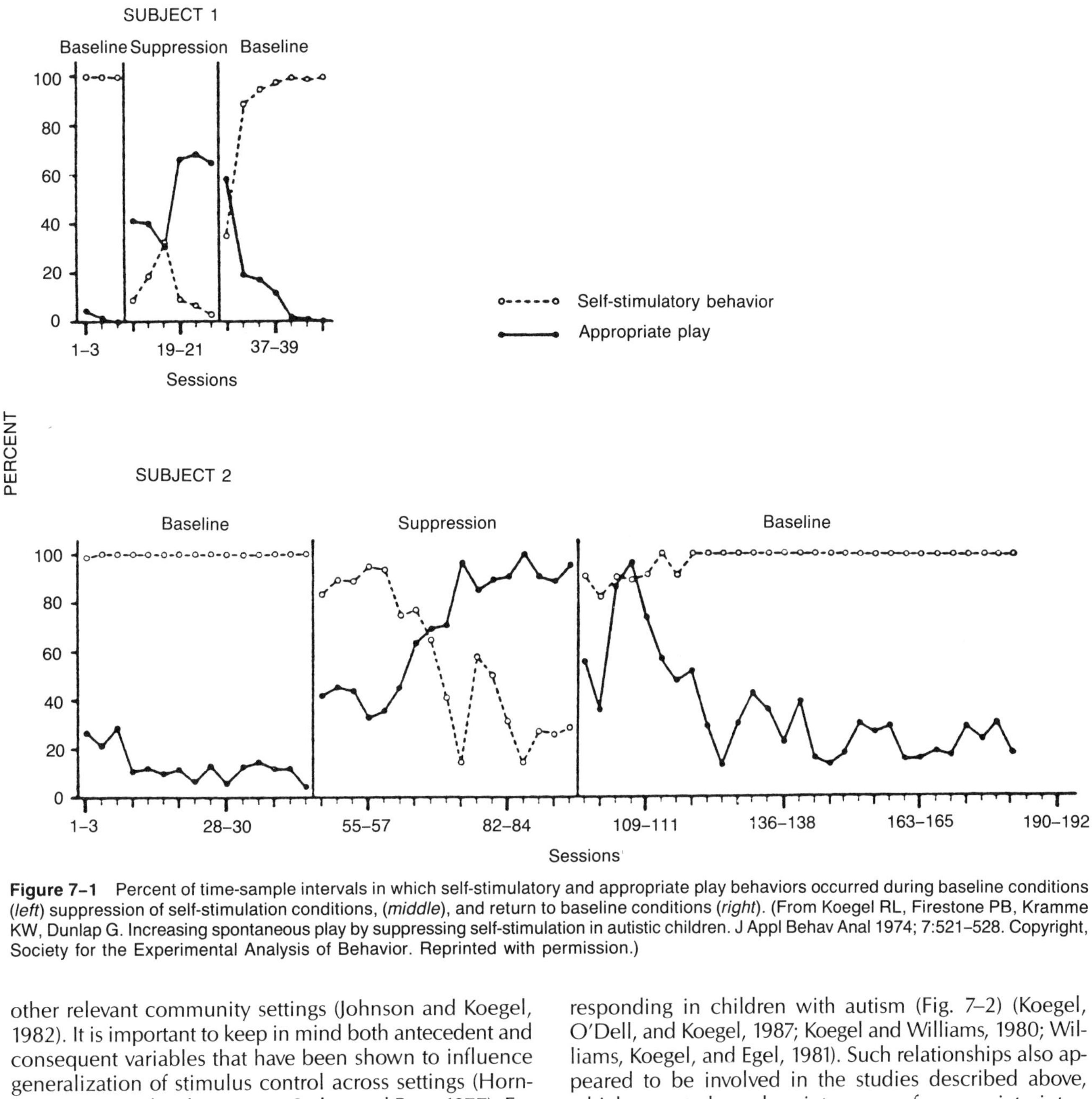

Figure 7–1 Percent of time-sample intervals in which self-stimulatory and appropriate play behaviors occurred during baseline conditions (*left*) suppression of self-stimulation conditions, (*middle*), and return to baseline conditions (*right*). (From Koegel RL, Firestone PB, Kramme KW, Dunlap G. Increasing spontaneous play by suppressing self-stimulation in autistic children. J Appl Behav Anal 1974; 7:521–528. Copyright, Society for the Experimental Analysis of Behavior. Reprinted with permission.)

other relevant community settings (Johnson and Koegel, 1982). It is important to keep in mind both antecedent and consequent variables that have been shown to influence generalization of stimulus control across settings (Horner, Sprague, and Wilcox, 1982; Stokes and Baer, 1977). For example, it would be important for training activities to sample the range of stimulus situations in which the behaviors are expected to occur (Albin, Horner, Koegel, and Dunlap, 1987; Horner, Bellamy, and Colvin, 1984).

The research reviewed above makes it clear that it would be necessary to consider carefully the type of stimulation and reinforcement employed in such training, especially initially. It may be necessary to schedule powerful preferred reinforcers contingent on desired behaviors. Making such reinforcers a natural consequence of engaging in the desired behavior would be ideal (e.g., opening a box to obtain and listen to a music toy, pushing a merry-go-round and riding it to receive visual or proprioceptive feedback). Research has demonstrated that such natural response-reinforcer relationships enhance appropriate responding in children with autism (Fig. 7–2) (Koegel, O'Dell, and Koegel, 1987; Koegel and Williams, 1980; Williams, Koegel, and Egel, 1981). Such relationships also appeared to be involved in the studies described above, which reported good maintenance of appropriate interactive behavior with toys (Eason, White, and Newsom, 1982; Rincover, Cook, Peoples, and Packard, 1979). Such direct training would almost necessarily involve some variation in the stimuli and consequences involved. Again, such variation has been shown to facilitate appropriate attention and responding in children with autism (Dunlap, 1984; Dunlap and Egel, 1982; Dunlap and Koegel, 1980).

The two approaches to treatment (both multiple cue and more direct training) may also have some reciprocal facilitative effects. For example, if multiple cue training is effective in increasing the number of cues or stimuli to which the children respond, it may facilitate the establishment of secondary or conditioned reinforcers during more direct training. That is, stimuli that are paired with the re-

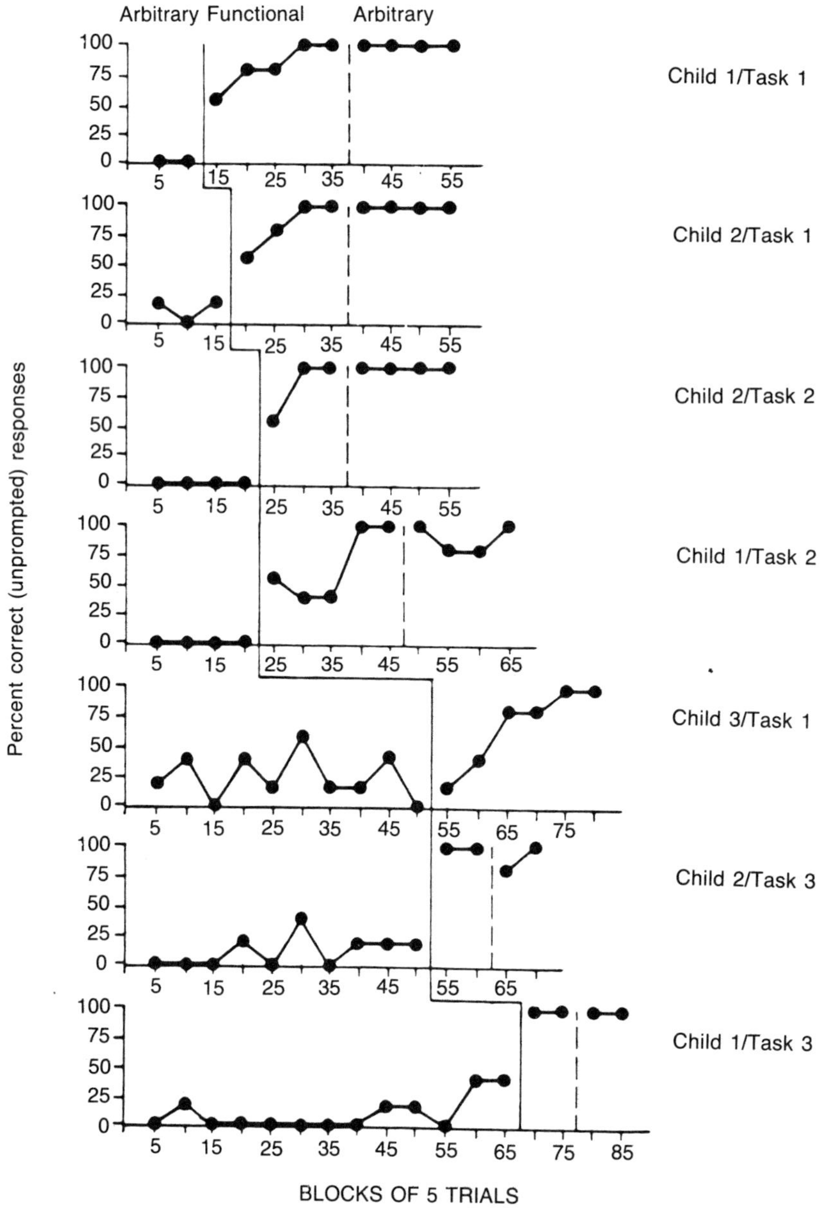

Figure 7–2 The results of a multiple baseline analysis of acquisition with functional versus arbitrary response-reinforcer relationships. (From Williams JA, Koegel RL, Egel AL. Response-reinforcer relationships and improved learning in autistic children. J Appl Behav Anal 1981; 14:53–60. Copyright, Society for the Experimental Analysis of Behavior. Reprinted with permission.)

inforcing stimulus may acquire some reinforcing properties. Such stimuli might include other available objects, children or adults who are present, and so on. Also, the direct training may have some effects on increasing the breadth of the children's attention to multiple cues or stimuli, depending on the type of interactions that are prompted and reinforced.

The section above is a general, speculative sketch of what might be possible based on the present knowledge. Other influential factors or variables may be delineated. For example, in the study by Koegel, Firestone, Kramme, and Dunlap (1974), increases in appropriate play were obtained by suppressing competing, inappropriate, perseverative behavior. Such an approach might be a useful first step in assessing a child's responsiveness and behavioral repertoire, and in determining the possible need for more complex or elaborate intervention procedures. Further research on the delineation of characteristics of subgroups of children with autism may also be influential, in that some children may be found to be more or less responsive to different types of interventions.

The influence of neurophysiologic variables may become clearer with continued research. Some of the children may have experienced very early neurologic dysfunction and may have been engaging in aberrant environmental interactions for long periods, which may have further adversely affected neurologic function. However, research has demonstrated that, in animals, the effects of environmental enrichment and interactions can overcome deficits caused by deprivation (Rosenzweig, 1971, 1976). Obviously, comparable studies with human subjects have not been done, but data from studies involving people with various types of brain insults (head trauma, cerebrovascular incidents, etc.) indicate that recovery of function can occur and may be facilitated by appropriate stimulation and training (Horton and Miller, 1984). This is supported by results presented in a study of central auditory processing deficits in children with autism (Wetherby, Koegel, and Mendel, 1981). Response data on the Staggered Spondaic Word (SSW) test, a test of central auditory processing, were gathered over a period of time while a child with autism was receiving behaviorally oriented treatment. The test scores improved in a systematic pattern over the course of treatment, which the authors speculated may have been due to an interaction of neural plasticity and treatment because such patterns of responding did not occur in older children. These results, as well as other issues discussed above, also point to the importance of beginning intervention as early as possible, in order to maximize the potential effects of such intervention (Bricker, 1986; Clunies-Ross, 1979; Wetherby, 1984).

Integrated Approaches Involving Multiple Variables

Along with the methods discussed above, a number of promising new avenues for increasing responsiveness to environmental stimuli have emerged in recent years. These procedures hold especially strong promise for promoting generalization because they focus on multiple variables, such as treatment in natural settings, programming common stimuli, use of multiple settings, and so on. In addition, these approaches incorporate and can supplement the direct and indirect training elements of methods discussed previously.

Delayed and Unpredictable Reinforcement

One approach is based on gradually removing the primary treatment personnel from the children's natural environments and then having the treatment providers deliver delayed (but contingent) consequences at unpredictable times (Fig. 7–3) (Dunlap and Johnson, 1985; Dunlap, Koegel, Johnson, and O'Neill, 1987; Fowler and Baer, 1981; Koegel and Rincover, 1977). Such delayed and intermittent schedules of reinforcement produce durable responding across multiple environments throughout the day, providing multiple opportunities for behavioral responses (and associated neurologic effects), which are then expected to enhance stimulus and response generalization further, as discussed above.

Parent and Teacher Training

Because persons with developmental disabilities may often engage in frequent interactions with untrained persons, one adjunct treatment has been to train significant others in the children's environment to respond favorably to the children's attempts to interact (cf. Koegel, Russo, and Rincover, 1977; Laski, Charlop, and Schreibman, in press). Such coordinated approaches (see also Dunlap, Koegel, and Koegel, 1984) result in especially powerful treatment changes across multiple settings and would be expected to increase the speed and breadth of change because of the large amount of productive environmental responding that would occur.

Self-Monitoring

One of the most promising approaches is based on principles and procedures of self-monitoring. It seems highly likely that many variables that promote generalization are also inherent in self-monitoring programs. For example, programming increased responding outside of a clinic setting may solicit reinforcers from the natural environment and thus bridge the delay that occurs between a behavior and a consequence, such as exchanging points for backup reinforcers (Ferster, Nurnberger, and Levitt, 1962). In addition, self-monitoring may involve sequential modification across multiple settings in the natural environment, which has been shown to result in increased generalization (Griffiths and Craighead, 1972; Murdock, Garcia, and Hardman, 1977). Also, monitoring outside of the clinic setting is likely to incorporate a range of familiar stimuli and more natural activities that are more likely to prompt and maintain appropriate responding (cf. Engel, Brandriet, Erickson, Gronhoud, and Henderson, 1966). Although these methods have been shown to be effective in promoting generalization individually, their combined influence may be especially powerful. Their relative individual and combined weights in an overall program's effectiveness have yet to be "teased out" and would be an interesting area for further research. For example, some authors (cf. Nelson and Hayes, 1981) have discussed the fact that the numerous components of the self-monitoring program, such as the therapist's instructions, the teaching per se, the self-recording device, and the actual self-monitoring responses may work together to prompt the external consequences that control behavior frequency. Advantages of a self-monitoring program are that it incorporates so many strategies into a single program that can be simple to implement, it is cost and time effective (Koegel, Koegel, and Ingham, 1986), and it can be programmed from a clinical setting with little need for additional assistance from significant others in the child's natural environment.

The sections above have discussed conceptual issues and data concerning the assessment and treatment of generalized responsive behavior of children with autism. In the next section we present case studies involving the application of some of the intervention procedures discussed above. This section illustrates how such procedures can be useful in promoting generalized appropriate behavior.

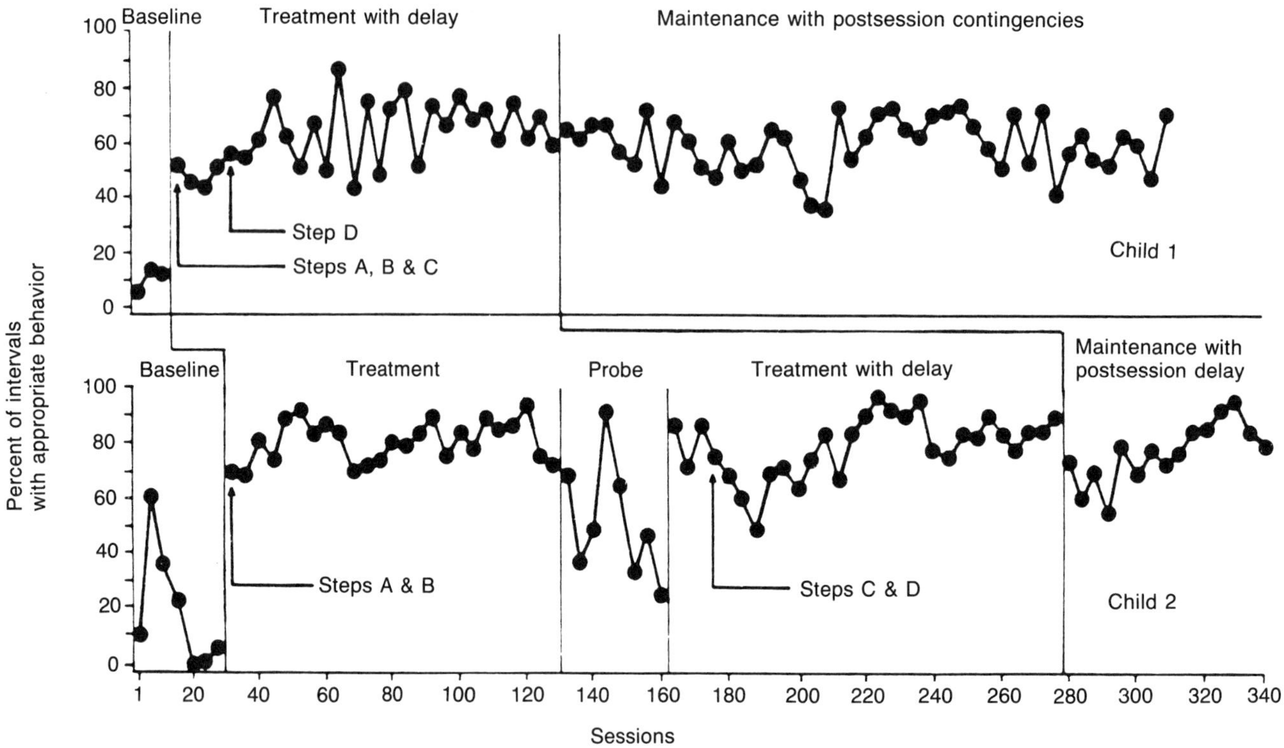

Figure 7–3 Appropriate responding in classroom settings. Sessions are plotted in blocks of four. The points at which the steps in the treatment process were initiated for each child are labeled (*steps A* through *D*). (From Dunlap G, Koegel RL, Johnson J, O'Neill RE. Maintaining performance of autistic clients in community settings with delayed contingencies. J Appl Behav Anal 1987; 20:185–191. Copyright, Society for the Experimental Analysis of Behavior. Reprinted with permission.)

CASE HISTORIES

In our research program we frequently encounter the type of problems discussed above. That is, pervasive unresponsiveness to the environment appears to be the rule rather than the exception for children with autism. The following case histories illustrate procedures that can be used to alter such unresponsiveness, thereby producing collateral changes in multiple responses across many environments, situations, and time.

Case 1: Self-Monitoring for Perseverative Responding

Nicholas (a pseudonym), a 12-year-old child, was diagnosed as having autism at age 3. When he began attending our after-school clinical program at the University of California at Santa Barbara, he had no expressive language skills and limited receptive skills. He also had a considerable amount of perseverative responding, including body-rocking, staring into space, and thumbsucking. He displayed negligible responding to other environmental stimuli.

After approximately 2 years of treatment, most of his perseverative responding had been reduced, but generalization of such suppression remained a significant problem. One type of perseverative responding, his thumbsucking, was especially problematic. Additionally, the thumbsucking had escalated to include biting his nails and small chunks of surrounding flesh off of each finger. The need for a treatment program that would result in widespread reduction was critical, because it appeared that this self-stimulatory behavior had been gradually increasing over the years to the point where it was becoming self-injurious (cf. Carr, 1977). Furthermore, the amount of clinician time spent attempting to reduce this behavior through the use of contingent response consequences was increasing, and a simultaneous decrease in on-task responding on the child's part was occurring. Similar problems of response covariation between perseverative and appropriate classes of responding have been well documented in the literature discussed above. We decided to develop a treatment program utilizing self-monitoring in the hope that the program could eventually be expanded to improve behavior both for extended periods of time and in settings where the clinician was not present. The steps of the self-monitoring program were based on principles described by Koegel and Koegel (1987).

The steps were implemented as follows. Preparation began with observing and operationally defining the target behavior. Any contact between hands and mouth was defined as inappropriate. Next, we determined that the perseverative responding was occurring at an extremely high rate at home and at a very low rate in school. We decided to begin treatment of the inappropriate perseverative behavior in the controlled clinical setting and to take generalization measures outside of the building in the presence of someone unknown to the child and at home in his mother's presence. Initial treatment sessions were begun with 5-second intervals; he was rewarded with a small star or sticker after each successful interval, with the ultimate behavioral objective of having him complete consecutive 1-hour, perseverative behavior-free intervals.

Training the self-monitoring in the treatment setting proved to be a challenge because of his limited language skills. However, his clinician observed that eating appeared to be incompatible with the target behavior. Thus, the child was given edibles during initial sessions to "prompt" short intervals of perseverative behavior-free responding. Following each 5-second interval, which was signaled by sounding the alarm-chime on a wristwatch, the clinician asked him (while demonstrating) about the success (or lack of success) of each interval. During this step Nicholas was trained to evaluate his own behavior prior to any feedback on the clinician's part, in order to begin the process of having him function as his own clinician (see discussion above).

Specifically, following each interval, he was trained to say "yes mouth," if he had put his fingers in his mouth, or "no mouth," if he had not. Then he was allowed to take a sticker following each successful interval, first of behaving appropriately, then of accurately evaluating that interval. Because great care had been taken in determining an initial interval that would be small enough to be likely for him to attain adequate reinforcement, he was able to move relatively quickly through the initial steps. Then, the clinician was gradually able to increase the length of the time interval. However, as the length of the time intervals increased, Nicholas did not always "remember" if he had engaged in persistent responding if it occurred during the first few seconds of the interval. Thus, the clinician needed to include an extra step in the program, which consisted of immediately pointing out that he did put his fingers in his mouth and that, therefore, when the chime would sound, he would not be able to take a sticker. This step was necessary only for a few sessions, and because the stepwise increase in the interval was so small and increased so gradually, the data showed that unsuccessful intervals were very infrequent.

Throughout this process of training the self-monitoring in the clinical setting, data were being collected in generalization environments, as mentioned above. These data showed some generalization of suppression outside of the building where treatment was taking place, but none to the home. After approximately 2 months of treatment (4 hours weekly), the time interval had been gradually increased to 20 minutes in the clinical setting, and Nicholas was wearing the wristwatch that was set to chime every 20 minutes to signal the end of the interval. Well above 90 percent of the intervals were completely free of any type of perseverative responding. Therefore, we thought that it would be an appropriate time to begin implementation of self-monitoring in natural settings (at home).

At home, the data had shown that between 3:00 PM and 4:00 PM, when Nicholas watched television, perseverative responding typically occurred during the entire hour. Therefore, we taught his mother to implement the same program we had been using in the clinic during that hour, except she began with 10-minute intervals (as opposed to the 20-minute intervals he had worked up to in the clinical setting). He wore his wristwatch at home set to chime every 10 minutes during the hour, and his mother sat with him and observed during that time period every day. She rewarded him with a sticker following each successful interval, just as we were doing in the clinical setting. After encountering success with the program in the afternoons, his mother began implementing the program before school in the mornings, when he also engaged in frequent perseverative responding.

As of this writing, Nicholas is successfully completing 40-minute intervals in the clinical setting and 30-minute intervals at home. We should mention here that, at one point during Christmas break, his mother called to inform us that Nicholas' perseverative responding was increasing and the self-monitoring did not appear to be working. In order to resolve this problem, we asked his mother to return temporarily to a shorter (15-minute) interval and then gradually work back up to the 40-minute interval, a procedure that worked very successfully.

It is important to note that as this perseverative responding is decreasing, Nicholas is showing increased responses to appropriate stimuli in his environment (cf. Koegel, Firestone, Kramme, and Dunlap, 1974) and in the number of correct responses to such stimuli during teaching sessions across a variety of settings. The intervention is thus resulting in increases in the breadth and type of his interactions. We hope these broadly generalized treatment gains will continue once we reach intervals long enough to permit natural consequences to have an impact. Similar types of covariation of classes of appropriate behavior have been found in recent studies (Parrish, Cataldo, Kolko, Neef, and Engel, 1986; Russo, Cataldo, and Cushing, 1981).

Case 2: Delayed and Unpredictable Reinforcement for the Treatment of Perseverative Responding

Amy, an 8-year-old child with autism, was relatively bright. That is, under optimal and modified testing conditions her IQ could be crudely estimated to be between 80 and 90. However, like many children with autism, her perseverative responding and tantruming made it impossible to test her under standardized conditions, and she was labeled "untestable" on all standardized tests. Furthermore, her parents had placed her in a foster home because they felt unable to deal with her inappropriate behavior, which was severely disrupting their family life. The personnel in Amy's school district placed her in a classroom for children with severe handicaps.

Our first step was to observe Amy in her classroom setting. During our initial observations we noted that, if Amy was left alone, she always went to the bookshelves, obtained one particular book, opened it, and stared at a small item on a page of the book. She appeared very content perseverating on the same item for lengthy periods of time. However, whenever the teacher made any type of demand, disrupted the perseverative responding, or made the particular book unavailable to her, a tantrum resulted that included screaming, bizarre language, biting, kicking, and crying. This severe failure to respond to other appropriate stimuli while engaged in perseverative responding is commonly observed in children with autism (cf. Lovaas, Litrownik, and Mann, 1971; Koegel, Firestone, Kramme, and Dunlap, 1974), and was seriously interfering with Amy's ability to function in a public-school classroom setting. Efforts to consequate the perseverative responding resulted in such frequent and extended periods of tantruming that response-contingent consequences required extensive vigilance and effort on the teacher's part; they were not always being administered contingently or consistently because of the lack of teacher time that could be dedicated to an individual child in a heavily populated classroom setting. Therefore, we decided to design a program that would focus on producing generalized gains across stimuli and time, so it would be effective in the absence of the teacher (such as when the teacher was working with another child in the classroom, or when Amy was outside at recess or lunch).

Our observations also revealed that her perseverative responding decreased, and simultaneous appropriate responding improved while she was in a one-on-one teaching situation. This decrease was particularly clear when she worked with one of the public school's speech-language specialists. It also was noted that after specified periods of appropriate responding, the speech-language specialist was permitting Amy to obtain the book that she perseverated on, as a reinforcer for a very short time. Utilizing self-stimulation as a reinforcer, as in this situation, has been discussed in the literature as an effective treatment technique (Devany and Rincover, 1982; Hung, 1978). Because of the already established successful relationship Amy had with the speech-language specialist, and because of that therapist's willingness to participate in a behavioral treatment program, her availability at the school sites, and her somewhat flexible schedule, we felt that she would make an ideal provider of primary treatment. An intensive behavioral program (1-hour daily sessions) was conducted during the initial steps and gradually faded to the therapist's regular 20-minute, twice-weekly sessions over a 3-month period.

The first step of the program was to ask the speech-language specialist to extend systematically and gradually the time period of appropriate responding in the one-on-one setting before Amy could earn her reinforcer (the book). Initial segments began at 2 minutes and were gradually increased to 20 minutes.

During this time, social reinforcers (praise and hugs) were constantly paired with the book. In addition, the period between administration of the social reinforcers and acquisition of the book as a reinforcer was increased, beginning with a few seconds and working up to a few minutes by the time the sessions reached 20 minutes. This process of using delayed reinforcers is frequently seen as a normal reinforcement procedure in classrooms for non-handicapped individuals. For example, children may be taken to get an ice cream cone after good behavior in school, or given privileges for a good report card. When utilized correctly, with systematically increased delays, this has been a successful technique for handicapped and non-handicapped children alike (Dunlap, Koegel, Johnson, and O'Neill, 1987 Fowler and Baer, 1981). Upon completion of six successive 20-minute intervals, the treatment setting was moved to the child's regular classroom. Additional children were included in the sessions in order to provide stimulus similarities related to the eventual goal of having Amy respond to appropriate stimuli in the classroom setting.

Finally, when she was successful in completing several 20-minute intervals with the speech-language specialist in a group setting without constant one-on-one attention, control was transferred to the classroom teacher. Transferring control to the classroom teacher was accomplished by first having the speech-language specialist sit immediately next to Amy in the classroom during the teacher's instructions. In order to begin implementation of unpredictable reinforcement (Dunlap and Johnson, 1985), the speech-language specialist provided social reinforcement (which by that time had become a very functional reinforcer for Amy) after random intervals of appropriate responding. The intervals varied from 15 seconds to 5 minutes and were gradually increased to 1 hour. After Amy was able to behave appropriately for 1-hour sessions, the speech-language specialist was "faded out." This was accomplished by having her very gradually move her chair further back in successive sessions and deliver the unpredictable social reinforcer from a distance. When the speech-language specialist was sitting a considerable distance behind the child so that her presence was not likely to be such a powerful discriminative stimulus, the teacher's assistance was incorporated.

The teacher gained stimulus control over the child's behavior by informing the child that the speech-language specialist had to leave the classroom for a little while and when she returned she was going to ask if Amy's behavior was good. Thus, by that point we were utilizing both delayed and unpredictable reinforcement. During the first few intervals, the speech-language specialist left for very short periods of time (e.g., 15 seconds). This interval was gradually increased until the child was able to go long periods of time responding to a variety of appropriate stimuli while the speech-language specialist was out of the room. Eventually, rather than having the therapist designate a specific hour daily, she was asked to reduce the necessary amount of child–clinician time by continuing to utilize unpredictable reinforcement throughout the entire day. Also, the aides began to participate in the program by reporting the child's behavior at recess. Eventually, Amy's teacher was able to administer the entire program. Although this program required some intensive training and coordination during the first few months, the eventual goal of being able to treat Amy as any other child by using delayed and unpredictable reinforcement was eventually achieved. Generalized appropriate responding to a myriad of appropriate classroom stimuli and teacher instructions was displayed throughout the day without any further need for the presence of a specialized treatment provider. Again, the program resulted in increases in Amy's attention and response to a greater variety of complex stimuli.

Case 3: Self-Monitoring for Intonation: Responding to Multiple Cues.

Sam, a 12-year-old child with autism, had been in a self-contained classroom since he entered school. During his initial years of schooling, he was extremely echolalic and had a considerable amount of perseverative responding. He was responsive to educational efforts and was showing consistent and steady gains in appropriate behaviors, including language skills. By the time he was 12, he typically answered questions appropriately, but he seldom initiated conversations. Additionally, all of his utterances lacked appropriate prosody, which is commonly observed in echolalic children (cf. Bagshaw, 1978; Schreibman, Kohlenberg, and Britten, 1986). As suggested earlier in this chapter, one of the reasons these children have difficulty with parts of language such as prosody may be because they do not respond to multiple components of a stimulus, but instead "overselect" to only one cue or a few cues involved in the complex stimuli of language (cf. Lovaas, Koegel, and Schreibman, 1979). We speculated that Sam was responding primarily on the basis of the content of speech stimuli and was not responding on the basis of the intonation cues. Therefore, our treatment plan focused on teaching him to be responsive to intonation cues.

In designing a treatment program for prosody, several issues needed to be considered. First, his parents were unwilling to participate or be involved in his educational program. They were in the process of locating a group home for handicapped children where he could be placed, because they felt he was disrupting their family life. Second, the speech-language specialist's case load was so large that her contact time with the child was limited to two 20-minute weekly sessions. Therefore, we decided that self-monitoring might provide a program in which the child would function as his own therapist, with the self-monitoring programmed to occur in the absence of the trainer (cf. Koegel and Koegel, 1987). This would be likely to result in a more widespread generalization of responding.

The first step of the program was to determine the target responses. We decided to begin with imitation of questions, in order to increase his initiation of conversational responses and to use a set of stimuli that provided an intonation *pattern* he could easily learn. The stimulus items consisted of 20 information questions and 20 yes–no questions, each printed on a separate index card. In addition, the intonation patterns (i.e., three steps going up for information, and three steps going up and then down for yes–no) were printed on separate cards. Next, Sam chose a functional reinforcer, going to the park with the clinician after school, to be earned contingent upon making appropriate responses to speech patterns.

Training the self-monitoring in the speech-language specialist's office began with placing the card with the intonation pattern in front of the child and then going through the first stack of 20 cards while having him imitate each question with appropriate intonation. After each of his responses, Sam was asked if his own intonation while repeating the question went up (or up and down) or if it was flat. If he answered (monitored) correctly, he received a point toward an intermediary reinforcer (a sticker). Once he was able to imitate all 40 questions with appropriate prosody and monitored those 40 utterances correctly, the procedure was repeated without a model. He was required to read the question, then look up at the clinician and ask her the question (whereupon she would answer it). At this point he was given a wrist counter to wear and was trained to depress it subtly (without looking down) each time he monitored a response. Following successful completion of these very structured steps, the clinician began to have Sam generate his own sentences in order to earn points. Language samples were taken weekly, and when naive listeners rated him as producing appropriate prosody on more than 90 percent of his questions, it was determined that he was ready to begin self-monitoring in natural settings. As we began this step of prompting his self-monitoring in natural settings, we were pleased to note that he had increased the number of conversation-initiating responses in his natural environment. As mentioned above, a common occurrence in children with autism is their lack of initiating conversations (Dyer, 1987). By carefully choosing the stimulus items (the questions) while working on prosody as a target behavior, an apparent by-product of greater initiation of conversational responses was emerging.

In order to begin the process of having Sam self-monitor his behavior in the natural environment, we began with careful planning of the questions he would ask and the individuals to whom he would ask them. This was done in order to facilitate our validation of his initial responses. His teacher, another speech-language specialist, and trained volunteers made it possible to validate Sam's responses and his self-monitoring. These sessions were arranged during Sam's regular speech-language treatment time. When Sam was able to complete these steps successfully, he was told that he could earn points by himself all day long by responding with appropriate intonation. During each subsequent speech session, Sam brought his points in to the clinician and continued to monitor during conversation with the clinician. Occasional covert language samples taken in the classroom indicated that Sam's appropriate prosody during questions generalized to unstructured speech in his classroom setting. Some additional appropriate generalization of prosody to other (nonquestion) utterances also was being evidenced. Thus, it seemed likely that Sam was beginning to increase his responsiveness to the numerous multiple cues required for appropriate intonation, as well as to situations in which question-asking was appropriate.

Case 4: Parent Training

Casy was a 9-year-old child who was diagnosed as having autism. When he entered our program his parents indicated that because of his severe behavior problems, he was only permitted to attend a special education self-contained classroom in the public schools for half of the full-day program. Initial observation of his behavior also demonstrated an extremely high rate of perseverative delayed echolalia in which elaborate stereotyped stories about cartoon characters were recited at great length in much the same manner each day. Other behavioral observations also revealed extremely restricted responding, i.e., an almost complete lack of spontaneous play with any toys other than ritualistic behavior with a few miniature plastic cartoon character replicas, and an almost complete lack of responding to instructions given by his parents. He also showed very little interest in interacting with others but was content sitting alone, either staring into space or manipulating the cartoon character replicas. Standardized testing and behavioral observations were consistent with the information above. He resisted responding to new stimulus materials, and whenever he was presented with a new stimulus item, he would cry, tantrum, and refuse to answer.

Our goal in Casy's treatment was to train his parents both to reduce his inappropriate behavior and to increase his responsiveness to appropriate environmental stimuli. Casy's initial treatment sessions began with training his parents to establish control over Casy's behavior. We began by showing them video tapes of various effective and ineffective behavioral treatment sessions with other children. Each tape was discussed in detail, and explanations of how examples were related to their own child were discussed. Discussions emphasized the use of easily discriminable instructional stimuli, use of effective within-stimulus prompts, use of contingent and functional reinforcers, and application of shaping and chaining procedures. His parents also read several texts (Baker, Brightman, Heifetz, and Murphy 1976; Koegel and Schreibman, 1982) that were discussed chapter by chapter each session. Upon completion of these steps, his parents were gradually brought into the clinic sessions and given feedback on their use of the treatment procedures with Casy. In order to do this, they observed the first portion of the session, then worked with him (beginning with a few minutes and gradually working up to 30 minutes) during the middle portion of the session, and received feedback in a general discussion during the last third of each session.

During the initial practice with feedback sessions, Casy frequently began to tantrum when he was presented with the first trial of a task. Under such conditions it was common for his care providers to tell him that he could play with the cartoon characters if he promised to work afterwards. However, by reversing this cycle through establishing extremely clear response-reinforcer contingencies by parent training, Casy now appears very eager to work for the necessary points needed to earn his reward. This result appears similar to that discussed in the learned helplessness literature (cf. Koegel and Mentis, 1985; Seligman, Maier, and Geer, 1968). Casy now appears to be relating task success to his behavior (on-task responding) instead of only relating task avoidance to his behavioral efforts (i.e., his previous tantrums, functioned as escape behavior leading to the termination of tasks) whereas now his attempts to respond appropriately to tasks result in successful termination of the task. Under these conditions his overall level of response attempts to appropriate environmental stimuli now is increasing greatly.

Our eventual goals are to continue teaching his parents to work on other similar pivotal target areas related to improved responding to environmental stimuli. These areas include the following:

1. Reducing the problem of overselectivity by training their child to respond on the basis of multiple cues (see discussions above)
2. Continuing to improve their child's environmental interactions by treating motivation to respond as a pivotal target behavior (see discussion above; Koegel, O'Dell, and Koegel, 1987; Koegel, O'Dell, and Dunlap, in press)
3. Enhancing response-reinforcer relationships and scheduling powerful preferred reinforcers in order to increase responding and improve maintenance (see above discussion; also see Dyer, 1987)
4. Utilizing such strategies as task and consequence variation (Dunlap, 1984; Dunlap and Egel, 1982; Koegel and Koegel, 1986) to improve overall motivation

Basing treatment on such "pivotal target behaviors," rather than focusing on individual behaviors, appears to us to result in increased responsiveness to the environment and in more widespread generalized treatment effects. These effects are expected to be further enhanced by training Casy's parents so that they can provide ongoing effective treatment for an increased number and variety of environmental interactions.

CONCLUSION AND SUMMARY

Over the years, researchers have established techniques that have resulted in steadily improved gains in the treatment of children with autism. The problem of generalization, which has been a major obstacle in even the finest state-of-the-art programs, is now increasingly understood and can often be overcome if considered as an integral part and necessary outcome of a treatment program. One of the best prospects for improving overall generalization may be in redefining the focus of the treatment techniques.

The techniques described in this article draw from the large existing literature on treatment procedures for children with autism. However, in this article, we focused not on establishing new appropriate behaviors singly, but rather on establishing greatly increased responsiveness to a variety of environmental stimuli. We hope that by teaching the children to respond more, to shift their responses among appropriate environmental alternatives, to respond to patterns and relationships between multiple stimuli, and to decrease perseverative stereotypic responding to restricted stimulus input, we can produce durable generalized behavioral gains with potential neurologic benefits. It is also our hope that the generalized increases in responsiveness we are observing may interact with and result in changes in the central nervous system (see above), which may function to promote long-term maintenance of behavioral change.

Preparation of this manuscript was supported in part by U.S. Department of Education, National Institute on Disability and Rehabilitation Research Cooperative Agreement No. G0087C0234; and by U.S. Public Health Service Research Grants MH28210 and MH39434 from the National Institute of Mental Health.

REFERENCES

Albin RW, Horner RH, Koegel RL, Dunlap G. Extending competent performances: applied research on generalization and maintenance. Specialized Training Program, University of Oregon, Eugene, OR: 1987.

Bagshaw N. An acoustic analysis of fundamental frequency and temporal parameters of autistic children's speech. Master's thesis, University of California at Santa Barbara, 1978.

Baker BL, Brightman AJ, Heifetz LJ, Murphy DM. Behavior problems. Steps to independence: a skills training series for children with special needs. Champaign, IL: Research Press, 1976.

Baldwin JD, Baldwin JI. Beyond sociobiology. New York: Elsevier North Holland, 1981.

Baldwin JD, Baldwin JI. Reinforcement theories of exploration, play, creativity, and psychosocial growth. In: Smith EO. Social play in primates. New York: Academic Press, 1978: 231.

Bambara LM, Spiegel-McGill P, Shores RE, Fox JJ. A comparison of reactive and nonreactive toys on severely handicapped children's manipulative play. Journal of the Association for Persons with Severe Handicaps 1984; 9:142–149.

Bettelheim B. The empty fortress. New York: Collier MacMillan, 1967.

Bijou SW. Exploratory behavior in infants and animals: a behavior analysis. Physchol Rec 1980; 34:525–535.

Bijou SW, Baer DM. Child development. II. Universal stage of infancy. New York: Appleton-Century-Crofts, 1965.

Bijou SW, Dunitz-Johnson E. Interbehavior analysis of developmental retardation. Psychol Rec 1981; 31:305–329.

Black M, Freeman BJ, Montgomery A. Systematic observation of play behavior in autistic children. J Child Psychol Psychiatry 1975; 18:67–72.

Boucher J. Alternation and sequencing behavior, and response to novelty in autistic children. J Child Psychol Psychiatry 1977; 18:67–72.

Bricker DD. Early education of at-risk and handicapped infants, toddlers, and pre-school children. Glenview, IL: Scott Foresman, 1986.

Burke JC, Koegel RL. The relationship of stimulus overselectivity to autistic children's responsiveness and incidental learning. Paper presented at the Association for Behavior Analysis; Milwaukee, WI, 1982.

Carr EG. The motivation of self-injurious behavior: a review of some hypotheses. Psychol Bull 1977; 84:800–811.

Catania AC. Learning. Englewood Cliffs, NJ: Prentice-Hall, 1984.

Cheyne JA, Rubin KH. Playful precursors of problem solving in preschoolers. Devel Psychol 1983; 19:577–584.

Ciaranello RD, VandenBerg SR, Anders TF. Intrinsic and extrinsic determinants of neuronal development: relation to infantile autism. J Autism Devel Disord 1982; 12:115–145.

Clunies-Ross G. Accelerating the development of Down's syndrome infants and young children. J Special Education 1979; 13:169–177.

Dansky JL, Silverman IW. Effects of play on associative fluency in preschool-aged children. Devel Psychol 1973; 9:38–43.

Dansky JL, Silverman IW. Play: a general facilitator of associative fluency. Devel Psychol 1975; 11:104.

DeMyer MK. Parents and children in autism. New York: John Wiley & Sons, 1979.

Devany J, Rincover A. Self-stimulatory behavior and sensory reinforcement. In: Koegel RL, Rincover A, Egel AL, eds. Educating and understanding autistic children. San Diego: College Hill Press, 1982:127.

Dunlap G. The influence of task variation and maintenance tasks on the learning and affect of autistic children. J Exp Child Psychol 1984; 37:41–64.

Dunlap G, Egel AL. Motivational techniques. In: Koegel RL, Rincover A, Egel AL, eds. Educating and understanding autistic children. San Diego: College Hill Press, 1982:106.

Dunlap G, Johnson J. Increasing the independent responding of autistic children with unpredictable supervision. J Appl Behav Anal 1985; 18:227–236.

Dunlap G, Koegel RL. Motivating autistic children through stimulus variation. J Appl Behav Anal 1980; 13:619–627.

Dunlap G, Koegel RL, Burke JC. Educational implications of stimulus overselectivity in autistic children. Except Educ Q 1981; 2:37–49.

Dunlap G, Koegel RL, Johnson J, O'Neill RE. Maintaining performance of autistic clients in community settings with delayed contingencies. J Appl Behav Anal 1987; 20:185–191.

Dunlap G, Koegel RL, Koegel LK. Continuity of treatment: toilet training in multiple community settings. J Assoc Persons Severe Handicaps 1984; 9:134–141.

Dyer K. The competition of autistic stereotyped behavior with usual and specially assessed reinforcers. Res Devel Disabil 1987; 8:607–626.

Dyer K. The competition of stereotyped behavior with external reinforcers in autistic children. Doctoral dissertation, University of California, Santa Barbara, 1985.

Eason LJ, White MJ, Newsom C. Generalized reduction of self-stimulatory behavior: an effect of teaching appropriate play to autistic children. Analysis and Intervention in Developmental Disabilities 1982; 2:157–169.

Engel DC, Brandriet S, Erickson K, et al. Carryover. J Speech Hear Disord 1966; 31:227–233.

Fantino E. Conditioned reinforcement: choice and information. In: Honig WK, Staddon JER, eds. Handbook of operant behavior. Englewood Cliffs, Prentice-Hall, 1977:319.

Ferster CB. Positive reinforcement and behavioral deficits of autistic children. Child Dev 1961; 32:437–456.

Ferster CB, Nurnberger J, Levitt E. The control of eating. J Mathematics 1962; 1:87–109.

Fowler S, Baer DM. Do I have to be good all day? The timing of delayed reinforcement as a factor in generalization. J Appl Behav Anal 1981; 14:13–24.

Freeman BJ. Behavior assessment of the syndrome of autism: behavior observation system. Unpublished manuscript, University of California, Los Angeles, 1984.

Goldstein H. Effects of modeling and corrected practice on generative language learning of preschool children. J Speech Hear Disord 1984; 49:389–398.

Griffiths H, Craighead WE. Generalization in operant speech therapy. J Speech Hear Disord 1972; 37:485–494.

Horner RH, Bellamy GT, Colvin GT. Responding in the presence of nontrained stimuli: implications of generalization error patterns. J Assoc Persons Severe Handicaps 1984; 9:287–295.

Horner RH, Sprague J, Wilcox B. General case programming for community activities. In: Wilcox B, Bellamy GT, eds. Design of high school programs for severely handicapped students. Baltimore: Paul H. Brookes, 1982:61.

Horton AM, Miller WG. Neuropsychology and behavior therapy. In: Hersen M, Eisler RM, Miller PM, eds. Progress in behavior modification. New York: Academic Press, 1984:2.

Hung DW. Using self-stimulation as reinforcement for autistic children. J Autism Childhood Schizophrenia 1978; 8:355–366.

Johnson J, Koegel RL. Behavioral assessment and curriculum development. In: Koegel RL, Rincover A, Egel AL, eds. Educating and understanding autistic children. San Diego: College Hill Press, 1982:1.

Kanner L. Autistic disturbances of affective contact. Nervous Child 1943; 2:217–250.

Kanner L. Follow-up study of eleven autistic children originally reported in 1943. J Autism Childhood Schizophrenia 1971; 1:119–145.

Kantor JR. Interbehavioral psychology. Chicago: Principia Press, 1959.

Kazdin AE. Symptom substitution, generalization, and response covariation: implications for psychotherapy outcome. Psychol Bull 1982; 91:349–365.

Koegel LK, Koegel RL. The effects of interspersed maintenance tasks on academic performance in a severe childhood stroke victim. J Appl Behav Anal 1986; 19:425–430.

Koegel LK, Koegel RL, Ingham JC. Programming rapid generalization of correct articulation through self-monitoring procedures. J Speech Hear Disord 1986; 51:24–32.

Koegel RL, Covert A. The relationship of self-stimulation to learning in autistic children. J Appl Behav Anal 1972; 5:381–388.

Koegel RL, Felsenfeld S. Sensory deprivation. In: Gerber S, ed. Audiometry in infancy. New York: Grune & Stratton, 1977:247.

Koegel RL, Firestone PB, Kramme KW, Dunlap G. Increasing spontaneous play by suppressing self-stimulation in autistic children. J Appl Behav Anal 1974; 7:521–528.

Koegel RL, Koegel LK. Generalization issues in the treatment of autism. Semin Speech Lang 1987; 8:241–256.

Koegel RL, Koegel LK. Generalized responsivity and pivotal behavior. In: Horner R, Dunlap G, Koegel RL, eds. Generalization and maintenance: lifestyle changes in applied settings. Baltimore: Brookes, 1988:41.

Koegel RL, Mentis M. Motivation in childhood autism: can they or won't they? J Child Psychol Psychiatry 1985; 26:185–191.

Koegel RL, O'Dell MC, Dunlap G. Producing speech use in nonverbal autistic children by reinforcing attempts. J Autism Devel Disord (in press).

Koegel RL, O'Dell MC, Koegel LK. A natural language teaching paradigm for nonverbal autistic children. J Autism Devel Disord 1987; 17:187–200.

Koegel RL, Rincover A. Research on the difference between generalization and maintenance in extra-therapy responding. J Appl Behav Anal 1977; 10:1–12.

Koegel RL, Russo DC, Rincover A. Assessing and training teachers in the generalized use of behavior modification with autistic children. J Appl Behav Anal 1977; 10:197–205.

Koegel RL, Schreibman L. Teaching autistic children to respond to simultaneous multiple cues. J Exper Child Psychol 1977; 24:299–311.

Koegel RL, Schreibman L. How to teach autistic and other severely handicapped children. Lawrence, KS: H & H Enterprises, 1982.

Koegel RL, Schreibman L, Britten K, et al. A comparison of parent training to direct child treatment. In: Koegel RL, Rincover A, Egel AL, eds. Educating and understanding autistic children. San Diego: College Hill Press, 1982:260.

Koegel RL, Schreibman L, O'Neill RE, Burke JC. The personality and family interaction characteristics of parents of autistic children. J Consult Clin Psychol 1983; 51:683–692.

Koegel RL, Williams JA. Direct vs indirect response-reinforcer relationships in teaching autistic children. J Abnorm Child Psychol 1980; 8:537–547.

Lane HL. The wild boy of Averyron. Cambridge, MA: Harvard University Press, 1976.

Laski KE, Charlop MH, Schreibman L. Training parents to use the natural language paradigm to increase their autistic children's speech. J Appl Behav Anal (in press).

Lovaas OI, Koegel RL, Schreibman L. Stimulus overselectivity in autism: a review of research. Psychol Bull 1979; 86:1236–1254.

Lovaas OI, Koegel RL, Simmons JQ, Long J. Some generalization and follow-up measures on autistic children in behavior therapy. J Appl Behav Anal 1973; 6:131–166.

Lovaas OI, Litrownik A, Mann R. Response latencies to auditory stimuli in children engaged in self-stimulatory behavior. Behav Res Ther 1971; 9:34–49.

Lovaas OI, Schreibman L, Koegel RL, Rehm R. Selective responding by autistic children to multiple sensory input. J Abnorm Psychol 1971; 77:211–222.

McAdoo GW, DeMyer MK. Personality characteristics of parents. In: Rutter M, Schopler E, eds. Autism: a reappraisal of concepts and treatment. New York: Plenum Press, 1978:251.

Miller LK. Principles of everyday behavior analysis. 2nd ed. Monterey, CA: Brooks/Cole, 1980.

Mullins M, Rincover A. Comparing autistic and normal children along the dimensions of reinforcement maximization, stimulus sampling, and responsiveness to extinction. J Exp Child Psychol 1985; 40:350–374.

Murdock JY, Garcia EE, Hardman ML. Generalization articulation training with trainable mentally retarded subjects. J Appl Behav Anal 1977; 10:717–733.

Murphy G, Callias M, Carr J. Increasing toy play in the profoundly mentally handicapped: I. Training to play. J Autism Devel Disord 1985; 15:375–384.

Murphy G, Carr J, Callias M. Increasing simple toy play in profoundly mentally handicapped children: II. Designing special toys. J Autism Devel Disord 1986; 16:45–58.

Nelson RO, Hayes SC. Theoretical explanations for reactivity in self-monitoring. Behav Modifm 1981; 5:3–14.

O'Neill RE. Environmental interactions of normal children and children with autism. Doctoral dissertation. University of California, Santa Barbara, 1987.

Ornitz EM. The functional neuroanatomy of infantile autism. Int J Neurosci 1983; 19:85–124.

Ornitz EM, Guthrie D, Farley AJ. The early development of autistic children. J Autism Childhood Schizophrenia 1977; 7:207–229.

Ornitz EM, Guthrie D, Farley AJ. The early symptoms of childhood autism. In: Sherban G, ed. Cognitive defects in the development of mental illness. New York: Brunner/Mazel, 1978: 24.

Pace GM, Invancic MT, Edwards GL, et al. Assessment of stimulus preference and reinforcer value with profoundly retarded individuals. J Appl Behav Anal 1985; 18:249–255.

Parrish JM, Cataldo MF, Kolko DJ, et al. Experimental analysis of response covariation among compliant and inappropriate behaviors. J Appl Behav Anal 1986; 19:241–254.

Rincover A, Cook AR, Peoples A, Packard D. Using sensory extinction and sensory reinforcement principles for programming multiple adaptive behavior change. J Appl Behav Anal 1979; 18:237–248.

Rincover A, Koegel RL. Setting generality and stimulus control

in autistic children. J Appl Behav Anal 1975; 8:235–246.
Rincover A, Newsom CD. The relative motivational properties of sensory and edible reinforcers in teaching autistic children. J Appl Behav Anal 1985; 18:237–248.
Ritvo ER. Autism: diagnosis, current research and management. New York: Spectrum, 1976.
Ritvo ER, Freeman BJ. National Society for Autistic Children definition of the syndrome of autism. J Autism Childhood Schizophrenia 1978; 8:162–167.
Romanczyk RG, Diament C, Goren ER, et al. Increasing isolate and social play in severely disturbed children: intervention and postintervention effectiveness. J Autism Childhood Schizophrenia 1975; 5:57–70.
Rosenberger-Debviesse J, Coleman M. Brief report: preliminary evidence for multiple etiologies in autism. J Autism Devel Disord 1986; 16:385–392.
Rosenzweig MR. Effects of environment on development of brain and behavior. In: Tobach E, Aronson L, Shaw E, eds. The biopsychology of development. New York: Academic Press, 1971:302.
Rosenzweig MR. Effects of environment on brain and behavior in animals. In: Schopler E, Reichler RJ, eds. Psychopathology and child development. New York: Plenum Press, 1976:33.
Russo DC, Cataldo MF, Cushing PJ. Compliance training and behavioral covariation in the treatment of multiple behavior problems. J Appl Behav Anal 1981; 14:209–222.
Rutter M, Schopler E, eds. Autism: a reappraisal of concepts and treatment. New York: Plenum Press, 1978.
Schopler E, Reichler RJ, DeVellis RF, Daly K. Toward objective classification of childhood autism: Childhood Autism Rating Scale (CARS). J Autism Devel Disord 1980; 10:91–103.
Schreibman L, Charlop MH, Koegel RL. Teaching autistic children to use extra-stimulus prompts. J Exp Child Psychol 1982; 33:475–491.
Schreibman L, Kohlenberg BS, Britten KR. Differential responding to content and intonation components of a complex auditory stimulus by nonverbal and echolalic autistic children. Anal Intervention Devel Disabil 1986; 6:109–125.
Seligman MEP, Maier SF, Geer J. The alleviation of learned helplessness in the dog. J Abnormal Soc Psychol 1968; 73:256–262.
Siegel B, Anders TF, Ciaranello RD, et al. Empirically derived subclassification of the autistic syndrome. J Autism Devel Disord 1986; 16:275–293.
Sigman M, Ungerer JA. Cognitive and language skills in autistic, mentally retarded, and normal children. Devel Psychol 1984; 20:293–302.
Smith PK, Dutton S. Play and training in direct and innovative problem solving. Child Devel 1979; 50:830–836.
Stokes TF, Baer DM. An implicit technology of generalization. J Appl Behav Anal 1977; 10:349–368.
Tilton JR, Ottinger DR. Comparison of the toy play behavior of autistic, retarded, and normal children, Psychol Rep 1964; 15:967–975.
Ungerer JA, Sigman M. Symbolic play and language comprehension in autistic children. J Amer Acad Child Psychiatry 1981; 20:318–337.
Voeltz LM, Evans IM. The assessment of behavioral interrelationships in child behavior therapy. Behav Assessment 1982; 4:131–165.
Weiner BJ, Ottinger DR, Tilton JR. Comparison of the toy-play behavior of autistic, retarded, and normal children: a reanalysis. Psychol Rep 1969; 25:223–227.
Wenar C, Ruttenberg BA, Kalish-Weiss B, Wolf EG. The development of normal and autistic children: a comparative study. J Autism Devel Disord 1986; 16:317–333.
Wetherby AM. Possible neurolinguistic breakdown in autistic children. Top Lang Disord 1984; 4:19–33.
Wetherby AM, Koegel RL, Mendel MI. Central auditory nervous system dysfunction in echolalic autistic individuals. J Speech Hear Res 1981; 24:420–429.
Williams JA, Koegel RL, Egel AL. Response-reinforcer relationships and improved learning in autistic children. J Appl Behav Anal 1981; 14:53–60.

Chapter Eight

MODEL OF GENERALIZATION

JOSEPH E. SPRADLIN, Ph.D.

The term *generalization* has been discussed in a variety of ways in the literature. At times the term has been introduced as a desired outcome of treatment (Costello Ingham, this book; Hughes, 1985; Kearns, this book; McReynolds, this book; Stokes and Baer, 1977; Thompson, this book; Warren, 1985). Sometimes it has been used to discuss behavioral processes (Hegde, 1985; Kearns, Costello Ingham, this book). At still other times, it has been discussed as an inadequate concept based on a behavioristic model (Connell, this book). Regardless of how one views the term generalization or the behavioristic model implied by the term, there is no doubt that the occurrence of behavior—under stimulus conditions that are different from those in which it was trained—is both an empirical fact and a desired outcome of therapy. It is also an empirical fact that sometimes behavior, that is different from the behavior being directly trained, changes as a function of training. This, too, is sometimes a desired outcome. Moreover, sometimes that behavior is maintained for long periods of time under conditions that are different from the conditions under which it was taught. And sometimes this, too, is a desired outcome. The previous chapters have discussed these outcomes as they related to therapy with persons with articulation problems, stuttering problems, aphasia, and general language problems.

It is indeed fortunate that not all new speech and language forms need to be taught in all of the conditions under which they are useful and that training conditions do not need to be maintained forever. Clinicians would never have the time for such a feat; and even if they had the time, they could never anticipate all of the situations under which speech and language would be useful. In spite of these fortunate sets of facts about behavior in general and language behavior as a special case, speech-language pathologists are faced with a difficult set of tasks. First, they must have some knowledge of the nature of language and language use if appropriate targets for therapy are to be selected. Second, clinicians must know something about the fundamental principles of behavior change—including the phenomena we call generalization. Finally, speech-language pathologists must know how to plan and arrange therapeutic programs so that the principles are applied in such a way as to result in improved language use. The current chapter focuses on procedures that result in generalization and how those procedures may be used in designing therapeutic programs to improve speech and language, and speech and language use.

PRIMARY STIMULUS GENERALIZATION

Primary stimulus generalization refers to stimulus generalization which is made possible by physical aspects that both training and generalization stimuli share.

Positive Stimuli

Often when stimulus generalization is discussed, the term *generalization gradient or curve* also occurs (Keller and Schoenfeld, 1950; Millenson and Leslie, 1979; Spence, 1956). According to the stimulus generalization reasoning, if a stimulus is brought to control a response through reinforcement, the probability of that response occurring in the presence of other stimuli varies according to how similar they are to the original stimulus used in conditioning. Hence, if the original stimulus used in conditioning was a 2,000-Hz tone, one would expect a slightly lower probability of response to a 1,500-Hz stimulus; a still lower probability of response, to a 750-Hz stimulus; and a very low probability, to a 250-Hz stimulus. The same generalization gradient could be illustrated using a specific value of the color spectrum and deviations from it. So one might get the impression that stimulus generalization always involved a gradual decrease in similarity of control as the test stimulus was faded from the original training stimulus. This has led to a hypothetical stimulus generalization curve as shown in Figure 8–1. This view of generalization is very neat and is occasionally found in experiments (Jenkins and Harrison, 1960).

There are also occasions when such gradients are not found. For example, if a training stimulus and a generalization stimulus both involve voice onset times that would ordinarily mark the same phoneme, normal adults generalize across markedly different voice onset times. If the two stimuli involve voice onset times that cross phoneme boundaries, they do not generalize so broadly. Interestingly, infants show similar responses to voice onset times (Eimas, 1974). There are many other instances when the generalization does not match the smooth hypothetical generalization gradient curves.

Most of the studies of generalization have varied stimuli along a single dimension such as frequency, intensity, wave length, voice onset time, and so on. However, any specific stimulus involves a combination of specific values along a number of dimensions (Spence, 1956). Suppose

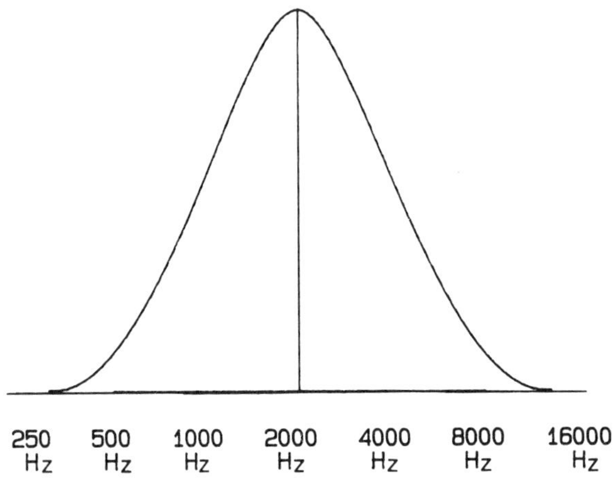

Figure 8–1 Hypothetical stimulus generalization gradient when the original training was 2,000 Hz and the test stimuli range from 250 to 16,000 Hz.

a child is taught to press a button when the consonant /f/ is presented and not to respond when no sound is presented. This can, of course, be accomplished by presenting a reinforcer when the child presses the button immediately after the /f/ sound has been presented, and by not presenting reinforcement if the child presses the button when no sound has been presented. If this behavioral sequence were accomplished, one would know very little about what the child had actually learned. Figure 8–2 demonstrates some of the dimensions along which generalization might occur.

The original /f/ sound is most often presented at a specific intensity for a specific duration, by a specific machine or person. Because that is the case, any one of these stimulus variables may gain control of the response. So it might turn out that the subject would fail to respond to the /f/ if any of these variables were changed. Moreover, the subject might generalize to any other consonant if it matched one of these variables. Given the limited training described above, there is no reason why the subject should come under the control of the specific variable designated as critical by the experimenter. Note that, since there was no contrasting sound, the child could have simply learned to respond to any sound that was presented. Or, the child may have learned to respond to any sound produced by the human voice. In fact, the child might have learned to respond on just about any basis ranging from responding to any noise to responding solely to the /f/ sound of a given intensity.

Fortunately, most children who come to the clinic know that certain aspects of the stimulus, such as loudness and duration, are not phonemic. However, a child's learning history is largely unknown to the clinician, and the clinician has no way of knowing exactly what aspects of the stimulus /f/ are controlling the response. The speech-language pathologist or experimenter can teach the child to respond to the /f/ alone by varying the values of the irrelevant dimensions of the /f/ stimulus. That is, the /f/ would be presented at different intensities and durations, with different voices, and responses to any /f/ sound would be reinforced. This procedure would ensure *generalization* to any /f/ stimulus presented in the session, but it would not ensure that the child would not also respond to any other stimulus.

Negative Stimuli

In order to be sure that the child does not respond to non-/f/ stimuli, a variety of negative stimuli would be presented in which the relevant dimensions were varied. (For a discussion of the importance of negative stimuli, see Englemann and Carnine, 1982). For example, the negative stimuli would include a sample of the consonants that /f/ is likely to be confused with, such as /v/ and /p/. When any of these stimuli are presented, the child's response would not be reinforced. Depending on one's interest, one might also present /fV/ items as negative stimuli. After such training, the child would very likely respond to any /f/ (generalization) in that situation and not to other consonants or the /f/ in a /fV/ context (discrimination).

Constant or Background Stimuli

Thus far, the discussion has focused on the positive and negative stimuli in the laboratory or training situation. However, there are also background or contextual stimuli (Goldiamond, 1962). These are stimuli that are constant. Some of the constant stimuli are the furniture or objects in the room, the color of the walls, the size of the room, the rug on the floor or the particular experimenter or trainer in the setting. If these background stimuli are constant, one might assume they are neutral and have no effect on the control exhibited by positive and negative stimuli. Ac-

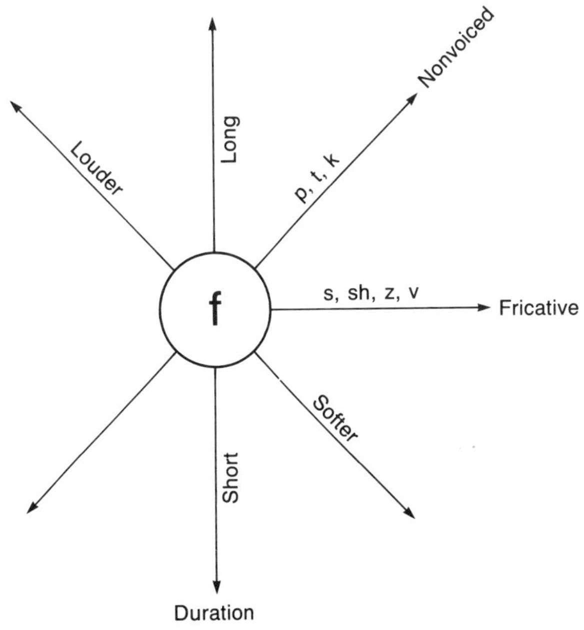

Figure 8–2 Dimensions along which generalization might occur if a child is taught to respond whenever a specific /f/ stimulus was presented and not to respond in the absence of that /f/ stimulus.

tually, this is not the case—constant stimuli often do affect control. The control of a discriminative stimulus over a response may break down if the constant or background stimuli are changed (Azrin, 1956). That is, the effective controlling stimulus is not simply the discriminative stimulus over a response that does not interact with background stimuli, one should vary irrelevant background stimuli. For example, a program to ensure that irrelevant background stimuli did not gain control over the articulation of a patient might vary such background stimuli as the clinician and settings.

Conditional Stimuli

On some occasions, control by contextual stimuli is undesirable. However, frequently such control is very helpful. The control exercised by a specific set of positive stimuli is not constant or permanent. That control depends on other conditional stimuli. For example, for the patient to say the word "red" when shown a red circle is not always acceptable. If the conditional stimulus is, "What is the shape of the figure?" the response "red" is inappropriate. The response "red" is an appropriate response to the red circle only if the accompanying conditional stimulus is "What color is the figure?"

In the hypothetical situation just described, procedures were suggested that would teach the child to respond only to the /f/ sound. In actual practice, the child is taught to respond to a number of specific values or dimensions. Which value or dimension controls responding at any given time depends on other contextual or conditional stimuli. For example, if the teacher says, "Press the button whenever you hear a consonant," a different set of contingencies is in effect than if the teacher says, "Press the button whenever you hear the /f/ sound." Furthermore, unless the child's repertoire is severely limited, the stimuli to which he or she responds would be very different under the two different conditions. How a person responds to a specific stimulus is determined by other conditional or contextual stimuli. No stimulus or aspect of a stimulus exercises the same control under all conditions.

PRIMARY RESPONSE GENERALIZATION

If the occurrences of a response with a specific topography are reinforced, not only does the frequency of that response increase but also responses with physically similar topographies (Keller and Schoenfeld, 1950). Response topographies vary across a number of dimensions including force, speed, form, and duration. The likelihood of responses occurring that exhibit a given aspect can be increased by reinforcing responses that exhibit that aspect and withholding reinforcement for responses that do not exhibit that aspect.

There are interesting effects of placing a contingency on a specific aspect of responses. Other aspects of the responses on which no contingencies are placed are likely to occur more frequently if they are present when the first response occurs that meets contingency criteria (Keller and Schoenfeld, 1950). For example, suppose a clinician decides to reinforce a severely nonvocal child each time he says /a/. Suppose, further, that the child's first /a/ was a brief loud utterance. It is likely that not only the frequency of /a/ would increase but also /a/s that are brief and loud. In other words, when the subject's first response is reinforced, there is no way to ensure that only the clinician's target aspect will be strengthened. There are, no doubt, many specific topographical aspects of speech that are determined by such accidental contingencies. If one desires to establish a certain aspect across a number of different topographies, one can withhold reinforcement for often repeated topographies and reinforce when the aspect occurs with new responses. Speech-language pathologists rarely attempt simply to shape responses involving specific topographic aspects in the absence of some type of stimulus control. Indeed, just as we attempt to establish conditional control over certain aspects of primary stimulus generalization, we also try to establish verbal control over specific dimensions of responding when we teach a child to respond appropriately to such words as "louder" or "slower."

GENERALIZATION BASED ON RECOMBINATION OF STIMULUS–RESPONSE UNITS

The term *response class* has been used widely in discussions of language (Costello Ingham, this book; Guess 1969; Guess, Sailor, Rutherford and Baer, 1968; Kearns, this book; McReynolds, this book; Peterson, 1968; Thompson, this book; Warren, 1985). This term has been used primarily descriptively to designate situations in which specific untreated behaviors have changed as a function of treatments applied to other behaviors. The question of what behaviors are members of the same response class is an empirical question and can be determined only after direct training and tests have been done. However, it may be possible to develop ways of doing training so that response classes are developed and generalization is predicted.

This section of the chapter attempts to describe a set of procedures that is very likely to generate response classes or allow the prediction of what behaviors are likely to be members of the same response class. These procedures primarily involve recombination of stimulus–response units.

Vocal Imitation

An important behavior for the speech-language pathologist is generalized imitation. One of the quickest ways to get most children to emit an approximation of the clinician's designated response is simply to provide a model and ask the child to repeat it. Ordinarily children acquire vocal imitation skills quite readily without structured training. However, there are a few children who do not. Lovaas, Berberich, Perloff, and Schaeffer (1966) described a procedure they used with mute schizophrenic children. Their first two phases involved increasing the child's rate of vocalizations and getting the child to vocalize immediately after the model vocalized. This was done using reinforcement and discrimination training procedures.

Lovaas and colleagues' third and fourth phases are most relevant to the discussion of generalization as a function of recombination of response units. They trained the children to imitate a number of sounds and words. Initially they taught syllables that began with bilabial consonants such as /b/ and /p/. The probability of the children's emitting the correct consonant was increased by the use of such physical prompts as holding the lips together then rapidly releasing them. Teaching the first few syllables required several days of training; however, after the first few syllables were taught, new words or syllables were learned much more rapidly. In fact, the children reached the point at which they correctly imitated new words without direct imitation training on the specific words. New words might initially be misarticulated, but correct articulation increased with repeated practice in the absence of reinforcement or punishment for these specific words. Reinforcement was maintained for correct imitation of other words.

It appears that if some imitative responses are reinforced, others may emerge and be maintained in the absence of observable reinforcement. A close look at syllables the children were taught to imitate indicates that many of the syllables contained some of the same aspects or components. Table 8–1 is derived from the syllables and words taught by Lovaas and associates (1966). It shows a breakdown of initial consonant or consonant blend and the vowel with which each was combined. The numbers in the table indicate the order in which the particular combination was introduced. As shown in the table, the consonant /b/ was introduced in combination with seven different vowels. The consonants /d/, /n/, /h/, and /m/ were all introduced in combination with at least two vowels each. Nine of the vowel sounds were taught in combination with at least two consonants. The article does not state specifically which syllables or words were correctly produced without training, nor whether they involved components that had been previously taught. However, I would speculate that the words correctly imitated without specific training involved previously taught components or aspects. If so, the study by Lovaas and colleagues is an example of generalization based on recombination of stimulus–response units. Note that the units are not simply responses; they consist of responses that bear a particular relation to specific stimuli or aspects of stimuli. The stimuli involved in vocal imitation are auditory and bear a point-to-point relationship to the response.

Fortunately, the speech clinician using an imitation procedure for remediating an articulation problem usually does not have to begin by teaching the child to imitate. Indeed, many children with articulation problems have elaborate speech and language systems. Those systems may be faulty in some ways, but they allow procedures for training that would be precluded by the speech system of children like the subjects in the study of Lovaas and associates. An approximation of the desired response can be obtained from a normal 6-year-old child not only by providing a spoken model, but also by presenting a picture, a spoken sentence frame, or perhaps written test.

The following pages contain a discussion of some previous speech and language research in terms of unit-combination.

Elbert and McReynolds (1975) selected 12 children between 5 and 12 years of age who misarticulated all /r/ allophones even when given a spoken model. The authors developed a test including combinations of the /r/ phoneme with ten different vowel sounds in four different positions—for example, initial position "rabbit"; consonant glide "train"; stressed vocalic "bird"; and unstressed "water." The specific items used in testing the subjects are presented in Table 8–2.

Note that the table involves a matrix with rows representing the various positions and columns representing the vowel combinations involved in the test. Each subject was given training on imitating only one allophone with one vowel—/e/. Note that the procedure allows a test of generalization across these three categories: combinations with different vowels with the /r/ phoneme in the same position as in the training syllable; different positions (allophones) with the same vowel as used in training; and syllables involving different vowels and different

TABLE 8–1 Matrix of Imitative Sounds Taught by Lovaas and Colleagues

Phoneme	*e*	*u*	*i*	*a*	*aI*	*I*	æ	ɛ	*o*	*aI*	ɛr	ʊ
—		2	3	28					14			
b	1			7/13	6	8		12		27		29
w			4									
p				5								
d				9			10					
t				11			32					
h			24	20			18				17	
m			23	19	21	22			25			
n									26	30		
k									31			
r												33
G									34			
Hw										15		
b								16				

TABLE 8–2 Test for Misarticulation of /r/

Glide consonant /r/ initial position	*Glide consonant /r/ initial blends*	*Stressed vocalic /ɝ/*	*Unstressed vocalic /ɚ/*
ri	tri	tɝt	itɚ
rɪ	drɪ	dɝd	ɪdɚ
rʌ	gre	gɝg	egɚ
rɛ	krɛ	kɝk	ɛkɚ
ræ	træ	kɝt	ætɚ
ru	dru	gɝd	udɚ
rʊ	grʊ	dɝg	ʊgɚ
ro	kro	tɝk	okɚ
rɔ	trɔ	dɝt	ɔtɚ
rɑ	drɑ	tɝd	ɑdɚ

Forty stimulus items used in baseline and probe tests. Ten items are included in each allophonic category: glide consonant /r/ in the prevocalic initial position, glide consonant /r/ in the prevocalic position in blends, stressed vocalic /ɝ/, and the unstressed /ɚ/ in a postconsonantal position. From Elbert M, McReynolds LV. Transfer of /r/ across contexts. J Speech Hear Disord 1975; 40:387.

positions. Elbert and McReynolds' study does not allow an independent analysis of position or allophonic generalization, because most items for tests of allophonic generalization involve new vowel combinations. The generalization obtained was highly variable across subjects. Nevertheless, most subjects showed some generalization.

Figure 8–3 shows some of the possible forms of recombination generalization that might have occurred for one type of training investigated. The figure shows that /r/ was tested in the context of vowels in addition to /e/. It also shows that the /r/ was tested in the context of consonant–/r/ clusters with various vowels, in final position in combination with a number of different consonants, and in the stressed vocalic position with a number of different consonants. The data provided by the authors on the three subjects who received training are interesting. All three performed at least as well on the consonant blend as on the /r/ vowel combinations. Each of the three children provided a different generalization pattern. Two subjects' responses demonstrated improved performance in imitating the /r/ sound in all contexts, but to different degrees. The third subject's responses improved only for /rV/ combinations and the /CrV/ combinations.

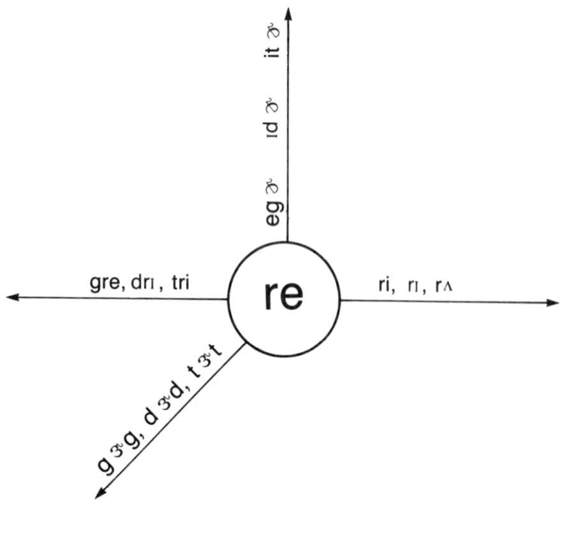

Figure 8–3 Possible generalization based on recombination of the /r/ phoneme with other phonemes and phoneme combinations in Elbert and McReynolds' 1975 study.

Table 8–3 shows the combinations of /rV/ actually taught in the current experiment. They include the /b/ and /m/ consonants with ten vowels and the /r/ with the /e/ vowel. The /b/ and /m/ were taught in pretraining and the /r/ in the experiment proper. It is likely, because the /r/ is one of the last consonants mastered, that the subjects also combined a number of other consonants with the vowels. It is my speculation that by teaching the /r/ in a small number of /rV/ combinations in addition to the /re/ combination, all of the current subjects would have mastered all /rV/ combinations. Literature on recombination of components suggests this (Goldstein, 1985; Wetherby, 1978; Wetherby and Striefel, 1978).

The procedure of teaching more than one vowel in combination with a target phoneme cluster has been used by McReynolds and Elbert (1981). One can look at the allophone generalization in the same way. It is likely that the subjects may have already mastered combinations of /n/, /m/ and /l/ in the various contexts prior to the experiment, as shown in Table 8–4. If so, then subjects had the basis for recombination generalization across allophones.

In this book, Elbert has made a major point that generalization is affected by the child's existing knowledge. Such prior knowledge may prove useful in predicting generalization. Moreover, the current discussion suggests that although generalization may occur after training involv-

TABLE 8–3 Matrix of Known and Trained Consonant–Vowel Combinations Involved in Elbert and McReynolds' (1975) Training Study

Phonemes	*e*	ɪ	ʌ	ɛ	æ	u	ʊ	o	ɔ	*a*
b	P	P	P	P	P	P	P	P	P	P
m	P	P	P	P	P	P	P	P	P	P
k	L	L	L	L	L	L	L	L	L	L
G	L	L	L	L	L	L	L	L	L	L
w	L	L	L	L	L	L	L	L	L	L
l	L	L	L	L	L	L	L	L	L	L
r	(T)	?	?	?	?	?	?	?	?	?

P = phonemes used in pretraining
L = likely to be exhibited or known already
(T) = trained in the current experiment

TABLE 8–4 Matrix of Possible Known and Trained Allophone Combinations Involved in Elbert and McReynolds' (1975) Allophone Training Study

Phoneme	*–e*	*C-e*	*C ə –*	*VC ə –*
l	L	L	L	L
m	L	L	L	L
n	L	L	L	L
r	(T)	?	?	?

L = likely to be exhibited or known already
(T) = trained in the current experiment

ing only one combination, to ensure that generalization across a specific dimension occurs, several combinations involving key units along a dimension in which generalization is desired should be taught. Note that this procedure might be a subclass of teaching sufficient examples (Stokes and Baer, 1977).

Generalization Across Phonemes As the Result of Teaching Distinctive Features

The research just discussed treated combinations of phonemes. However, generalization may also occur across sounds if the various sounds include a common feature or aspect. McReynolds and Bennett (1972) conducted a study with children who exhibited errors in several phonemes that involved the same distinctive feature. One subject exhibited errors on /b/, /g/, and /d/ sounds. In each case the voicing feature was absent. The subject was given imitation training with /b/ and /p/ in combination with /a/ in both the arresting and releasing position. After training he was given a test in which the /b/, /p/, /d/, /t/, /g/, and /k/ were tested in both the arresting and releasing positions. His performance on all sounds in the releasing position was completely accurate; there were some errors in the arresting position. The generalization involved in this study is very complex, because the change in an aspect or feature of one sound is recombined with other aspects to form new sounds. Moreover, there is generalization from two simple syllables to words spoken in response to pictures. There can be no doubt that the child's already existing speech and understanding of speech played a major role in his achievement. It is possible that the child discriminated between voiced and unvoiced stops prior to training even though he did not produce voiced stops in a way that distinguished them for a listener.

Generalization of Phoneme Production Across Evoking Stimuli

McReynolds and Bennett's study also involves establishing both imitation and picture control over correct articulation. The control of correct articulation by different stimuli is of considerable interest, and a study by McLean (1970) is quite suitable for the discussion of the generalization involved in the extension of control. McLean's study involved training mentally retarded subjects who mispronounced specific phonemes in a variety of vowel contexts and in a number of different stimulus contexts. The study tested specifically for four types of generalization: first, generalization to new words with the trained phoneme in the initial position; second, generalization to new words with the trained phoneme in a different position; third, generalization of the trained phoneme when a different stimulus mode was used to evoke the stimulus; and fourth, generalization to words in which the initially substituted phoneme would have been correct.

None of the subjects emitted the target phoneme correctly on any item when tested for picture, printed word, or intraverbal control. All but one subject correctly produced the phoneme on some occasions when it was evoked in imitation. Interestingly, McLean was unable to teach a subject (who never correctly produced the phoneme in imitation) to imitate the target sound correctly during the experiment. McLean taught each of the other subjects to emit the correct response in the echoic condition then he presented the vocal model stimuli paired with a picture. After a few trials he omitted the model, eventually getting the subject to respond correctly to the pictures alone. The pictures were then presented paired with printed words. After a few trials he presented the printed words alone. When the printed words evoked correct phonemes, he then paired the printed words with intraverbal stimuli and repeated the procedure. The subjects were tested prior to training on the printed words and intraverbal stimuli. All four subjects showed some generalization on these tests. Three of the four subjects generalized to new words when they were evoked by pictures and overgeneralized to words in which the previously substituted phoneme would have been correct. (*Note* when McReynolds and Bennett taught their subject the voicing feature, they taught /b/ in contrast to /p/; then when they tested for generalization, the + and – voicing distinction was maintained.) There was no generalization across positions by any of the McLean subjects. Of course, the phoneme was trained only in one position. It is likely that McLean's subjects would not have overgeneralized if the contrast between the initially substituted phoneme and the trained phoneme had been included in training. It is also possible that not all children who made errors of the type found in the McLean study would need to be taught the contrast. Some children might already discriminate the two phonemes as listeners but simply be unable to produce one.

McLean's finding that there was no across-position generalization is in marked contrast to the results of Powell and McReynolds (1969), who found considerable across-position generalization with normal children between 4 years 9 months, and 6 years 7 months of age. Once again, the difference in generalization probably depends on the child's initial repertoire of speech and language skills (Elbert's knowledge) when he or she enters the training situation.

Recombination of Larger Units

Tables 8–1, 8–2, 8–3 and 8–4 above all show combinations of phonemes presented in a matrix form, and I have attempted to explain generalization or failure in generalization by the training of several of the correct combinations, or failure to train enough combinations or the correct type of combinations. Wetherby (1978) and Wetherby and Striefel (1978) have presented a rather complete discussion of miniature language systems and the use of the matrices in organizing and analyzing the results of language training. Striefel and his colleagues (Striefel, Bryan and Aikens, 1974; Striefel and Wetherby, 1973; Striefel, Wetherby and Karlan, 1976) conducted a series of studies in which they taught retarded children to follow simple verb–noun commands. Initially each command consisted of a single verb and noun such as "Push glass." In one of their earlier studies (Striefel and Wetherby, 1973), they taught a subject to follow a series of commands, as shown in Table 8–5. As can be seen, each verb is nearly always presented with the same unique noun. When the subjects were tested on new combinations, they showed no generalization in following commands. However, when Striefel and coworkers (1976) trained in a way that involved systematic recombination of verbs and nouns, the subjects all generalized to untrained combinations. Table 8–6 shows the results of the data for one of Striefel and coworkers' subjects. Note that it is not simply responses that are being recombined but complex stimulus–response units. This same recombination of units has also been demonstrated with simple productive speech (Whitehurst, 1971; Wetherby, 1978; Goldstein, 1984).

Thompson (this book) has noted in her work with aphasics that after training on several exemplars of a sentence type, the subject can often produce new examples of that same sentence type but not examples of other sentence types. It is very likely that the training involved recombinations of units. However, it is also quite likely that there would be generalization beyond the specific words trained in therapy, because the aphasic client would have had a wealth of prior experience with those words. The fact that generalization did not occur with nontrained sentence types suggests once again that, if you want to obtain generalization of a particular type, you should teach several examples involving recombination of units along the dimensions for which generalization is sought.

Acquired Stimulus Classes

One area involving unit recombinations that is currently being extensively investigated is the development of acquired stimulus classes. Acquired stimulus classes consist of stimuli that have similar or related controlling properties but that have no physical properties in common. For example, the spoken word "five," the printed word *five*, the Arabic numeral 5, the set of five objects or events, all share some controlling relations. Yet they have no defining physical properties in common. These stimuli have developed related controlling properties on some other basis than primary physical similarity.

Early researchers, who studied the development of stimulus classes, trained children to give two different stimuli the same name. Then the children were taught a discrimination using one of the stimuli. When these children were tested with the remaining stimulus, they tended to respond to it in a manner more similar than did children in a control group who had received training in which the two stimuli had been given distinctive names (Birge, 1949 [as cited in Miller and Dollard, 1941]; Kendler, 1972; Reese, 1972). This finding led a number of researchers to believe that such common functions had

TABLE 8–5 Striefel and Wetherby (1973) Training and Generalization Combinations Used in Their Instruction-Following Experiment

	Glass	*Hand(s)*	*Spoon*	*Ball*	*Car*	*Knee*	*Arms*	*Block*	*Mouth*	*Feather*	*Scissors*	*Glove*	*Cheek*	*Ear*	*Shoe*	*Nose*	*Tongue*	*Hair*	*Shoe*
Drink from	T																		
Raise		T																	
Clap your		T																	
Eat with			T																
Drop				T						G–									
Push					T			G–											
Touch your						T							G–						
Fold your							T												
Lift					G–			T											
Open your									T										
Blow on				G–						T									
Hold out		G–									T								
Fold							T												
Put on												T							
Wave your		T									G–								
Rub your						G–							T						
Point to														T	T	T			
Nod head yes																		G–	
Shake head no																			
Stick out																	T		
Brush																			G–

T = trained
G– = generalization failure

TABLE 8–6 Matrix Derived from Data Presented for Striefel, Wetherby, and Karlan's (1976) Subject 1 on Following Instructions

	Nouns											
Verbs	*Glass*	*Scissors*	*Car*	*Ball*	*Comb*	*Plane*	*Glove*	*Spoon*	*Feather*	*Fork*	*Banana*	*Block*
Push	T	T	T	T	T	G	G	G	G	G	G	G
Drop	T	T	T	T	T	T	T	T	T	T	G	G
Blow on	T	T	T	G	G	G	G	G	G	G	G	G
Hold out	T	T	T	G	G	G	G	G	G	G	G	G
Point to	T	T	G	G	G	G	G	G	G	G	G	G
Wave	T	G	G	G	G	G	G	G	G	G	G	G
Tap	T	T	G	G	G	G	G	G	G	G	G	G
Pound with	T	G	G	G	G	G	G	G	G	G	G	G
Smell	T	G	G	G	G	G	G	G	G	G	G	G
Elevate	T	G	G	G	G	G	G	G	G	G	G	G
Turn	T	G	G	G	G	G	G	G	G	G	G	G
Encircle	T	G	G	G	G	G	G	G	G	G	G	G

T = trained
G = generalized

to be mediated verbally (Miller and Dollard, 1941; Jenkins, 1963). The early research was conducted with groups, so it was difficult to determine what a specific child did. More recently, procedures have been developed for studying the development of stimulus classes that allow a rather precise determination of the classes of individual children (Sidman, 1971; Spradlin, Cotter, and Baxley, 1973). The basic procedure used by these investigators is one in which the child is taught two or more conditional discriminations. For example, a child might be presented the capital letters "A" and "B" as choice stimuli and sometimes the spoken stimulus "a" and sometimes the spoken stimulus "b." The child's task is to select *A* when "a" is spoken and *B* when "b" is spoken. After acquiring this conditional discrimination, the child might be presented the lower case letters *a* and *b* as choices, and the spoken "a" and the spoken "b" at other times. Now, the child could simply learn the two conditional discriminations and no more. However, after this training, this child is typically able to match lower case *a* with capital *A* and lower case *b* with capital *B*. Moreover, in some cases, the child is able to name the lower case and capital letters appropriately. Essentially, the training establishes two three-member classes, any one of which can, under certain conditions, be substituted for another without a change in functional control. The development of such stimulus classes has been demonstrated by a variety of investigators under a variety of conditions (Dixon, 1978; Dixon and Spradlin, 1976; Lazar, 1977; Lazar, Davis-Lang and Sanchez, 1984; Sidman and Cresson, 1973; Sidman, Cresson and Willson-Morris, 1974; Sidman, Kirk and Willson-Morris, 1985; Sidman and Tailby, 1982; Spradlin and Dixon, 1976; Spradlin and Saunders, 1986).

Sidman's first experiment involved teaching a 17-year-old microcephalic man to select 20 printed words in response to their spoken names (Sidman, 1971). This man could name and select pictures of common objects. Prior to training, the man had been unable to select printed words in response to spoken names, to read printed words, or to match printed words to the pictures the words represented. After training on only the one task, he was able to perform all three tasks he had previously been unable to do. In a sense, Sidman established twenty three-member classes consisting of the spoken word, the picture, and the printed word. Any one of the stimuli could, under certain conditions, be substituted for any other. One could question whether the class formation is dependent on training in which the subject is taught to select the printed word in response to its spoken name, or whether it could be established by teaching the child to select the printed word in response to its representative picture.

Hollis (1987) used three procedures to develop the reading classes taught by Sidman. In one procedure, he taught the subjects to name the printed words; in another, he taught the child to select the printed words in response to spoken words; and in the third, he taught the children to select printed words in response to pictures. In all cases the subjects had near-perfect performance on all tasks after training. Moreover, they were approximately 85 percent correct on all tasks after 5 months without additional training.

Gast, VanBiervliet, and Spradlin (1979) taught children to select printed number names in response to their spoken names (the children were able to count, name numerals, and select a numeral in response to a spoken number). When they were able to do this, they were also able to do all the remaining tasks involving spoken number names, printed numbers, printed number words, and sets of objects. Gast and colleagues established a four-member class in which any member could, under certain conditions, be substituted for any other. Both Sidman's and Gast and colleagues' studies involved conventional classes that were at least partially developed on the basis of nonexperimental history. Other researchers have used stimuli in their experiments that have no conventional relationship to one another, to demonstrate these procedures for establishing classes (Devany, Hayes and Nelson, 1986; Dixon, 1978; Dixon and Spradlin, 1976; Sidman, Creson and Willson-Morris, 1974; Sidman, Kirk and Willson-Morris, 1985; Sidman, Willson-Morris and Kirk, 1985;

Wetherby, Karlan and Spradlin, 1983). Classes of stimuli with as many as nine members have been reported in the literature (Saunders, Wachter and Spradlin, 1988). There may be a limit to the number of stimuli that can enter such classes, but there is no indication that that limit has yet been reached.

Although the procedures for establishing stimulus classes described above all involved conditional discriminations, such procedures are not necessary for establishing stimulus classes. In our laboratory severely retarded, nonverbal subjects were conditioned to press a button when either a tone or a light was presented. They were then conditioned to pull a chain when the tone was presented. Without additional training, the subjects then pulled the chain when the light was presented. In other words, the tone and the light, when given a common function through direct training, exhibited a second common function even though only one stimulus was directly involved in conditioning.

This led Spradlin and Dixon to hypothesize that if two or more stimuli could be substituted for each other in one context without changing contingencies, there was an increased probability they would exhibit similar functions in contexts in which not all stimuli had been involved in direct training (Spradlin and Dixon, 1976). This position is not too different from Nelson's position that particular objects may be members of the same class by virtue of being substitutable in certain scripts or routines (Nelson, 1983).

The concept of acquired stimulus classes also has implications for understanding generalization of behavior among people. The concept of primary stimulus generalization has long been invoked to explain generalization among people. For example, if a child learned to obey her mother and to disobey her father, then because of physical similarities the child might obey women and not men. Such primary stimulus generalization may be involved initially; however, after a few interactions, behavior may be more nearly determined on the basis of similarities in contingencies applied by the people than on the basis of physical similarities.

Haavik, Spradlin, and Altman (1984) conducted a study in which a trainer taught a number of performances to severely retarded preschool children. The child's performances were rarely correctly performed at home for the mother. However, when the mother started home training with reinforcement, the child's other home performances began to improve when tested by the mother. In other words, the mother became a member of the stimulus class "teach" with regard to these performances. Silverman, Anderson, Marshall, and Baer (1986) conducted a study that demonstrated that audiences could be established as members of a stimulus class using procedures similar to those used in laboratory studies of stimulus class development.

Now consider McLean's (1970) study in the light of the acquired stimulus class discussion presented above. McLean used four different stimulus conditions for teaching his subjects initial phonemes. The first was an echoic model (a test or use of the ability to stimulate), the second was a picture, the third was a printed word, and the fourth was a verbal sentence which the subject was to complete with a specific word.

During training, McLean first presented the target phoneme in spoken words and had the subject repeat them. Then he paired the spoken words with pictures and continued training until the subject's production of the target phoneme was 100 percent correct for two 10-trial sessions. Then the pictures were presented alone. One subject showed almost no decrement when the pictures were presented alone; a second subject's performance dropped to 0 percent correct but rapidly recovered; and two subjects required extended training prior to reaching criteria level. McLean then paired the pictures and printed words. Three subjects' performances remained high. The fourth subject's performance decreased. Finally, McLean presented sentence frames requiring completion with words that included the target phoneme. This was at the point at which the words were required when the printed word was presented. No subject required more than three sessions to reach criteria level, and no subject's response dropped below 90 percent correct when the printed word was removed. McLean's study suggests the role that stimulus classes may play in speech and language learning.

McLean presented pairs of stimuli simultaneously. In each case, one type of stimulus already resulted in the production of the target phoneme on some occasions. Presumably the control of the second type of stimulus was minimal. No questions were asked in McLean's study to determine whether any relationships had been learned other than those involved with productive speech. However, it would not be surprising if at least some of the subjects (after training) could have selected the picture and printed words in response to the spoken words or selected the pictures in response to printed words, and printed words in response to sentence frames. Because these stimulus pairs had been presented contiguously, there is reason to believe that some relationship might have been learned.

What if a different mode of training had been used? Suppose that the subject had only been trained to produce the correct phonemes in response to spoken words and pictures, as shown in Figure 8–4. Suppose, further, that the subject had been trained to select printed words in a match-to-sample task, and to select the printed words

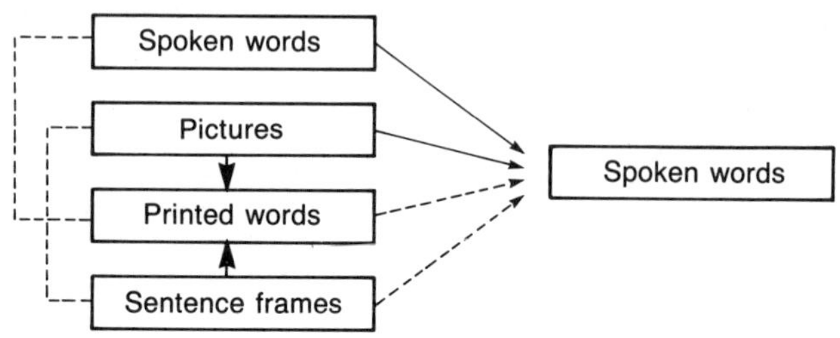

Figure 8–4 This diagram shows what McLean's subjects might have learned if they had been taught in a slightly different fashion. The solid lines with arrows indicate the trained relations. The broken lines indicate the relations that might emerge without training.

in response to sentence frames. Would the subjects then be able to produce the correct phonemes in response to printed words and sentence frames? Would they also be able to select pictures in response to the sentence frame and to select printed words in response to spoken words? If the original target phonemes are maintained in response to the pictures, the remainder of the performances may emerge. That is essentially what literature on stimulus class development shows. Of course, subjects in stimulus class experiments also exhibit individual differences in generalization.

Stimulus Control in Speech Context

Thus far most of the discussion has involved the control over speech by clinician- or experimenter-presented stimuli. However, much of the control over misarticulated or stuttered utterances may be exercised by the client's own speech. The errors are not solely under the control of some externally produced stimulus but under the control of stimuli produced by the client's own behavior. These are essentially Skinner's intraverbals or autoclitics (Skinner, 1957). These are the stimuli that are maintained across settings and they are the stimuli that come to exercise the greatest control. Costello Ingham has proposed that the procedure for getting clients to speak fluently is first to teach the subject to speak fluently in brief utterances, then to extend the fluent speech to larger utterances, then still larger, and finally to connected speech. No doubt the speech is first emitted slowly, then speed is increased in the same manner as length of utterance. Although the studies of recombination of units involved in articulation described above did not extend the investigation to the complex units occurring in conversation, there is no doubt that the probability of obtaining correct phoneme production in conversational units would have decreased, especially if those larger units were produced rapidly. So some of the aspects of control of fluent articulate speech must be involved in the speech in which the specific erroneous speech is embedded. That is, there is intraverbal control over both correct and incorrect production.

Diedrich and Bangert (1980) have proposed a 3-minute connected-speech sample as a way of evaluating articulation. Moreover, they suggest that speech in such samples is somewhat stable across samples. It is doubtful that this brief test would be adequate for evaluating stuttering. However, if stuttering occurred in such a sample, it would no doubt predict stuttering in conversational settings. The point made here is that many of the stimuli controlling correct production are intraverbal and, if the correct productions are not strongly controlled by these intraverbal stimuli, one should not expect broad generalization of correctly produced new speech. Note that all other stimuli that potentially control speech vary across settings; however, the stimuli produced by the subject's own speech are more likely to be constant. Hence, control by these stimuli offer the greatest possibility of bridging speech situations.

Speech pathologists have long made the point that correct articulation involved internalization or automatization. How does this fit with the training programs that teach the subject to pronounce the target sound when evoked by a model, then a picture, then a printed word, then a carrier phrase? Each of these procedures decreased the chances that correct articulation will come under the restrictive control of irrelevant stimuli and makes it more likely that it will come under the control of relevant stimuli. Some of these relevant stimuli are produced by the client's own speech. Varying the size of the unit in which a production is embedded and varying the speed of speaking are ways of increasing the chances that correct productions will come under the control of the relevant speech-produced stimuli.

Elimination of Unwanted Response Components

Not every speech or communication problem involves missing components or recombination failures. Stuttering often involves the addition of unwanted response components such as hesitations, prolongations, repetitions, and tremor disfluencies. These components have come to be combined with other speech components in such a way as to interfere with communication under certain circumstances.

According to Costello Ingham (this book), a variety of punishment techniques have been successful in reducing the rate of specific stuttering behavior. Just as not all combinations need to be taught in teaching new speech behavior, the unwanted behavior does not need to be punished in all of the combinations in which it occurs. This is fortunate, because one would probably never treat all of the combinations into which the unwanted component intrudes. Interestingly, sometimes different components (such as hesitations, tremor disfluencies, and repetitions) covary; when one is punished, the other also decreases in frequency. Why this occurs is not understood; however, it seems likely that these components may have become members of the same response class because each of these behaviors had the same effect on a listener.

ISSUES REGARDING USE OF LEARNED SKILLS IN THE NATURAL ENVIRONMENT

The first section of this chapter was devoted to the presentation of principles and procedures for predicting and promoting generalization. This section is devoted to teaching speech and language in such a way that it is used and its use is reinforced in natural environments. The issue of getting "correct" speech and language used in the natural environments involves more than generalization. It may involve prompting and reinforcing speech and language in the environments in which it is to be used. In this case, the issue is not generalization but training. It may also involve ensuring that there is some differential reinforcement for correct speech and language when it does occur in the natural environment, that is, maintenance. Although Baer, Wolf, and Risley (1968) and Stokes and Baer (1977) have considered maintenance a type of generalization—generalization across time—maintenance is not considered generalization in the current chapter. Indeed, Baer and associates' reconceptualization was unfortunate because it focused practitioners away from a massive amount of literature designated by the terms "resistance to extinction" and "maintenance." There are numerous factors that determine whether taught speech and language skills are used in the natural environment. These are discussed briefly below.

Selection of Skills

The first issue to be addressed is selection and characterization of the skill to be taught. Is it a skill that allows the person to do more things or do things better in his natural environment? This may have a considerable impact on the success in getting that skill used in the natural environment. There are numerous examples in which a skill or set of skills of no value in the natural environment was taught in the training setting. The people who have developed language training programs for severly retarded persons in institutions are painfully aware of the issue of teaching something in training sessions that is not supported back on the wards (Warren, 1985). Many of the early language training attempts involved teaching retarded people to name or describe pictures. When the retarded subjects named or described pictures in teaching sessions, their actions were reinforced with edibles, tokens, or social attention. It is not surprising that these skills did not generalize back to the wards. A busy caretaker with 15 severely retarded people simply does not have enough time to provide pictures to name and describe. Moreover, this skill does not make the changes in the environment that are necessary to maintain it. Even a skill as apparently useful as requesting may not be generalized to the environment if things are not provided when requests occur or if they are consistently provided in the absence of requests. So, if skills are to be maintained, they must be useful in the person's natural environment.

In some cases when people who stutter are taught fluent speech or people who misarticulate are taught proper articulation, these new skills may fail to make much difference in the person's day-to-day communication. For example, an otherwise normal child or adult who has a mild to moderate articulation problem may communicate in normal social situations in very effective ways. He or she can issue directives, make requests, tell about last evening's ball game, and do all of the things speech is supposed to do. If the person learns clearly articulated speech and uses it, it also does all of those things for the person. Of course, periodically the misarticulating person may be misunderstood or socially embarrassed, but these experiences are likely to constitute only a very small percentage of the social exchanges. In short, in most situations it does not make much difference whether the person misarticulates or not. Because the old misarticulated speech serves the person well, what are the contingencies that result in giving up an old familiar and effective behavior to develop a new one? For some people with what we call a speech problem, not having that speech problem simply does not make enough difference in the situation in which misarticulation was learned and maintained over many years. This may be one of the reasons why it is so much more difficult to change speech patterns in adults than in children. Perhaps teachers, parents, and others are also more likely to aid in teaching correct articulation to children by pointing out that an error has occurred. In any case, when targets are selected for change, it is important to make sure that the changes actually make a difference in the natural environment of the client.

Role of Settings in Speech and Language Skill Use

Settings are essentially a set of background stimuli, as discussed under primary stimulus generalization in the first section of this chapter. Historically, speech therapy has been conducted within the confines of a small room in the clinic or school with a speech or language therapist. The speech or language skills being taught are to be exhibited in the classroom, on the playground, at home, around the dinner table, in the work setting, and so on. None of these settings resembles the training situation very much. In view of the massive differences between the background stimuli of the training setting and the background stimuli of the settings in which the skills are to be exhibited, it is not surprising that speech or language therapy sometimes fails. To ensure use in relevant natural environments, one might simultaneously institute training in each of the various environments in which use of the taught speech and language is desirable. However, that would be impractical and might not be effective even if it were possible. The natural environment contains many background stimuli that may have gained control over incorrect speech and language. Hence, there may be a greater amount of interference from the old speech patterns that would occur in the rather novel background stimuli found in the speech clinic.

For that reason, it might prove more effective to teach new speech and language within the clinic and then to extend use systematically into other settings. Suppose there are a number of aspects of the child's speech that need training and extension into natural environments. One might consider a hypothetical training sequence such as that shown in Table 8–7. The clinician would start by teaching skill #1 within the clinic therapy room. Then one would test to see if skill #1 were used outside the therapy room but still within the clinic. If it were not, then it would be trained in that setting. This procedure would be continued until skill #1 was occurring in new settings without direct training. Skill #2 would be taught and evaluated in the same manner. One would, of course, continue to review skill #1 in a variety of settings to ensure that it was maintained. After skill #2 was established across a number of settings, the clinician would introduce skill #3 in the same fashion. It is likely that after training and tests across three or four skills, a skill would only need to be taught in the clinic therapy room to generalize to other settings.

One may look at the training described above as training that extends the stimulus control from the clinical therapy room to the outside clinic, to the home livingroom, and to the school playground. This is probably a misleading way of looking at generalization. Probably a better way to look at the training is that by teaching the client a skill in a variety of settings, the client is taught that the setting is not a relevant controlling variable. Hence, the skill is no longer controlled by setting variables.

By teaching a number of speech skills across a number of settings, the client learns that any skill taught in the clinic therapy room is applicable across any of a variety of settings. This is essentially what is predicted by the current literature on stimulus class development. Note that although skills #1 through #6 may have initially been independent after the type of training illustrated in Table 8–7, they would function as a response class by the time training had been completed. So in the training illustrated by Table 8–7, there is the simultaneous development of a stimulus class (setting) and a response class (skills).

Role of People or Trainers in Speech and Language Usage

Different natural environments often involve different people. So even though the speech-language pathologist may teach speech skills in a number of situations, one set of background stimuli that may gain control over correct responding is the set associated with the specific person doing the training or therapy. In order to ensure that speech skills are used with different people, it may be necessary to have a number of different people teaching, or at least requiring, the speech skills. To ensure that a child uses speech skills with different people, therapy might be planned in accordance with the same matrix organization as suggested with natural environments. For example, it might be necessary for special therapy procedures to be used by several people when the first skill is taught, in order for the skill to generalize to a new person (Table 8–8).

TABLE 8–7 Training Sequence for Ensuring that a Set of Speech and Language Responses are Used in all Relevant Natural Settings

	Skills					
Settings	*1*	*2*	*3*	*4*	*5*	*6*
Clinic therapy room	T	T	T	T	T	T
Outside clinic	T	T	T	G	G	G
Home livingroom	T	T	G	G	G	G
School classroom	T	G	G	G	G	G
School playground	T	G	G	G	G	G

T = trained
G = generalized

TABLE 8–8 Matrix of Training Skills and Persons Who Might Engage in Training the Expected Generalization

	Skills					
Trainer	*1*	*2*	*3*	*4*	*5*	*6*
Clinician 1	T	T	T	T	T	T
Clinician 2	T	T	G	G	G	G
Parent 1	T	T	G	G	G	G
Parent 2	T	G	G	G	G	G
Teacher	T	G	G	G	G	G

T = trained
G = generalized

However, after three or four skills have been taught by more than one person, additional skills might need to be taught by only one person for that skill to be demonstrated in the presence of other people. Note once again that this reduces control by what is essentially an irrelevant stimulus (a person). Once again, by the time training has been completed, the various skills would probably form a response class and the people, a stimulus class.

Client As a Therapeutic Agent

Most frequently in discussions of generalization, the person who is being taught speech or communication skills is viewed as a somewhat passive participant. It is the clinician, the parent, the teacher, or peers who serve as listeners and provide the feedback that modifies the child's speech, and the physical and social contexts that control production. These discussions overlook one rather obvious fact about the stimuli controlling the production of correct speech production, namely that many stimuli are produced by the client's own behavior. These stimuli may accompany the client across settings. These stimuli may exercise primary control over the speech in context or they may interact with other situational or background stimuli. In the case of misarticulation, the stimuli that are constant to the person seem to exercise primary control, because misarticulations tend to occur across nearly all contexts. In the case of stutterers, the constant or internal stimuli seem to interact with other situational stimuli, because the person's stuttering varies greatly across contexts (Costello Ingham). Clinicians in practice and the authors of chapters in this book have recognized this in a variety of ways. For example, few clinicians would teach a client to produce a specific sound only in isolation. Rather, they initially get the client to produce it in isolation, then in the context of smaller unit words, then perhaps in sentences, and finally in the contexts of combination of sentences and continued speech or conversation (Costello Ingham). If this training is successful, the correctly articulated sound will occur, not in response to some prompt by a teacher or parent, but in response to the continuous flow of stimuli produced by the child's own speech. Diedrich's evaluation of 3-minute-talk tasks seems designed in many ways to determine the degree of this kind of stimulus control over articulation. McLean (personal communication) has long maintained that most of the control of articulation is internal and it is not until the child controls it that generalization can be expected. So what is being said here is not new. The nature of the stimulus control exercised by the speaker's own behavior and how it interacts with contextual control is not a simple matter. One might assume that the internal control by people with articulation errors is rather constant across contexts. However, the stuttering of people with stuttering problems varies in severity from situation to situation.

Perhaps these forms of stimulus control produced by the client's own speech also explain why articulation or stuttering therapy seems so much more successful with children than with adults. By the time an adult enters therapy, there have been years of reinforced practice. Misarticulated or stuttered speech is largely successful in communication; hence, with increasing years, internal stimulus control becomes more powerful and more resistant to change. It is not surprising that there are not enduring changes produced as a function of relatively brief periods of practice in a therapy session. Additionally, significant others are less likely to give feedback to the adult than to the child concerning misarticulations or stuttering.

Although it is appropriate for the speech-language pathologist to enlist the aid of the parent, teacher, and peers in teaching and providing the conditions for maintaining skills with children, it is probably less appropriate and practical for the clinician to engage significant others directly in therapy with normal adults.

However, there are procedures that might be used to aid an adult in coming to use newly trained communication skills in natural environments.

While the primary therapeutic agents for working with a child's articulation or stuttering problem may be the speech clinician, parent, and teacher, the primary therapeutic agent for working with a normal adult with an articulation or stuttering problem must be the client himself or herself. Presumably the adult client who comes to a communication specialist has some motivation to change his or her speech pattern in some way, at least under specified conditions. The speech clinician may want to explore with the client the possibility of the client's enlisting the aid of other significant people such as a spouse, friend, or children in the treatment. If the client is willing to enlist these significant people in the treatment and they are willing to help, greater success may be achieved. Of course, that is an empirical question. In any case, the key person ensuring that treatment gets done is the client.

As noted above, the client's self-produced stimuli in some ways control the problem speech aspects. The client, in addition to being a speaker, also listens to his own speech. Although initially clients may not be able to discriminate misarticulations or hesitations in their own speech, with training they can, no doubt, do this. If a specific consequence or stimulus condition is effective in reducing the rate of hesitation, then the client might also be taught to apply those contingencies (see Costello Ingham). Simply having the subject count or monitor those incidents may be enough of a punisher and enough of a controlling stimulus to reestablish quickly whatever speech pattern was developed in the clinic.

Research on "self-control" is relatively recent, and empirical knowledge of principles is limited. However, changing one's own behavior may involve many of the issues of changing another person's behavior. Just as the clinician (from lack of time or energy) would not attempt to apply a specific treatment procedure across a client's entire day, the client (as his or her own change agent) may not want to begin by trying to change behavior across all settings. For example, initially an adult receiving speech therapy might decide to practice the new speech patterns acquired in the clinic during only a relatively brief period in a specified setting (for example, at breakfast). During this time, the client would apply to speech abnormalities whatever contingencies had been determined previously. In the case of a person who stutters, a 5-second delay in talking might be self-imposed for each stuttering act. The client would maintain meticulous adherence to the program during this period. When there were almost no hesitations in speech in this situation, the client might stop such careful monitoring of his or her speech to see if the rate of stuttering occurrences remained low. In other words, are the situation stimuli and the person's intraverbal stimuli enough to maintain low rates? If so, the client might initiate the procedures in a second setting. When the new speech patterns are produced without the extra monitoring procedures in this situation, treatment could be extended to a third setting. By conducting treatment in this way, it is likely that at some point the client might find this new speech pattern generalizing into new settings in the absence of the careful monitoring procedures. At this point, the speech might be considered unconscious and we might talk of speech automatically occurring. The comments on self-control and extending speech across settings are totally speculative. However, because similar procedures seem to be successful in getting behaviors to generalize across settings, the suggested procedures merit an empirical test.

SUMMARY

This chapter began by reviewing primary stimulus and primary response generalization, and made the following points:

1. If one reinforces a response in the presence of a specific stimulus and withholds reinforcement in the absence of the stimulus, there is no way of predicting what dimensions of that stimulus would gain control over the response and hence no way of predicting generalization to other stimuli.
2. By reinforcing responses to a variety of stimuli that vary on a given dimension, the probability that generalization will occur along that dimension is increased.
3. By presenting stimuli that vary along a specific dimension and withholding reinforcement for responses to

all values along that dimension but one, the probability of generalization occurring across that dimension can be reduced.

4. Background stimuli may develop controlling properties such that stimulus control is maintained only in the context of a given background.
5. Such background control can be reduced by varying background conditions during discrimination training.
6. Typical stimulus control is *conditional*. That is, the control exercised by a particular stimulus is affected by other stimuli. For example, the probability that a pencil (primary stimulus) will be picked up depends on other conditional stimuli such as, "Pick up the pencil," or, "Don't pick up the pencil."
7. When one places a contingency on one aspect of a response, other aspects of the response besides the criterial aspect are also "accidentally" reinforced and increased in strength.
8. Many instances of generalization, often discussed in terms of response classes, are based on recombination of previously learned stimulus–response units. Examples of such recombination are found in articulation training, instruction following, and grammatical production.
9. Optimal training combinations for the development of generalization can often be readily seen when components are organized in terms of matrices.
10. Many of our techniques for producing generalization in language conditions actually involve varying stimuli along irrelevant dimensions so that responding is controlled by appropriate stimulus dimensions. In short, desired generalization often depends on teaching the appropriate discrimination.
11. Many of the desired stimuli for controlling speech are stimuli produced by the person's verbal and nonverbal behavior. No doubt, internal locus of control and the way speech becomes automatic involve such control.
12. The same matrix arrangement that is useful in visualizing and organizing training or combinations of speech units is also useful in organizing and planning for generalization across settings and persons.

REFERENCES

Azrin, NH Some effects of noise on human behavior. J Exp Anal Behav 1956; 1:183–200.

Baer DM, Wolf MM, Risley TR. Some current dimensions of applied behavior analysis. J Appl Behav Anal 1968; 1:91–97.

Devany JM, Hayes SC, Nelson RO. Equivalence class formation in language-able and language-disabled children. J Exp Anal Behav 1986; 46:243–258.

Diedrich W, Bangert S. Articulation learning. San Diego: College Hill Press, 1980.

Dixon MH. Teaching conceptual classes with receptive label training. Acta Symbolica 1978; 9:17–35.

Dixon MH, Spradlin JE. Establishing stimulus equivalence among retarded adolescents. J Exp Child Psychol 1976; 21:144–164.

Eimas PD. Linguistic processing of speech by young infants. In: Schiefelbusch RL, Lloyd LL, eds. Language perspectives: acquisition, retardation, and intervention. Baltimore: University Park Press, 1974.

Elbert M, McReynolds LV. Transfer of /r / across context. J Speech Hear Disord 1975; 40:380–387.

Engelmann S, Carnine D. Theory of instruction: principles and applications. New York: Irvington Publishers, 1982.

Gast DL, VanBiervliet A, Spradlin JE. Teaching number–word equivalences: a study of transfer. Am J Ment Defic 1979; 83:524–527.

Goldiamond I. Perception. In: Bachrach AJ, ed. Experimental foundations of clinical psychology. New York: Basic Books, 1962: 280.

Goldstein H. Effects of modeling and corrected practice on generative language learning of preschool children. J Speech Hear Disord 1984; 49:389–398.

Goldstein H. Enhancing language generalization using matrix and stimulus equivalence training. In: Warren S, Rogers-Warren A, eds. Teaching functional language. Baltimore: University Park Press, 1985:225.

Guess D. A functional analysis of receptive language and productive speech: acquisition of the plural morpheme. J Appl Behav Anal 1969; 2:55–64.

Guess D, Sailor W, Rutherford G, Baer D. An experimental analysis of linguistic development. The productive use of the plural morpheme. J Appl Behav Anal 1968; 1:297–306.

Haavik SF, Spradlin JE, Altman KI. Generalization and maintenance of language responses: a study across trainers, schools, and home settings. Behav Modif 1984; 8:331–359.

Hegde MN. Treatment procedures in communicative disorders. San Diego: College Hill Press, 1985.

Hollis JH. Reading vocabulary acquisition and retention in developmentally disabled children. Working Paper in Child Development 1987; 2: Child Language Program, University of Kansas.

Hughes DL. Language treatment and generalization: a clinician's handbook. San Diego: College Hill Press, 1985.

Jenkins HM, Harrison RH. Effects of discrimination training on auditory generalization. J Exp Psychol 1960; 59:246–253.

Jenkins JJ. Mediated associations: paradigms and situations. In: Cofer CN, Musgrave BS, eds. Verbal behavior and learning: problems and processes. New York: McGraw-Hill, 1963: 210.

Keller FS, Schoenfeld WS. Principles of psychology. New York: Appleton-Century-Crofts, 1950.

Kendler TS. An ontogeny of mediational deficiency. Child Dev 1972; 43:1–17.

Lasar R. Extending sequence-class membership with matching to sample. J Exp Anal Behav 1977; 27:381–392.

Lazar RM, Davis-Lang D, Sanchez L. The formation of visual stimulus equivalences in children. J Exp Anal Behav 1984; 41:251–266.

Lovaas OI, Berberich JP, Perloff BF, Schaeffer B. Acquisition of imitative speech by schizophrenic children. Science 1966; 151:705–707.

McLean JE. Establishing stimulus control of phoneme articulation by operant techniques. In: Girardeau FL, Spradlin JE, eds. A functional analysis approach to speech and language. ASHA Monograph 1975; 14:24–48.

McLean JE. Personal communication, 1976.

McReynolds LV, Bennett S. Distinctive feature generalization in articulation training. J Speech Hear Disord 1972; 37:462–470.

McReynolds LV, Elbert MF. Generalization of correct articulation in clusters. Applied Psycholinguistics 1981; 2:119–132.

Millenson JR, Leslie JC. Principles of behavioral analysis. New York: Macmillan, 1979.

Miller NE, Dollard J. Social learning and imitation. New Haven: Yale University Press, 1941.

Nelson K. The derivation of concepts and categories from event representation. In: Scholnick E, ed. New trends in conceptual representation: challenges to Piaget theory. Hillsdale, NJ: Erlbaum, 1983:129.

Peterson RF. Some experiments on the organization of a class of imitative behaviors. J Appl Behav Anal 1968; 1:225–235.

Powell J, McReynolds LV. A procedure for testing position generalization from articulation training. J Speech Hear Res 1969; 12:629–645.

Reese HW. Acquired distinctiveness and equivalence of cues in young children. J Exp Child Psychol 1972; 13:171–182.

Saunders RR, Wachter J, Spradlin JE. Establishing auditory stimulus control over an eight-member equivalence class via conditional discrimination procedures. J Exp Anal Behav 1988; 49:195–221.

Sidman M. Reading and auditory–visual equivalences. J Speech Hear Res 1971; 14:5–13.

Sidman M, Cresson O, Jr. Reading and crossmodal transfer of stimulus equivalences in severe retardation. Am J Ment Defic 1973; 77:515–523.

Sidman M, Cresson O Jr, Willson-Morris M. Acquisition of matching-to-sample via mediated transfer. J Exp Anal Behav 1974; 22:261–273.

Sidman M, Kirk B, Willson-Morris M. Six-member stimulus classes generated by conditional-discrimination procedures. J Exp Anal Behav 1985; 43:21–42.

Sidman M, Tailby W. Conditional discriminations vs matching-to-sample: an expansion of the testing paradigm. J Exp Anal Behav 1982; 37:5–22.

Sidman M, Willson-Morris M, Kirk B. Matching-to-sample procedures and the development of equivalence relations: the role of naming. Analysis and Intervention of Developmental Disabilities 1985; 6:1–20.

Silverman K, Anderson SR, Marshall AM, Baer DM. Audience control of language repertoires: a stimulus class analysis. Analysis and Intervention of Developmental Disabilities 1986; 6:21–40.

Skinner BF. Verbal behavior. New York: Appleton-Century-Crofts, 1957.

Spence K. Behavior theory and conditioning. New Haven: Yale University Press, 1956.

Spradlin JE, Cotter VW, Baxley NR. Establishing a conditional discrimination without direct conditioning: a study of transfer with retarded adolescents. Am J Ment Defic 1973; 77:556–566.

Spradlin JE, Dixon MH. Establishing conditional discriminations without direct training: stimulus classes and labels. Am J Ment Defic 1976; 80:555–561.

Spradlin JE, Saunders RR. The development of stimulus classes using match-to-sample procedures: sample classification vs comparison classification. Analysis and Intervention in Developmental Disabilities 1986; 6:41–58.

Stokes TF, Baer DM. An implicit technology of generalization. J Appl Behav Anal 1977; 10:349–367.

Striefel S, Bryan KS, Aikins DA. Transfer of stimulus control from motor to verbal stimuli. J Appl Behav Anal 1974; 7:123–135.

Striefel S, Wetherby B. Instruction-following behavior of a retarded child and its controlling stimuli. J Appl Behav Anal 1973; 6:663–670.

Striefel S, Wetherby B, Karlan G. Establishing generative verb–noun instruction-following skills in retarded children. J Exp Child Psychol 1976; 22:247–260.

Warren SF. Clinical strategies for the measurement of language generalization. In: Warren SF, Rogers-Warren AK, eds. Teaching functional language: language intervention series. Baltimore: University Park Press, 1985:197.

Wetherby B. Miniature languages and the functional analysis of verbal behavior. In: Schiefelbusch RL, ed. Bases of language intervention. Baltimore: University Park Press, 1978:397.

Wetherby B, Karlan GR, Spradlin JE. The development of derived stimulus relations through training in arbitrary-matching sequences. J Exp Anal Behav 1983; 40:69–78.

Wetherby B, Striefel S. Application of miniature linguistic system or matrix training procedures. In: Schiefelbusch RL, ed. Language intervention strategies. Baltimore: University Park Press, 1978:317.

Whitehurst GJ. Generalized labeling on the basis of structural response classes by two young children. J Exp Child Psychol 1971; 12:59–71.

INDEX